Antimicrobial Agents and Immunity

Antimicrobial Agents and Immunity

Edited by

J. Jeljaszewicz
National Institute of Hygiene,
Warsaw, Poland

and

G. Pulverer
Hygiene Institute, University of Cologne,
Federal Republic of Germany

1986

ACADEMIC PRESS
Harcourt Brace Jovanovich

London Orlando San Diego New York
Austin Boston Sydney Tokyo Toronto

ACADEMIC PRESS INC. (LONDON) LTD.
24/28 Oval Road, London NW1 7DX

United States Edition published by
ACADEMIC PRESS. INC.
Orlando, Florida 32887

British Library Cataloguing in Publication Data

Antimicrobial agents and immunity.
1. Anti-infective agents 2. Immunology
I. Jeljaszewicz, J. II. Pulverer, G.
615'.329 RM267

ISBN 0-12-383830-4

Phototypeset by
Dobbie Typesetting Service, Plymouth, Devon

Printed in Great Britain by
St Edmundsbury Press, Bury St Edmunds, Suffolk

Contributors

J. BELSHEIM
Department of Clinical Bacteriology, Gävle Central Hospital, S-801 17 Gävle, Sweden

G. P. BODEY
Section of Infectious Diseases, Department of Internal Medicine, University of Texas, M.D. Anderson Hospital and Tumor Institute, 6723 Bertner Avenue, Houston, TX 77030, U.S.A.

E. de CLERCQ
Rega Institute for Medical Research, Katholieke Universiteit Leuven, 10 Minderbroedersstraat, B-3000 Leuven, Belgium

V. FAINSTEIN
Section of Infectious Diseases, Department of Internal Medicine, University of Texas, M.D. Anderson Hospital and Tumor Institute, 6723 Bertner Avenue, Houston, TX 77030 U.S.A.

H. GNARPE
Department of Clinical Bacteriology, Gävle Central Hospital, S-801 17 Gävle, Sweden

P. J. HEIDT
Radiobiological Institute TNO, Rijswijk, The Netherlands

J. JELJASZEWICZ
National Institute of Hygiene, 24 Chocimska, 00-791 Warsaw, Poland

G. PULVERER
Institute of Hygiene, University of Cologne, Goldenfelstrasse 19, 5000 Cologne 41, Federal Republic of Germany

K. V. I. ROLSTON
Section of Infectious Disease, Department of Internal Medicine, University of Texas, M.D. Anderson Hospital and Tumor Institute, 6723 Bertner Avenue, Houston, TX 77030, U.S.A.

K. ROSZKOWSKI
National Institute of Lung Diseases and Tuberculosis, Plocka 26, PL-01138, Warsaw, Poland

W. ROSZKOWSKI
National Institute of Lung Diseases and Tuberculosis, Plocka 26, PL-01138, Warsaw, Poland

R. P. SILLETTI
Bronx-Lebanan Hospital Center, Microbiology Division, 1276 Fulton Avenue, Bronx, NY10456, U.S.A.

Y. H. THONG
Department of Child Health, University of Queensland, Mater Children's Hospital, South Brisbane 4101, Australia

D. van der WAAIJ
Laboratory for Medical Microbiology, University Hospital, Groningen, The Netherlands

D. P. WEST
College of Pharmacy, University of Illinois, P.O. Box 6998, Chicago, IL 60680, U.S.A.

K. W. WITTE
College of Pharmacy, University of Illinois, P.O. Box 6998, Chicago, IL 60680, U.S.A.

Preface

Antimicrobial agents represent one of the most commonly used groups of drugs. Their saving influence on human and animal health are well known. Typical side effects of antimicrobials are investigated and reported in the literature in great detail. However, the interaction of these drugs with the immune system has long escaped attention which at first was only directed towards simple inhibition of antibody production. It appears that antimicrobials interact in many ways with the humoral and cellular immune system, and can even influence antitumour activity.

This volume presents a section of contributions on these fascinating phenomena. Some chapters are prepared as reviews of the literature, while others detail the authors' own results.

We believe that this volume covers a very important area of modern medicine.

Gerhard Pulverer *Janusz Jeljaszewicz*

May 1986

Contents

Chapter 1

Antibacterial Agents and the Immune System

Waldemar Roszkowski,[1] Kazimierz Roszkowski,[1] Janusz Jeljaszewicz[2] and Gerhard Pulverer[3]

[1]National Institute of Lung Diseases and Tuberculosis, Warsaw, Poland, [2]National Institute of Hygiene, Warsaw, Poland and [3]Institute of Hygiene, University of Cologne, Cologne, F.R.G.

From the time of the introduction of penicillin into clinical practice, antibiotics have become one of the most commonly used pharmacological agents. By definition, they are used in situations in which the host immune system is, or at least should be, mobilized for antimicrobial defence. Until recently, the main avenue of research was centred on investigating the relations between microorganisms and antibiotics. It is surprising that studies on the interactions of antimicrobial agents with the immune system were not initiated until quite recently. The possibility of such interactions is generally ignored in clinical practice, although the number of primary and secondary defects of the immune system is increasing.

All the components of the immune system participate in resistance against infectious agents and their toxins. Certain compartments of immunity are more important for particular microorganisms than others. These include B and T subpopulations of lymphocytes, neutrophils and mononuclear phagocytes, probably natural killer (NK) cells, antibody-dependent cytotoxic cells (K-cells) and the complement system. Even subtle impairment of the above components may lead to a potent facilitation of bacterial or viral infections. It seems obvious that a therapy directed against infectious agents may at the same time affect any of these immune mechanisms.

Antimicrobial agents and immunity
ISBN 0-12-383830-4

The first line of host defence during bacterial infections is based on the function of phagocytes. These include neutrophils, monocytes and macrophages. The main abnormalities of neutrophil function are listed in Table 1. Inherited or acquired defects of neutrophils and agranulocytosis result in greatly increased susceptibility to infections, even with microorganisms of low virulence. Patients with such diseases have recurrent and chronic infections with bacteria that are usually well tolerated by normal patients (e.g. *Escherichia coli* or *Serratia marcescens*). Prolonged chemotherapy is required to keep these infections under control. Defects of macrophage function are much less recognized. It is known that these cells play an important role in resistance against mycobacterial and other intracellular infections. Activation of macrophages may result in increased natural resistance to bacteria, viruses, fungi and tumours or facilitate recovery from infection (Fauve, 1975). Macrophage and monocyte activation occurs in a variety of circumstances, for example after treatment with BCG or *Corynebacterium parvum*. All phagocytic cells possess several potent antimicrobial systems which are oxygen-dependent and independent. They are activated during the contact of the microorganism with the cell membrane. This contact may occur directly between the bacteria and phagocyte as is the case with several non-encapsulated bacteria. The character of this direct interaction is unknown. In the case of encapsulated bacteria, the presence of opsonins is necessary for the interaction and subsequent phagocytosis. However, it should be mentioned that the process of internalization of bacteria by phagocytes is not always essential for their

Table 1
Defects of polymorphonuclear leucocyte function

1.	Agranulocytosis
2.	Chronic granulomatous disease
3.	Chediak-Higashi syndrome
4.	Myeloperoxidase deficiency
5.	Myeloid leukaemia
6.	Phosphate deficiency
7.	Copper deficiency
8.	Virus infections
9.	Crohn's disease
10.	Sarcoidosis
11.	Malignancies
12.	Scurvy
13.	Burns

Infectious complications: high susceptibility to bacterial infections, including microorganisms of low virulence.

killing. There is evidence that killing of bacteria may occur outside the activated phagocyte (Okamura *et al.*, 1979).

Non-specific killing is an attribute not only of phagocytes. A subclass of human or animal lymphocytes can lyse target cells coated with small amounts of antibodies. These cells have surface receptors for the Fc region of immunoglobulin and for complement (C3), although complement is not required for lysis. These K-cells seem to be involved in resistance against *Cryptococcus neoformans*. Another subpopulation of lymphocytes named NK cells can kill targets without sensitization by antibody. The role of these cells in natural resistance to bacterial or parasitic infection is not known. The phenomenon of direct killing of bacteria by lymphocytes was demonstrated under experimental conditions (Nencioni *et al.*, 1983). Defective NK activity, together with other immune abnormalities, is characteristic for acquired immune deficiency syndrome (AIDS). The clinical picture of this disease consists of opportunistic infections and/or neoplasia. Gram-negative bacteria can be killed not only by the cells but also by serum. This is based on the interaction of complement with the outer membrane of the bacteria as the first point of attack, followed by the action of lysosyme on the peptidoglycan layer.

On the other hand, complement and serum antibodies have three major effects in bacterial infections:

(1) direct lysis of bacteria,
(2) opsonization for phagocytosis,
(3) neutralization of bacterial toxins.

Lysis of Gram-negative bacteria occurs in the presence of antibodies to cell wall antigens. These antibodies usually belong to IgM and IgG class, but secretory IgA may also participate in this reaction. However, unlike IgG and IgM, IgA antibodies do not activate complement by the classical pathway but by the alternative pathway. Defects of antibody production may occur in different B-lymphocytes immunodeficiencies (Table 2),

Table 2
B-cell immunodeficiencies

1. Sex-linked hypogammaglobulinaemia (lack of B lymphocytes, affects male relatives)
2. Sex-linked deficiency of IgG and IgA
3. Variable hypogammaglobulinaemia with or without B cells
4. Transient hypogammaglobulinaemia
5. Isolated IgA deficiency

Infectious complications: recurrent and chronic upper and lower respiratory tract infections, digestive tract infections, viral infections.

Table 3
Combined immunodeficiencies

1.	Swiss-type agammaglobulinaemia (stem-cell deficiency)
2.	Adenosine daminase deficiency
3.	Hypogammaglobulinaemia with functional T-cell deficiency
4.	Wiskott–Aldrich syndrome
5.	Ataxia-telangiectasia

Table 4
Selective immunodeficiencies

1.	Inability to produce specific antibodies despite the presence of normal immunoglobulin levels
2.	Lack of cellular immune response to a particular antigen despite the presence of normal responses to other antigens and a normal non-specific mitogen response

combined immunodeficiencies (Table 3) or selective defects (Table 4). The importance of this arm of host defence is well demonstrated by the increased susceptibility of patients with severe hypogammaglobulinaemia to infections with pneumococci, *Haemophilus influenzae* and other bacteria. Also, selective deficiencies of IgG, IgM and IgA can have similar effects even when immunoglobulin levels are in the normal range. As stated above, killing of microorganisms by antibodies also involves the action of complement. Defects of the components of complement (Table 5), in addition to increased susceptibility to lupus-like syndromes, glomerulonephritis and angioneurotic oedema, also lead to increased susceptibility to bacterial infections. Recurrent upper and lower respiratory tract infections are associated with a deficiency of C3. This can result from the failure to synthesize C3 or to an increased breakdown of C3 secondary to a deficiency of C3b inhibitor. Lack of the inhibitor results in continuous feedback activation of the alternative pathway, reducing C3 and factor B to very low levels. According to a widely held view, specific cellular immunity is combined with resistance to intracellular bacteria. The spectrum of diseases produced by defects in cellular immunity as well as major T-lymphocyte deficiencies are listed in Table 6. In this type of specific host defence, macrophages play the final role as bacteria-killing cells. As previously mentioned, activated macrophages possess potent antimicrobial activities. In this case the stimulus for the activation of macrophages comes from specifically sensitized T lymphocytes responding to bacterial antigens and liberating products which activate the phagocytes. The borderline between cellular and humoral immunity is not sharp.

Table 5
Defects of complement

1.	Severe primary or secondary C3 deficiency
2.	Impaired alternative pathway activation
3.	Moderate secondary C3 deficiency
4.	C6 deficiency
5.	Clr, C2, C4 deficiencies
6.	C3 nephritic factor
7.	Cl esterase deficiency

Manifestations: recurrent, chronic upper and lower respiratory tract infections, diarrhoea, allergy, infections with *Neisseria meningitis*, lupus-like syndromes, dermatomyositis, angioneurotic oedema.

Table 6
T-cell immunodeficiencies

1.	di George syndrome
2.	Inosine phosphorylase deficiency
3.	Nezelof syndrome
4.	AIDS

Infectious complications: myobacterial infections, viral infections, opportunistic bacterial, fungal and protozoal infections, neoplasms, possibly of viral aetiology (Kaposi's sarcoma, lymphoma, squamous cell carcinoma).

Macrophages can also be activated through immune complexes or the complement system. The best example of the complexity of immune reaction to one individual agent is the clinical picture and variety of immunological phenomena in leprosy. In this case, the diversity of immune reactions becomes one of the factors in the classification of this disease (Ridley and Jopling, 1966).

Taking into consideration all the above-mentioned antimicrobial immune mechanism, two major questions arise: do antibiotics influence the antimicrobial potential of the immune system and do they modify bacteria by changing their interaction with the host defence system. A number of investigators have studied these problems analysing both bactericidal and bacteriostatic drugs and considering the importance of phagocytes as the first line of host defence. Various functions of these cells were analysed, including all the steps of phagocytosis, e.g. chemotaxis, internalization of microbes and their killing. In addition, the metabolic events occurring during these processes were examined under the influence of antibiotics.

Mandell (1982) evaluated the effects of commonly used antibacterial, antifungal and antiviral agents on the chemotactic function of human polymorphonuclear phagocytes. The majority of substances tested by Mandell inhibited the chemotactic response. In many cases the inhibition was dependent on the chemoattractant used in the experiment. When fraction C5a of complement was applied, cell movement was impaired by erythromycin, chloramphenicol, tetracycline, penicillin, cephalothin and rifampicin. However, when bacterial filtrate was used as a chemoattractant, only vancomycin, tetracycline, penicillin and rifampicin inhibited chemotaxis. Similarly, Forsgren and Schmeling (1977) analysed the effects of 20 antibiotics on the chemotaxis of human neutrophils using agarose gel techniques. Markedly reduced migration was observed for the cells incubated with clinically obtainable concentrations of rifampicin and sodium fusidate. A more slightly reduced migration was detected at high concentrations of chloramphenicol, erythromycin and tetracycline, but there was no inhibition of chemotaxis for penicillin, gentamicin and cephalosporins. Inhibition of leucocyte movement under the influence of tetracyclines was also observed by other investigators (Martin *et al.*, 1974; Gnarpe *et al.*, 1978). All of the authors cited above observed significant effects of aminoglycosides on chemotaxis. However, Seklecki *et al.* (1978) noted that five antibiotics of this pharmacological group including gentamicin produce a modest decrease of leucocyte migration.

Apart from all these finally inconclusive observations, there is no explanation for the mechanism of the effects of the drugs on leucocyte movement except in the case of the tetracyclines. For these antibiotics it was suggested that the inhibitory effect is attributed to complex formation with membrane-bound divalent cations (Gnarpe and Leslie, 1974). These ions are known to be necessary for chemotaxis (Wilkinson, 1975). Using scanning electron microscopy Gnarpe and Leslie (1974) could detect distinct surface alterations in human granulocytes exposed to tetracyclines. In addition to disturbances in locomotion, the cells also exhibited a decreased phagocytic capacity (Forsgren *et al.*, 1974). Furthermore, leucocytes obtained from healthy volunteers as well as from patients with postoperative wound infections treated with tetracyclines also demonstrated impaired phagocytosis (Belsheim *et al.*, 1979). On the other hand, Hoeprich and Martin (1970) could not find any effect of tetracyclines nor of polymyxin B and rifampicin on the phagocytic and microbicidal activity of leucocytes. In an early study with various tetracycline preparations Forsgren and Gnarpe (1973*a*) also found no adverse effect of these antibiotics on phagocytic function. This did not confirm findings of Munoz and Geister (1950) and Altura *et al.* (1966). However, it should be noted that Forsgren *et al.* (1974), after changing assay techniques, did observe inhibition of phagocytosis of yeasts and bacteria by human neutrophils under the influence of both doxycycline and tetracycline. The opposite effect was observed with tetracycline by Mandell (1982): he noted that this antibiotic, as well as erythromycin, chloramphenicol, penicillin and cephalothin, potentiates whereas gentamicin and rifampicin inhibit human granulocyte phagocytosis. It is interesting that the study showed opposing effects of the antibiotics on the processes of ingestion and cell movement. The drugs inhibiting chemotaxis showed enhanced phagocytosis. However, all the antibacterial substances examined showed an effect on nitro blue tetrazolium reduction. This would suggest that all the substances examined do not affect the bactericidal function of leucocytes. Other investigators also noted a change in phagocytosis under the influence of antibiotics; however, their results are sometimes conflicting. Downey and Pisano (1965) found that bacitracin and polymyxin B impaired phagocytosis of *Staphylococcus aureus* and latex particles by guinea pig leucocytes. This effect was observed at drug concentrations 10 times higher than the bactericidal level. On the other hand, they did not observe any influence by penicillin G, streptomycin, neomycin, chloramphenicol and sulphonamides in the experiment. In a similar experimental model, Zalman *et al.* (1963) did observe enhanced phagocytosis with penicillin. In the study by Pickering *et al.* (1978), examining the effects of different penicillins on the phagocytosis and killing of *E. coli*, the antibiotics had no effect on human polymorphonuclear cell fuction. Similarly our own study has not shown any significant modification of granulocyte and monocyte function under the influence of penicillins (Roszkowski *et al.*, 1985*b*). We also analysed the chemiluminescence of human phagocytes in the presence of or after 1 h preincubation of the cells with mezlocillin, amikacin and cefotaxime. Even with the highest concentrations used of the antibiotics (comparable with that obtained after therapeutic intravenous application of the drugs) the metabolic activity of the cells was not influenced.

On the other hand, the respiratory burst of human polymorphonuclear cells was significantly reduced by chloramphenicol in the studies by Kaplan *et al.* (1969) and Lehrer (1973). Also Limbert *et al.* (1982) examined the respiratory burst of neutrophils measured by phagocytosis-associated chemiluminescence under the influence of antibiotics. The authors observed that β-lactam drugs either have no influence on luminescence or slightly reduce it at very high concentrations. In contrast, both erythromycin and clindamycin showed a significant negative influence on this reaction. Similar observations were made with tetracycline, doxycycline, gentamicin and tobramycin. However, it has to be pointed out that the authors analysed the above activity of the antibiotics in arbitrarily chosen concentrations not corresponding to those obtained in serum under therapeutic conditions.

Duncker *et al.* (1984) also observed a potent inhibition of neutrophil chemiluminescence by several antibiotics. However, they used a very unstable experimental system based on incubation of the cells at different, rapidly changing temperatures. A more conclusive system was applied by Kowolik *et al.* (1982). They analysed the influence of ampicillin and cefaclor on neutrophil myeloperoxidase activity as well as on chemiluminescence after drug administration to healthy human volunteers and to four adult patients with chronic bacterial infections. Cefaclor clearly enhanced myeloperoxidase activity while ampicillin generally depressed this enzyme's activity in the blood neutrophils. Luminol-dependent luminescence assay supported these findings.

What seems to be of particular importance is a marked drop in myeloperoxidase levels, which was observed in patients with chest infections after each administration of ampicillin, followed by a slow recovery after completing the treatment. Myeloperoxidase is an important component of the oxidative bactericidal system of neutrophils (Klebanoff and Clark, 1978) and is also responsible for the phenomenon of chemiluminescence (Dahlgren and Stendahl, 1983). Thus, the results of this study strongly suggest the possibility of impairment of phagocyte function by antibiotics *in vivo*. Patients with chronic granulomatous disease show a lack or a significant reduction of the level of this enzyme. In 1975 Johnson *et al.* reported a favourable clinical experience with sulphisoxazole in this disease. They also showed an enhanced bactericidal activity of leucocytes after addition of sulphisoxazole. However, the study by Seger *et al.* (1982) indicates that this is due to the accumulation of sulphamethoxazole and trimethoprim in the cells rather than an enhancement of bactericidal activity of the cells. Removal of the phagocytosed material, the last stage of phagocytosis, was investigated by Midtvedt *et al.* (1982): They observed a reduced elimination of ^{32}P-labelled *E. coli* by human polymorphonuclear cells under the influence of doxycycline. On the other hand, fusidic acid and rifampicin enhanced this phase of phagocytosis.

Interaction between phagocytes and antibiotics was investigated not only on granulocytes but also on macrophages. Brunner and Undeutsch (1982) analysed the effects of cephalothin and gentamicin on the phagocytosis of *Klebsiella pneumoniae* by guinea pig alveolar macrophages. Gentamicin inhibited the uptake of opsonized bacteria only at high concentrations which can be reached in serum during intensive antimicrobial therapy. On the other hand, cephalothin affected the bacterial uptake in concentrations never obtained in clinical chemotherapy.

Reviewing the papers cited above, it is striking how conflicting the reported data are. This is mainly due to the differences in the methods used by the various investigators and also to arbitrarily chosen doses of the drugs examined which did not correspond to *in-vivo* conditions. In analysing the possible effects of antimicrobial drugs on phagocytosis, we should also consider changes in microbial structure facilitating or impairing the above process. As mentioned, the bacteria can be taken up either directly by phagocytes or with the participation of opsonins. Theoretically, antibiotics may change the surface protein M or A content, modify the bacterial capsule or shape and thereby influence the process of phagocytosis. It is known that some microbes produce chemotactic factors stimulating phagocyte activity (Webster and Leyden, 1980). Production of such factors can also be influenced by antibiotics. Dierich and Weikel (1982) found that *Pseudomonas aeruginosa*, growing in subinhibitory concentrations of gentamicin, generates about 50% less chemotactic factor. Obviously this effect of gentamicin would not assist the host's defence efforts; however, the real biological significance of the finding is difficult to evaluate. On the other hand, subinhibitory concentrations of antibiotics can enhance phagocytic killing as was shown for *S. aureus* by Root *et al.* (1981). A similar phenomenon was observed by Easmon and Desmond (1982). In their experiments, subinhibitory concentrations of benzylpenicillin halved bacterial survival as compared with untreated group B streptococci. Intriguingly, the authors observed that other antibiotics like clindamycin, rifampicin and chloramphenicol could modify *S. aureus*, *E. coli* or group B streptococci, leading to significant changes in human neutrophil chemiluminescence. However, this was not accompanied by changes in bacterial ingestion. The results suggest modified cell–cell interactions with subsequent changes in light production by the granulocytes. In this study opsonized bacteria were used. A similar phenomenon was observed by us. In our experiments, we used *S. aureus* (strain SG 511) grown overnight at 37°C in the presence of subinhibitory concentrations of different antibiotics. When this particular strain of *S. aureus* was cultivated without antibiotics and added to a suspension of human granulocytes a rather moderate chemiluminescence was induced (see Fig. 1). A pronounced increase of light production was noted when amikacin-treated bacteria were used, whereas a decrease was observed with cefotaxime. The results of the chemiluminescence assay were confirmed by bactericidal tests (Table 7). Amikacin significantly increased killing of *S. aureus* by neutrophils even without the participation of opsonins. This may lead to the conclusion that amikacin is able to modify the *S. aureus* cell wall in a way which facilitates direct interaction with phagocytes. It is interesting that Easmon and Desmond (1982) observed some discrepancy between the results of chemiluminescence and phagocytosis assays but not between light production and killing effect. It can be explained by the possibility of extracellular killing which may occur during activation of phagocytes

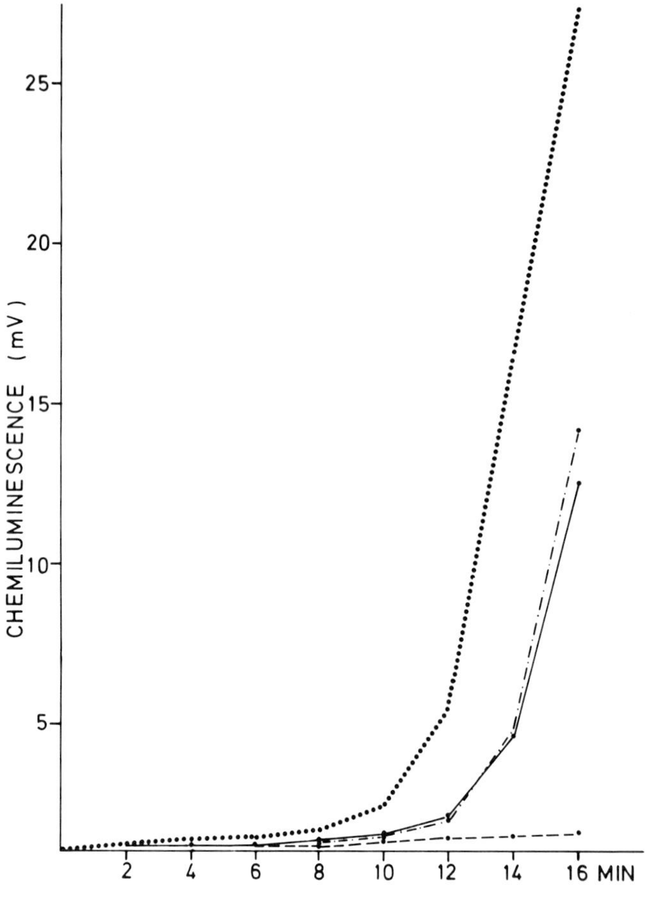

Fig. 1. Chemiluminescence induced by *Staphylococcus aureus* precultured in control medium (—) and with subinhibitory concentrations of cefotaxime (0·8 μg/ml; — — — —), mezlocillin (0·8 μg/ml; — · — · —) and amikacin (0·2 μg/ml; . . . .).

without the uptake of bacteria (Okamura *et al.*, 1979). However, increased susceptibility of bacteria to bactericidal activity must also be considered.

It was observed that previous exposure of bacteria to several different antibiotics increases their susceptibility to the bactericidal activity of neutrophils (Pruul and McDonald, 1979; McDonald *et al.*, 1981). It is proposed that the bacteria are rendered more susceptible to intracellular leucocyte killing mechanisms as a result of structural damage to the cell wall (Pruul *et al.*, 1981). Pruul *et al.* (1982) tested granules of human neutrophils for their bactericidal activity against strains from several genera

Table 7
Granulocyte and monocyte killing of *Staphylococcus aureus* strain SG 511 cultured in subinhibitory concentrations of antibiotics.

		Non-opsonized bacteria killed (%)	Opsonized bacteria killed (%)
S. aureus cultured without the antibiotics (control)	granulocytes	0	57
	monocytes	0	42
S. aureus cultured in medium with amikacin (0·2 μg/ml)	granulocytes	62	80
	monocytes	48	75

of Gram-negative bacteria. The results of this study confirm the above proposition. Similarly Ginsburg *et al.* (1982) observed that penicillin G makes resistant strains of staphylococci and streptococci susceptible to lysis induced by leucocyte extracts. These authors showed that brief non-lethal exposure to chloramphenicol, gentamicin, tetracycline and streptomycin increased the susceptibility of the bacteria to the granules by an average of 50%. They also found that such induced killing was inhibited by divalent cations and anionic polyelectrolytes. Enhanced susceptibility of antibiotic-treated bacteria to killing by phagocytes was also observed by other investigators (Friedman and Warren, 1974; Efrati *et al.*, 1976; Lorian and Atkinson, 1980; Gemmel *et al.*, 1981). Furthermore, low concentrations of the drugs can enhance the phagocytosis of bacteria by macrophages (Ginsburg *et al.*, 1982) and monocytes (Gemmel and Abdul Amir, 1979).

However, the mechanisms are still not clear by which antibiotics render bacteria more susceptible to phagocyte killing. It seems that this cannot be attributed only to increased ingestion of bacteria as was reported for penicillin-treated streptococci (Home and Tomasz, 1981; Ginsburg *et al.*, 1982). The results of Gemmell *et al.* (1981) and other investigators suggest the importance of facilitated opsonization of the drug-treated bacteria by complement. This is supported by the fact that trypan blue, which has been shown to block the C3 receptor on phagocytes (Harper *et al.*, 1981), prevents the killing of both antibiotic-treated and untreated bacteria (Pruul *et al.*, 1981; Lam *et al.*, 1982). Moreover, subinhibitory concentrations of the antibiotics may weaken the tight integrity of the bacterial membranes. This may also facilitate the access of phagocyte factors to their targets in drug-treated bacteria. The above hypothesis may also be applicable for non-opsonized bacteria.

In addition to an increased susceptibility to phagocyte activity, a change in the susceptibility of drug-treated bacteria to serum was observed. It was shown that combination of chloramphenicol and normal human serum is antagonistic in the killing of *E. coli* (Traub and Sherris, 1970) and additive in the killing of *Salmonella typhi* (Treffers and Muschel, 1954). Forsgren and Gnarpe (1973*a*,*b*) reported on the antagonism between tetracycline and the killing effect of normal human serum for *E. coli*. However, Dutcher *et al.* (1978) observed an opposite effect for tetracycline on *E. coli* killing. The study of Hart *et al.* (1982) with tetracyclines, chloramphenicol and rifampicin shows that these antibiotics can alter the susceptibility of *E. coli* to the bactericidal activity of serum and to the classical complement pathway. Moreover, they also observed a change in the expression of antigenicity under the influence of rifampicin and nalidixic acid. Bacterial surface modifications by subinhibitory concentrations of antibiotics were also noted by Opferkuch (1982). His study shows that *E. coli* exposed to different β-lactam antibiotics can bind even 900 times more C1 than can non-treated bacteria. However, it is interesting that one of strains examined possessed opposite properties: the binding of C1 was markedly reduced by pretreatment with antibiotics as compared to control cells.

All the studies cited above referred to interactions of antibiotics with the first line of host defence, namely phagocytes or serum antimicrobial activity. There is a significant lack of information on other functions of monocytes and macrophages, particularly with respect to cooperation with other cells of the immune system. It is not known to what extent the antibiotic-altered antimicrobial activity of these cells is related to the antigen-presenting function of the phagocytes. It is also not known if antibiotics can modify the production of kinins like IL-1 playing an important role in the induction of immune responses. The study on the influence of antibiotics on specific immune responses started from investigations on lymphocyte function *in vitro*. It is well known that specific cellular and humoral immune responses include the proliferative phase of lymphoid cells. It is also generally accepted that substances affecting the proliferation usually possess immunosuppressive activity *in vivo*. Thus, it was obvious to examine the effects of antibiotics on lymphocyte proliferation in an *in-vitro* system. A wide range of antibiotics was tested by Forsgren and Banck (1978) for their influence on ^{3}H-thymidine incorporation by stimulated human T lymphocytes. Of the 20 substances tested, fusidic acid and rifampicin had a pronounced inhibitory effect at therapeutic concentrations. At concentrations above the therapeutic level a marked inhibition was detected by the authors for tetracyclines, erythromycin, clindamycin and nitrofurantoin. There was no apparent inhibitory effect on the proliferative response of human lymphocytes with penicillins, cephalosporins, chloramphenicol and aminoglycoside antibiotics. Similar phenomena were noted for stimulated human B cells. The authors postulated that some antibiotics acting by inhibition of protein synthesis also affect protein synthesis and function of human lymphocytes. The results of these investigators support earlier findings concerning rifampicin (Nilsson, 1971; Grassi and Pozzi, 1972). However, it has to be mentioned that Smith *et al.* (1972) and Dajani *et al.* (1972) found that rifampicin itself had no effect on lymphocyte proliferation while other rifampicin derivatives gave a slight depression. There are also contradictory data concerning the effects of cephalosporins on lymphocyte function *in vitro*. The experiments of Forsgren and Banck (1978) did not show any effect of the cephalosporins (cefazolin, cephalothin) on lymphocyte proliferation, whereas Chaperon and Sanders (1978) and Chaperon *et al.* (1980) did observe suppressive effects of several antibiotics of this pharmacological group. The results of these investigators show that the inhibition of lymphocyte stimulation is not due to a direct effect of the drugs on the lymphoid cells.

Inhibition of lymphocyte response to phytohaemagglutinin by cephalosporins can be partially reversed by adding low concentrations of indomethacin to the cell culture. This strongly suggests that the suppression is at least partially mediated by prostaglandin E_2, which points to the role of activated monocytes in these experiments (Schuelke and Chaperon, 1981). It has to be pointed out that not all cephalosporins produce this effect. In our experiments cefotaxime did not affect the lymphocyte stimulation (Roszkowski *et al.*, 1985*a*). However, attempts to correlate the physical or chemical properties of different drugs of this group with theirs effects on lymphocyte response have been generally unsuccessful. A similar diversity of pharmacological effects was found in the group of penicillins. Among different penicillins known not to affect lymphocyte proliferation, we found that mezlocillin produces a significant suppression (Roszkowski *et al.*, 1985*a*). Obviously the question arises as to what extent these observations from *in-vitro* experiments can be transferred to *in-vivo* conditions. Such simple factors like albumin binding may reduce or even abolish the *in-vivo* effect of the drug. Thus the next steps in looking for the biological relevance of *in-vitro* findings were studies performed on animals. The most established data obtained *in vivo* concern the effects of rifampicin. Rifampicin given to experimental animals produces a significant depression of the cellular immune response to dinitrochlorobenzene, BCG and PPD (Paunescu, 1970; Grassi and Pozzi, 1972; Dajani *et al.*, 1973). With this antibiotic, the primary antibody response to BSA in guinea pigs and rabbits was suppressed (Paunescu, 1970), as was the response in mice and guinea pigs to erythrocytes (Paunescu, 1970; Bassi *et al.*, 1973; Dajani *et al.*, 1973). It was also shown that rifampicin significantly prolongs allograft survival (Serrou *et al.*, 1972) and impairs antitumour immunity (Roszkowski *et al.*, 1984).

Data concerning the influence of antibiotics on the experimental humoral response come from a limited number of studies. Gillissen (1982) reported that several cephalosporins enhanced the formation of IgM-producing murine spleen cells when up to 30 mg/kg body weight were injected in a single dose. Higher doses of up to 300 mg/kg induced either a further stimulation or a decrease of the humoral immune response depending on the substance examined. Thong and Ferrante (1980) demonstrated diverse effects of tetracycline on humoral and cellular immune responses in mice. Animals treated with tetracycline had an unchanged humoral response to sheep erythrocytes; however, their capacity to establish delayed-type hypersensitivity was significantly reduced. Our recent studies show that two penicillins, mezlocillin and piperacillin, as well as cefotaxime can produce a significant reduction of both humoral and cellular immune responses in mice when given for 7 consecutive days (Roszkowski *et al.*, 1985*a*). This effect was observed when the treatment was performed either before or after challenge with antigen. This study shows that the depression of immune reactions is not limited only to the period of treatment but lasts after completing drug administration. The most striking observation was that penicillins that are commonly believed to be neutral for immune functions can produce potent and long-lasting effects. The results of Gillissen (1982) and Roszkowski *et al.* (1985*a*) concerning the immunopharmacological effects of cephalosporins clearly show that there is a difference between the effects of single administration of a drug and prolonged treatment. Similar phenomena were observed for amphotericin B. The antibiotic given in a single dose enhanced the immune response, whereas repeated injections of the drug resulted in depression of the immune reaction (Blanke *et al.*, 1977; Little *et al.*, 1978; Shirley and Little, 1979; Rosette and Kauffman, 1980).

Another very important but not well recognized problem was studied by Kasamaki *et al.* (1979). They analysed cellular and humoral immunological phenomena in rabbits treated with tetracycline and found that administration of this drug can induce cellular and humoral immunity not only against the antibiotic but also against autologous gammaglobulin and tissue antigens. This points to another possible adverse effect of antibiotics, as a potential agent for the induction of autoimmune disease.

The number of studies referring to the influence of antibiotic therapy on the human immune system is also very limited. Among the many antimicrobial agents used in clinical practice, rifampicin again attracted most attention. This is mainly due to the fact that treatment with rifampicin is long-lasting and the consequences of therapy can be evaluated more easily than in the case of other antibiotics used in acute infections. The effects of rifampicin on antibody response in man are variable. It was observed that seroconversion to smallpox vaccination is suppressed when rifampicin is applied (Moshkowitz *et al.*, 1971). Oral administration of rifampicin also interferes with the antibody response to keyhole limpet haemocyanin (Graber *et al.*, 1972). However, Bassi *et al.* (1973) and Ruben *et al.* (1974) reported that antibody response to influenza and cholera vaccines was not affected. In patients receiving rifampicin for tuberculosis, skin reactivity to PPD is progressively yet reversibly reduced (Ruben *et al.*, 1974) which supports earlier observations from animal studies.

Other antibiotics have not been examined so extensively for their immune effects in humans. In general, the recognition of immunomodulating effects of antibacterial drugs during therapy of bacterial infection is very difficult if possible at all. Thus under these circumstances the only way to get objective information is to perform studies on volunteers as it was done for cotrimoxazole (Arvilommi *et al.*, 1972). Our own experience as well as that of others strongly suggests that it is difficult to draw conclusions concerning a whole pharmacological group of antibiotics based on the data obtained for one or a few drugs. To obtain a real picture for the interaction of antibacterial drugs with the immune system and to know the major adverse and positive effects, each individual drug should be examined. Then it should be possible to develop more efficient regimens for antibacterial therapy.

REFERENCES

Altura, B. M., Hershey, S. G., Ali, M. and Thaw, C. (1966). *J. Reticuloendothel. Soc.* **3**, 447-457.

Arvilommi, H., Vuori, M. and Salami, A. (1972). *Br. Med. J.* **iii**, 761-762.

Bassi, L., Di Bernardino, I., Arioli, V., Silvestri, L. G. and Cherie Ligniere, E. L. (1973). *J. Infect. Dis.* **128**, 736-744.

Belsheim, J., Gnarpe, H. and Persson, S. (1979). *Scand. J. Infect. Dis.* **11**, 141-145.

Blanke, T. J., Little, J. R., Shirley, S. F. and Lynch, R. G. (1977). *Cell. Immunol.* **33**, 180.

Brunner, H. and Undeutsch, C. (1982). *In* "The Influence of Antibiotics on the Host-Parasite Relationship" (Eickenberg, H. U., Hahn, H. and Opferkuch, W., eds), pp. 129-138. Springer-Verlag, Berlin.

Chaperon, E. A. and Sanders, W. E. (1978). *Infect. Immun.* **19**, 378-384.

Chaperon, E. A., Degen, M. and Sanders, W. E. (1980). *In* "Current Chemotherapy and Infectious Diseases" (Nelson, J. D. and Grassi, C., eds), pp. 836-838. American Society for Microbiology, Washington, D.C.

Dahlgren, C. and Stendahl, O. (1983). *Infect. Immun.* **39**, 736-741.

Dajani, B. M., Canady, M. S., Thompson, J. S. and Kasik, J. E. (1972). *Lancet* **ii**, 1094.

Dajani, B. M., Kasik, J. E. and Thompson, J. S. (1973). *Antimicrob. Agents Chemother.* **3**, 451-455.

Dierich, M. P. and Weikel, W. (1982). *In* "The Influence of Antibiotics on the Host-Parasite Relationship" (Eickenberg, H. U., Hahn, H. and Opferkuch, W., eds), pp. 139-140. Springer-Verlag, Berlin.

Downey, R. J. and Pisano, J. C. (1965). *J. Reticuloendothel. Soc.* **2**, 75-88.

Duncker, D., Ullmann, U. and Reese, G. (1984). *Zbl. Bakt. HygA,* **256**, 433-434.

Dutcher, B. S., Reynard, A. M., Beck, M. E. and Cunningham, R. K. (1978). *Antimicrob. Agents Chemother.* **13**, 820-826.

Easmon, C. S. F. and Desmond, A. M. (1982). *In* "The Influence of Antibiotics on the Host-Parasite Relationship" (Eickenberg, H. U., Hahn, H. and Opferkuch, W., eds), pp. 202-207. Springer-Verlag, Berlin.

Efrati, C., Sacks, T., Ne'eman, N., Lahav, M. and Ginsburg, I. (1976). *Inflammation* **1**, 371-407.

Fauve, R. M. (1975). *In* "*Corynebacterium parvum*: Application in Clinical and Experimental Oncology" (Halpern, B., ed.), pp. 77-83. Plenum Press, New York.

Forsgren, A. and Banck, G. (1978). *Infection* **6** (*Suppl. 1*), 91-97.

Forsgren, A. and Gnarpe, H. (1973*a*). *Antimicrob. Agents Chemother.* **3**, 711-715.

Forsgren, A. and Gnarpe, H. (1973*b*). *Nature New Biol.* **244**, 82-83.

Forsgren, A., Schmeling, D. (1977). *Antimicrob. Agents Chemother.* **11**, 580-584.

Forsgren, A., Schmeling, D. and Quie, P. (1974). *J. Infect. Dis.* **130**, 412-415.

Friedman, H. and Warren, G. H. (1974). *Proc. Soc. Exp. Biol. Med.* **146**, 707-711.

Gemmell, C. G. and Abdul Amir, M. K. (1979). *In* "Pathogenic Streptococci" (Parker, M. T., ed.), pp. 67-68. Reedbooks, Chertsey, Surrey, U.K.

Gemmell, C. G., Peterson, P. K., Schmeling, D., Kim, Y., Mathews, J., Wannamaker, L. and Quie, P. G. (1981). *J. Clin. Invest.* **67**, 1249-1256.

Gillissen, G. J. (1982). *In* "The Influence of Antibiotics on the Host-Parasite Relationship" (Eickenberg, H. U., Hahn, H. and Opferkuch, W., eds), pp. 5-11. Springer-Verlag, Berlin.

Ginsburg, I., Lavah, M., Bergner-Rabinowitz, S. and Ferne, M. (1982). *In* "The Influence of Antibiotics on the Host-Parasite Relationship" (Eickenberg, H. U., Hahn, H. and Opferkuch, W., eds), pp. 219-227. Springer-Verlag, Berlin.

Gnarpe, H. and Leslie, D. (1974). *Microbios* **10A**, 127-138.

Gnarpe, H., Belsheim, J. and Persson, S. (1978). *Infection* **6** (*Suppl. 1*), 98-101.

Graber, C. D., Jebailey, J., Galphin, R. L. and Doering, E. (1972). *Am. Rev. Resp. Dis.* **126**, 542-544.

Grassi, G. G. and Pozzi, E. (1972). *J. Infect. Dis.* **126**, 542-544.

Harper, B. L., Fine, D. P., Guckian, J. C. and Cavallo, T. (1981). *Immunology* **42**, 61-66.

Hart, R. F., Reynard, A. M. and Cunningham, R. K. (1982). *In* "The Influence of Antibiotics on the Host-Parasite Relationship" (Eickenberg, H. U., Hahn, H. and Opferkuch, W., eds), pp. 255-262. Springer-Verlag, Berlin.

Hoeprich, P. D. and Martin, C. H. (1970). *Clin. Pharmacol. Ther.* **11**, 418-422.

Horne, D. and Tomasz, A. (1981). *Antimicrob. Agents Chemother.* **19**, 745-753.

Johnson, R., Wilfert, C., Buckley, R., Webb, L., DeChatelet, L. and McCall, C. (1975). *Lancet* **i**, 824-827.
Kaplan, S. S., Perillie, P. E. and Finch, S. C. (1969). *Proc. Soc. Exp. Biol. Med.* **130**, 839-843.
Kasamaki, A., Furuya, K. and Kanamitsu, H. (1979). *J. Toxicol. Sci.* **4**, 389-404.
Klebanoff, S. J. and Clark, R. A. (1978). "The Neutrophil: Function and Clinical Disorders". North Holland, Amsterdam.
Kowolik, M. J., Raeburn, J. A. and Grant, M. (1982). *In* "The Influence of Antibiotics on the Host-Parasite Relationship" (Eickenberg, H. U., Hahn, H. and Opferkuch, W., eds), pp. 56-66. Springer-Verlag, Berlin.
Lam, C., Georgopoulos, A., Laber, G., Schütze, E. and Wenzel, A. (1982). *In* "The Influence of Antibiotics on the Host-Parasite Relationship" (Eickenberg, H. U., Hahn, H. and Opferkuch, W., eds), pp. 242-254. Springer-Verlag, Berlin.
Lehrer, R. I. (1973). *J. Infect. Dis.* **127**, 40-48.
Limbert, M., Seibert, G. and Schrinner, E. (1982). *In* "The Influence of Antibiotics on the Host-Parasite Relationship" (Eickenberg, H. U., Hahn, H. and Opferkuch, W., eds), pp. 74-86. Springer-Verlag, Berlin.
Little, J. R., Blanke, T. J., Valeriote, F. and Madoff, G. (1978). *In* "Immune Modulation and Control of Neoplasia by Adjuvant Therapy" (Chrigos, M. A., ed.), p. 381. Raven Press, New York.
Lorian, V. and Atkinson, B. (1980). *Antimicrob. Agents Chemother.* **18**, 807-813.
Mandell, L. A. (1982). *In* "The Influence of Antibiotics on the Host-Parasite Relationship" (Eickenberg, H. U., Hahn, H. and Opferkuch, W. eds), pp. 40-55. Springer-Verlag, Berlin.
Martin, R. R., Warr, G. A., Couch, R. B., Yeger, H. and Knight, V. (1974) *J. Infect. Dis.* **129**, 110-116.
McDonald, P. J., Wetherall, B. L. and Pruul, H. (1981). *Rev. Infect. Dis.* **3**, 38-44.
Midtvedt, T., Lingaas, E. and Melby, K. (1982). *In* "The Influence of Antibiotics on the Host-Parasite Relationship" (Eickenberg, H. U., Hahn, H. and Opferkuch, W., eds), pp. 118-128. Springer-Verlag, Berlin.
Moshkowitz, A., Goldblum, N. and Heller, E. (1971). *Nature* **229**, 422-424.
Munoz, J. and Geister, R. (1950). *Proc. Soc. Exp. Biol. Med.* **75**, 367-370.
Nencioni, L., Villa, L., Boraschi, D., Berti, B. and Tagliabue, A. (1983). *J. Immunol.* **130**, 903-907.
Nilsson, B. S. (1971). *Lancet* **ii**, 374.
Okamura, N., Ishibashi, S. and Takano, T. (1979). *J. Biochem.* **86**, 469-475.
Opferkuch, W. (1982). *In* "The Influence of Antibiotics on the Host-Parasite Relationship" (Eickenberg, H. U., Hahn, H. and Opferkuch, W., eds), pp. 236-266. Springer-Verlag, Berlin.
Paunescu, E. (1970). *Nature* **228**, 1188-1190.
Pickering, L. K., Ericsson, C. D. and Kohl, S. (1978). *Cancer* **42**, 1741-1746.
Pruul, H. and McDonald, P. J. (1979). *Antimicrob. Agents Chemother.* **16**, 695-700.
Pruul, H., Wetherall, B. L. and McDonald, P. J. (1981). *Antimicrob. Agents Chemother.* **19**, 945-951.

Pruul, H., Wetherall, B. L. McDonald, P. J. (1982). *In* "The Influence of Antibiotics on the Host-Parasite Relationship" (Eickenberg, H. U., Hahn, H. and Opferkuch, W., eds), pp. 208-218. Springer-Verlag, Berlin.
Ridley, D. S. and Jopling, W. H. (1966). *Int. J. Lepr.* **34**, 255-273.
Root, R. K., Istunz, R., Molavi, A., Metcalf, J. A. and Melech, H. L. (1981). *J. Clin. Invest.* **67**, 247-259.
Roselle, G. A. and Kauffman, C. A. (1980). *Clin. Exp. Immunol.* **40**, 186-192.
Roszkowski, W., Lipinska, R., Roszkowski, K., Jeljaszewicz, J. and Pulverer, G. (1984). *Med. Microbiol. Immunol.* **172**, 197-205.
Roszkowski, W., Ko, H. L., Roszkowski, K., Jeljaszewicz, J. and Pulverer, G. (1985*a*). *In* "Chemotherapy and Immunity" (Pulverer, G. and Jeljaszewicz, J., eds), *Zbl. Bakt. Suppl.* **13**, 59-72. Gustav Fischer Verlag, Stuttgart.
Roszkowski, W., Ko, H. L., Roszkowski, K., Jeljaszewicz, J. and Pulverer, G. (1985*b*). *Med. Microbiol. Immunol.* **173**, 279-289.
Ruben, F. L., Winkelstein, A. and Fotiadis, I. G. (1974). *Antimicrob. Agents Chemother.* **5**, 383-387.
Schuelke, G. and Chaperon, E. A. (1981). *Am. Soc. Microbiol. Abstracts* **81**, 58.
Seger, R. A. Baumgartner, S. and Gmünder, F. K. (1982). *In* "The Influence of Antibiotics on the Host-Parasite Relationship" (Eickenberg, H. U., Hahn, H. and Opferkuch, W., eds), pp. 96-105. Springer-Verlag, Berlin.
Seklecki, M. M., Quintiliani, R. and Maderazo, E. G. (1978). *Antimicrob. Agents Chemother.* **13**, 552-554.
Serrou, B., Solassol, A., Joyeux, H., Pujol, H. and Romieu, C. (1972). *Transplantation,* **14**, 654.
Shirley, S. F. and Little, J. R. (1979). *J. Immunol.* **123**, 2878-2882.
Smith, R. G., Whang-Peng, J. and Gallo, R. C. (1972). *Nature New Biol.* **236**, 166-171.
Thong, Y. H. and Ferrante, A. (1980). *Clin. Exp. Immunol.* **39**, 728-732.
Traub, W. H. and Sherris, J. C. (1970). *Chemotherapy* **15**, 70-83.
Treffers, H. P. and Muschel, L. H. (1954). *J. Exp. Med.* **99**, 155-165.
Webster, G. F. and Leyden, J. J. (1980). *Inflammation* **4**, 261-269.
Wilkinson, P. C. (1975). *Exp. Cell Res.* **93**, 420-426.
Zalman, M. V., Frasinel, N. and Neagoe, N. (1963). *Arch. Roumaines Pathol. Exp. Microbiol.* **22**, 919-930.

Chapter 2

Antiviral Agents and the Immune System

Erik de Clercq
Rega Institute for Medical Research, Katholieke Universiteit Leuven, 10 Minderbroedersstraat, B-3000 Leuven, Belgium

I. INTRODUCTION

For a long time the development of selective antiviral agents has been considered a tantalizing task because of the close alliance between the virus replication cycle and normal cell metabolism. As a result of this alliance it would seem hard, if not impossible, to design a strategy that would allow us to destroy the virus without adversely affecting the normal cell. The advent of such potent and selective antiherpes agents as acyclovir (ACV), bromovinyldeoxyuridine (BVDU) and fluoroiodoaracytosine (FIAC) has made it clear that the specific treatment of virus infections is no longer a utopian ideal.

Since viruses depend heavily—more than bacteria—on the host cell for their replication, and since host defence mechanisms are essential for the recovery from virus infections, it is obvious that if antiviral agents are to be used successfully in the chemotherapy of virus infections, they should not interfere with the host's immune responses toward the infection. This is even more important in those patients where the immune system has been compromised, i.e. cancer patients or recipients of bone marrow or kidney transplants who are treated with strong immunosuppressants. That an antiviral drug used to combat an intercurrent herpesvirus infection in such patients should be devoid of immunotoxicity is clearly demonstrated

Antimicrobial agents and immunity
ISBN 0-12-383830-4

by the adverse effects noted for cytosine arabinoside, which was found to protract rather than suppress the dissemination of herpes zoster in immunocompromised patients (Stevens *et al.*, 1973).

As a routine precaution and safety assessment, all antiviral agents, and in particular those that are scheduled for use in the treatment of virus infections in immunocompromised patients, should be evaluated for their potential immunotoxic and myelotoxic side effects. A wide variety of immuno- and myelotoxicity assay systems are now available, e.g.

(a) the primary and secondary plaque-forming cell (PFC) responses of lymphocytes to either T-cell-dependent antigens (e.g. sheep erythrocytes) or T-cell-independent antigens (e.g. bacterial lipopolysaccharide);
(b) the mixed lymphocyte reaction, which measures the proliferation of helper and cytotoxic T cells after recognition of foreign antigens on other lymphocytes;
(c) mitogen-induced blastogenesis or the proliferative response of peripheral blood mononuclear cells (PBM) to the mitogens phytohaemagglutinin (PHA), concanavalin A (ConA) or pokeweed mitogen (PWM);
(d) antigen-stimulated blastogenesis or the proliferative response of PBM cells to specific antigens such as herpes simplex virus type 1 (HSV-1) or type 2 (HSV-2) or varicella-zoster virus (VZV);
(e) cell-mediated lympholysis, which represents killing of target lymphocytes by sensitized T lymphocytes;
(f) the natural killer (NK) activity of lymphocytes (which do not express T- or B-cell surface markers) against tumour cells or virus-infected cells without prior sensitization;
(g) the killer (K) activity or antibody-dependent cell-mediated cytotoxicity of lymphocytes (which also do not express T- or B-cell surface markers but possess Fc receptors on their surface) against target cells sensitized with antibody;
(h) the phagocytic activity of macrophages;
(i) the release of lymphokines [e.g. interleukin-2 (T-cell growth factor), B-cell growth factor or IFN-γ (immune interferon)] by T lymphocytes in response to mitogens (e.g. PHA) or specific antigens; and
(j) the growth of bone marrow (granulocyte–monocyte) progenitor cells, also referred to as CFU-c (colony-forming unit cells).

It is striking how little attention has been paid to the interaction of antiviral agents with the immune system. Only in a few instances were antiviral agents evaluated for their inhibitory effects on some of the systems mentioned above, and no antiviral compound has been submitted to the whole battery of the immune response assays. Yet, a thorough investigation of all potential antiviral drugs in these test systems seems warranted, not only to rule out that the compounds are deleterious for the immune response but also to detect possible immunostimulatory effects. Together with the antiviral effects, such effects may contribute to the host's recovery from a virus infection.

This chapter is not aimed at describing all known antiviral agents. It is focused on a selected number of compounds which are either in clinical use (or considered for clinical use) or subject to extensive experimental investigations. The compounds which will be discussed are:

(A) amantadine and rimantadine, which are recommended for the prophylaxis and (early) therapy of influenza A virus infection;

(B) ribavirin, a broad-spectrum antiviral agent which offers some promise for the tropical or systemic treatment of influenza, respiratory syncytial and arenavirus infections;

(C) the 'classical' or 'first-generation' antiherpes compounds, idoxuridine (5-iodo-2′-deoxyuridine, IDU), trifluridine (5-trifluoro-2′-deoxythymidine, TFT), cytarabine (araC, cytosine arabinoside, 1-β-D-arabinofuranosyl-cytosine) and vidarabine (araA, adenine arabinoside, 9-β-D-arabinofuranosyl-adenine), which were used some time ago (araC) or are still in use (IDU, TFT, araA) for the tropical (IDU, TFT, araA) or systemic (araA) treatment of herpesvirus infections, although these compounds exhibit little, if any, selectivity in their antiviral action;

(D) 'transition' compounds, which span the bridge from the classical to the selective antiherpes compounds and which have to some extent served as models for the development of the latter, e.g. 5′-amino-5-iodo-2′,5′-dideoxyuridine (AIU), 5-ethyl-2′-deoxyuridine (EDU), 5-iodo-2′-deoxycytidine (IDC) and thymine arabinoside (araT, 1-β-D-arabinofuranosylthymine);

(E) the selective or 'second-generation' antiherpes compounds, such as acyclovir [ACV, acycloguanosine, 9-(2-hydroxyethoxymethyl)guanine], dihydroxypropoxymethylguanine [DHPG, 9-((2-hydroxy-1-hydroxymethyl)ethoxymethyl)guanine], bromovinyldeoxyuridine [BVDU, (*E*)-5-(2-bromovinyl)-2′-deoxyuridine), bromovinylarauracil [BVAU, 1-β-D-arabinofuranosyl-(*E*)-5-(2-bromovinyl)uracil], fluoroiodoaracytosine [FIAC, 1-(2′-fluoro-2′-deoxy-β-D-arabinofuranosyl)-5-iodocytosine], fluoromethylarauracil [FMAU, 1-(2′-fluoro-2′-deoxy-β-D-arabinofuranosyl)-5-methyluracil], fluoroiodoarauracil [FIAU, 1-(2′-fluoro-2′-deoxy-β-D-arabinofuranosyl)-5-iodouracil], which all share a common mechanism of action based upon a specific phosphorylation by the viral 2′-deoxythymidine (dThd) kinase followed by a preferential interaction with the viral DNA polymerase;

(F) interferon and interferon inducers which cannot be regarded as truly antiviral agents since they display a variety of biologic activities including immunostimulatory effects (on T lymphocytes) as well as immunosuppressive effects (on B lymphocytes);

(G) isoprinosine (inosiplex, a 3:1 mix of N,N-dimethylamino-2-propanol *p*-acetamidobenzoate and inosine), a rather controversial substance which has been advocated as an antiviral agent acting through stimulation of the host immune response.

Compounds A–G will be analysed from the following viewpoints:

(1) spectrum of antiviral activity;
(2) mechanisms of action;
(3) effects on the immune system *in vitro*;
(4) effects on the immune system *in vivo*, including efficacy against virus infections in immunosuppressed patients.

From the discussion of the data in the literature, it will become clear that for most compounds only limited information is available on their interaction with the immune system. For interferon, however, the interaction with the immune system is so complex that a full account of this topic falls beyond the scope of the present chapter. Instead, the immunomodulatory role of interferon (inducers) will be presented in a highly simplified manner.

II. VIRUS INFECTIONS IN THE IMMUNOCOMPROMISED HOST

As a consequence of the steadily increasing number of allograft (kidney, bone marrow etc.) transplantations requiring the use of strong immunosuppressants and the more aggressive treatment of cancer with combinations of cytotoxic agents, opportunistic infections have become alarmingly frequent and severe in such patients. Generally speaking, immunocompromised patients are more vulnerable to any viral infection than are healthy persons in the general population, but this principle does not hold to the same extent for all viruses. By far, the most serious viral infections in immunosuppressed patients are those caused predominantly by members of the herpesvirus family, HSV, VZV and cytomegalovirus (CMV) (Ho, 1977; Shannon and Schabel, 1980) (Table 1). Among the immunosuppressed, those with malignant lymphoma or Hodgkin's disease

Table 1
Increased frequency and/or severity of virus infections in immunocompromised patients

Virus	Disease
Herpes simplex virus (HSV)	Mucocutaneous herpes (e.g. herpetic stomatitis) Visceral herpes (hepatitis, pneumonia, oesophagitis)
Varicella-zoster virus (VZV)	Varicella (and visceral complications) Zoster (localized or disseminated)
Cytomegalovirus (CMV)	CMV disease (e.g. pneumonitis)
Papova virus	
Papovavirus JC	Progressive multifocal leucoencephalopathy
Papilloma virus	Warts
Vaccinia virus	Vaccinia gangrenosa
Measles virus	Measles (and visceral complications)

Inoculation
↓
Incubation period (10–21 days)
↓
Acute infection (3–7 days): VARICELLA
↓ Rash: face→trunk→extremities
Mild hepatitis, transient pneumonitis
Resolution of acute infection
↓ Humoral immunity (IgG, IgM)
Cellular immunity (lymphocyte transformation, interferon production)
Resolution of the acute infection is delayed and the illness may be fatal in immunosuppressed patients
Latent infection
↓
Incubation period
↓
Recurrent infection: ZOSTER
↓ Localized neuralgia and rash, confined to a single dermatome
Resolution of recurrent infection
↓ Humoral immunity (IgG)
Cellular immunity (lymphocyte transformation, interferon production)
Zoster tends to disseminate in immunosuppressed patients
Latent infection

Fig. 1. The pathogenesis of Varicella-zoster as a typical example of a virus infection.

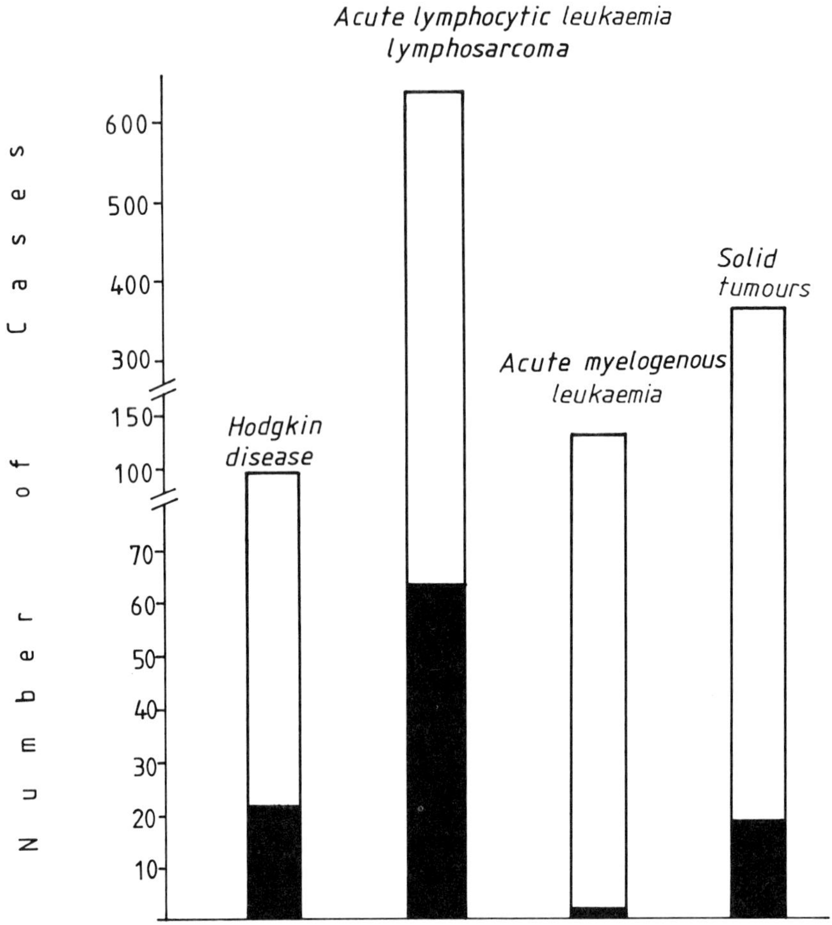

Fig. 2. Incidence of herpes zoster among 1132 children with malignant neoplasias (Feldman *et al.*, 1973).

are most susceptible to viral infections, primarily because of the deficiency in cell-mediated immunity that is associated with the disease. Radio- or chemotherapy may further impair the immune response and thereby amplify the severity of the infection.

One of the most representative examples of a viral infection that is quite mild and benign in healthy individuals, but often serious and occasionally fatal in immunosuppressed children, is varicella (Fig. 1). In children undergoing cancer chemotherapy, varicella may be rapidly progressive and disseminate to the gastrointestinal tract, liver, lungs, pancreas, brain and adrenals. The lesions may become haemorrhagic and necrotic, and death may ensue due to circulatory collapse, generalized intravascular coagulation or visceral complications such as pneumonitis (Bodey, 1975). Herpes zoster, the recurrent form of varicella, occurs in 0·2–2% of the general adult population, but it occurs in 20% of patients with Hodgkin's disease and 10% of patients (primarily children) with acute lymphocytic leukaemia (ALL) (Schimpff *et al.*, 1972; Bodey, 1975). Since the incidence of ALL in children is significantly greater than the incidence of Hodgkin's disease, the majority of the children presenting with herpes zoster have ALL as the underlying disorder (Fig. 2). While usually confined to the infected dermatome, herpes zoster often disseminates in immunosuppressed patients. This dissemination may not only involve the skin but also the gastrointestinal tract, liver, lungs, pancreas, brain and adrenals (as noted above for varicella). The severity and duration of the cutaneous and visceral dissemination of the VZV lesions depend directly on the level of viraemia, which in turn is related to the host's deficiency in mounting an adequate cell-mediated or humoral immune response (Fig. 1). As a rule, the risk of developing generalized varicella or herpes zoster increases substantially with any decrease in immunologic competence, whether this decrease is due to advanced disease, chemotherapy, radiotherapy or combinations thereof.

For HSV and CMV infections in immunosuppressed patients, the same principles prevail as those discussed for VZV infections. In particular, transplant recipients and patients with lymphoproliferative malignancies are at risk for severe HSV and CMV infections (Ho, 1977). The source of the infection appears to be the reactivation of a latent, rather than a primary, infection. The HSV infection may start as a localized infection of the oral mucosa or skin, and then spread to the respiratory and digestive tract, thereby causing tracheobronchitis, oesophagitis and occasionally pneumonia. Generalized vesicular lesions of the skin and mucous membranes, resembling Kaposi's varicelliform eruption, may also occur. CMV infections may present as pneumonitis, mononucleosis, fever and rash and these infections may eventually evolve into fatal visceral disease with involvement of the lungs, liver, gastrointestinal tract, kidneys etc. The most common form of disseminated CMV infection is pneumonia, which may by itself be fatal or be accompanied by a more serious bacterial or fungal infection (e.g. *Pneumocystis carinii*).

Since VZV, CMV and, to a lesser extent, HSV often represent life-threatening infections in immunosuppressed patients, there exists a real and urgent need for effective antiviral drugs to combat these viral infections. Other viruses (e.g. measles and vaccinia) are less important as the source of infection in immunocompromised patients, the former because the widespread use of measles vaccine has caused a marked drop in the incidence of this highly contagious virus infection, the latter because vaccination against smallpox has been abandoned. Obviously, no live virus vaccine, be it smallpox, measles or varicella, should ever be administered to patients with an impaired immune system, since they are prone to develop a severe generalized infection upon contact with the vaccine virus.

III. ANTIVIRAL AGENTS

A. Amantadine and Rimantadine

1. Antiviral spectrum

Amantadine and rimantadine (Fig. 3) possess antiviral activity against influenza A, rubella, measles, respiratory syncytial and parainfluenza virus. They are not active against influenza B virus. Laboratory and clinical studies have clearly established that all known subtypes of human influenza A viruses (H_1N_1, H_2N_2 and H_3N_2) are inhibited by amantadine and rimantadine, and the prophylactic efficacy of these drugs against influenza A virus infections appears to be equivalent to that of influenza vaccines (Oxford, 1984).

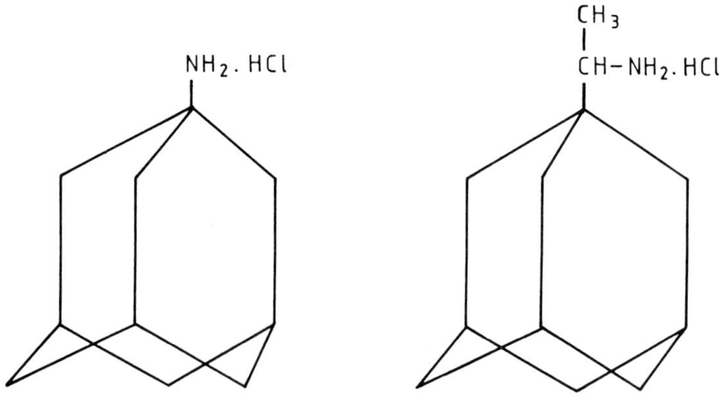

1 - adamantanamine hydrochloride (amantadine HCl, Mantadix®, Amantan®, Symmetrel®)

α - methyl-1-adamantanemethylamine hydrochloride (rimantadine HCl, Remantadine®)

Fig. 3. Amantadine and rimantadine.

2. *Mechanism of action*

The exact mode of action of amantadine and rimantadine remains enigmatic. The drugs seem to affect virus penetration or uncoating, steps in the virus replication cycle which follow the attachment of the virus to the host cell but which precede the initiation of RNA transcription (Skehel *et al.*, 1978; Koff and Knight, 1979). Most of the cell-associated amantadine does not contribute to the antiviral action of the drug. Only that portion of the cell-associated amantadine which is rapidly exchanged with the extracellular medium may account for the antiviral activity of amantadine (Richman *et al.*, 1981).

3. In-vitro *interaction with the immune system*

There are only limited data on the interaction of amantadine or rimantadine with the host immune response. At a concentration range [25–100 μg/tube (17–70 μg/ml?)] which is inhibitory to the response of sensitized lymphocytes to specific antigens (tetanus toxoid or purified protein derivative, amantadine rather stimulates the lymphocytes' response to mitogens (e.g. PHA) (Mardiney and Bredt, 1971). It is not clear whether other adamantane derivatives (such as rimantadine) also exhibit such ambivalent immunomodulatory effects. Further studies on the effects of amantadine and rimantadine on different manifestations of the cell-mediated immune response seem warranted. Amantadine has been advocated for topical use by an aerosol in order to avoid central nervous system (CNS) side effects which are frequently observed following oral administration of the drug (Hayden *et al.*, 1979; Knight *et al.*, 1979). The cell-mediated immune response of the respiratory tract mucosa is assumed to play a major part in the host defence against influenza virus infection, and it would seem particularly fitting to evaluate the extent to which amantadine or rimantadine may influence this response, if these drugs are to be administered by aerosol.

4. In-vivo *interaction with the immune system*

After it had been the subject of considerable controversy for some time (Jackson, 1978; Sabin, 1978), amantadine has been recognized since 1979 as a useful drug for both prophylaxis and early treatment (i.e. within 48 h after onset of the clinical symptoms) of influenza A virus infections. According to the recommendations, amantadine should be used for prophylaxis for periods of 4–6 weeks (in case of an influenza A epidemic):

(a) in children and elderly adults at high risk of morbidity or mortality because of other diseases such as pulmonary, cardiac, metabolic and immunologic deficiencies;

(b) adults whose activities are essential to community functions and who have not been vaccinated;
(c) individuals in semi-enclosed environments, especially older persons who have not been vaccinated.

Several studies have indicated that prophylactic administration of amantadine (200 mg/day p.o. for 6 weeks) significantly reduces the incidences of influenza A, as verified by a number of parameters such as clinical illness, virus isolation and rise in serum antibody to influenza A virus (Petterson *et al.*, 1980; Dolin *et al.*, 1982). Rimantadine is equally efficacious for this purpose, but since rimantadine leads to fewer CNS side effects, it may be preferable over amantadine (Dolin *et al.*, 1982). These CNS side effects are related to the plasma drug levels achieved by amantadine and rimantadine (Hayden *et al.*, 1983*a*) and consist primarily of insomnia, nervousness, dizziness, 'jitteriness' and difficulty in concentrating (Bryson *et al.*, 1980; Dolin *et al.*, 1982).

To what extent amantadine or rimantadine interact with the immune system when given orally at a dose of 200 mg/day is not known. The therapeutic effects of oral amantadine are not striking and its toxic side effects on the CNS preclude an increase in oral dosage. Therefore other delivery forms have been attempted: as an aerosol (at 1 g/100 ml distilled water) amantadine appears to be reasonably well tolerated and moderately effective in reducing the clinical symptoms of naturally acquired influenza A virus infection (Hayden *et al.*, 1980). Hayden *et al.* (1980) speculated that 'topically applied amantadine could theoretically alter host cellular immune response and nonspecifically affect the course of illness'. However, whether amantadine via an aerosol actually interacts (stimulates or inhibits) with the host immune response to influenza A virus infection has not been established.

B. Ribavirin

1. Antiviral spectrum

The antiviral activity spectrum of ribavirin (Fig. 4) is the broadest ever reported for a chemical agent that does not act via interferon induction. It includes all major virus families, i.e. adeno-, pox-, herpeto-rhabdo-, arena-, bunya-, orthomyxo-, paramyxo-, toga-, picorna- and retroviridae (Sidwell *et al.*, 1972*b*; for respiratory syncytial virus, see Hruska *et al.*, 1980). Ribavirin has been found to be effective in the treatment of influenza, parainfluenza and respiratory syncytial virus infections in animals (mice, rats, hamsters or ferrets) (Sidwell *et al.*, 1975; Hruska *et al.*, 1982). In addition, life-threatening virus infections such as those caused by Lassa

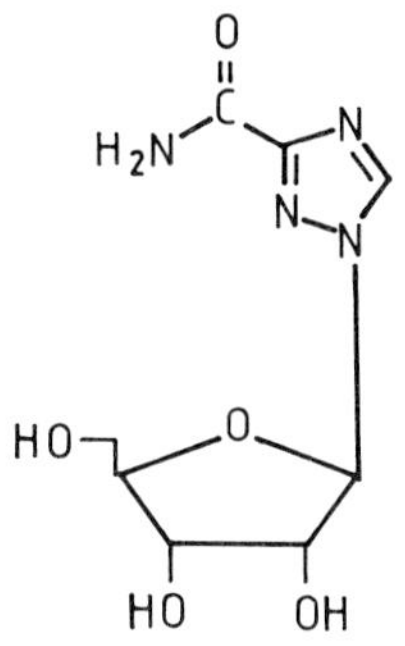

1-β-D-ribofuranosyl-1,2,4-triazole-3-carboxamide
(ribavirin, Virazole®)

Fig. 4. Ribavirin.

virus (Jahrling *et al.*, 1980) and Rift Valley fever virus (Canonico *et al.*, 1982) also react favourably to ribavirin treatment, at least in animal models. From a clinical viewpoint, ribavirin has been pursued primarily for topical (i.e. aerosol) treatment of influenza A and B virus infections (Knight *et al.*, 1981; McClung *et al.*, 1983) and respiratory syncytial virus infections (Hall *et al.*, 1983*a*, *b*; Taber *et al.*, 1983).

2. Mechanism of action

The mechanism of action of ribavirin is polymodal. It inhibits viral and cellular nucleic acid biosynthesis, apparently as a consequence of a perturbation of the nucleotide pools (Browne, 1978; Drach *et al.*, 1981). The prime event may well be an inhibition by ribavirin 5′-monophosphate (formed within the cell from ribavirin through the action of purine nucleoside kinases) of the enzyme inosine 5′-monophosphate dehydrogenase that converts IMP to XMP, the immediate precursor of GMP (Streeter *et al.*, 1973). This would then lead to a depletion of the pool size of GTP and, indirectly, of all other nucleoside 5′-triphosphates linked to GTP by feedback control reactions. Such depletion of GTP may account for most of the biological effects of ribavirin, i.e. broad-spectrum antiviral activity, antimetabolic activity and immunosuppressive activity (see below), since all these effects are fully reversible by exogenous guanosine or xanthosine. However, the rather specific inhibition of influenza virus synthesis by ribavirin is not achieved via a depletion of the GTP pool (Scholtissek, 1976) and, indeed, addition of guanosine only partially overcomes the inhibitory effect of ribavirin on influenza viral RNA synthesis (Wray *et al.*, 1984*b*). The latter effect can be attributed to a direct interference of ribavirin 5′-triphosphate with influenza viral RNA polymerase (Eriksson *et al.*, 1977). As has recently been ascertained by Wray *et al.* (1984*a*), ribavirin 5′-triphosphate would interact with influenza RNA synthesis by a dual mechanism: (i) primarily by blocking RNA chain elongation, but also (ii) by preventing primer generation, this is cleavage of 5′-capped oligonucleotides from cellular mRNAs for use as primers for transcription of the influenza RNA genome.

3. In-vitro *interaction with the immune system*

Ribavirin can generally be considered as an immunosuppressive agent. At concentrations of ⩾5 μg/ml it inhibits PHA-, ConA- and PWM-induced proliferation of human peripheral blood lymphocytes (Peavy *et al.*, 1980). At a concentration of ⩾2·5 μg/ml, ribavirin also inhibits the murine spleen T-cell response to ConA stimulation and the B-cell response to *Escherichia coli* lipopolysaccharide (LPS) (Powers *et al.*, 1982). In addition, ribavirin inhibits the primary and secondary sheep erythrocyte-specific, plaque-forming cell (PFC) responses of murine spleen cells (Powers *et al.*, 1982). Since it is equally effective on the PFC response of T-cell-depleted spleen cell cultures, ribavirin may owe its immunosuppressive activity to a direct action on B cells. The immunosuppressive effects of ribavirin can be completely reversed by exogenous guanosine, indicating that they are based on a depletion of GTP (see above).

Whereas ribavirin inhibits the primary and secondary PFC response of murine spleen cells at a concentration of 5–10 μg/ml, it enhances these responses at a concentration of 0·1–1 μg/ml. This enhancement has been ascribed to a selective inhibition of suppressor T cells (Powers *et al.*, 1982). The molecular basis for the differences in the effects of ribavirin on different lymphocyte subpopulations is not clear, but may be related to the relative importance of the *de-novo* pathway of GTP formation.

4. In-vivo *interaction with the immune system*

The immunosuppressive activity of ribavirin *in vivo* has been demonstrated in a number of test systems, based on:

(a) inhibition of the serum antibody response to inactivated influenza virus vaccine in guinea pigs (Potter *et al.*, 1976);
(b) increase in the rejection time for skin allografts in rabbits (Jolley *et al.*, 1977);
(c) suppression of the PFC responses to both T-cell-dependent (sheep erythrocyte) and T-cell-independent (LPS) antigens in mice (Peavy *et al.*, 1981);

(d) reduction of antibody formation to DNA in female NZB/W F_1 mice, a particular mouse strain that develops an autoimmune disease resembling systemic lupus erythematosus in humans (Klassen *et al.*, 1977). In fact, ribavirin treatment was effective in prolonging the survival of NZB/W F_1 mice and this beneficial effect may have been related to the immunosuppressive action of the compound.

When given orally at a dose of 1 g/day for 5 days, ribavirin did not appear effective in the treatment of naturally occurring influenza A virus infections, even if treatment was initiated within 24–48 h after onset of the clinical symptoms (Smith *et al.*, 1980). However, ribavirin offers greater promise when applied as an aerosol. Ribavirin treatment by aerosol seems to have a beneficial effect on the outcome of influenza A and B and respiratory syncytial virus infections, as judged by a reduction in the severity of systemic illness and/or virus shedding in the respiratory secretions (Knight *et al.*, 1981; Hall *et al.*, 1983*a*, *b*; McClung *et al.*, 1983; Taber *et al.*, 1983).

Upon oral use of ribavirin (1 g/day for 5 days), a significant reduction in the antibody rise due to influenza A was observed, as determined by the complement-fixation test (Smith *et al.*, 1980). Applying ribavirin by aerosol, the antibody response was enhanced in one study (Knight *et al.*, 1981) but depressed in another (Taber *et al.*, 1983). What is urgently needed now, especially if aerosol ribavirin were to be used on a large scale in the treatment of respiratory tract virus infections, are further studies on the effects of ribavirin on the cellular immune responses towards the viruses concerned (e.g. influenza and respiratory syncytial viruses).

C. 'First-generation' Antiherpes Compounds

1. Antiviral spectrum

Of the 'classical' or 'first-generation' antiherpes compounds (Fig. 5), idoxuridine (IDU) and trifluridine (TFT) have been licensed, e.g. as 0·1% (IDU) or 1% (TFT) eye drops, for the topical treatment of herpetic keratitis, and vidarabine (araA) has been marketed for both topical use (as a 3% eye ointment) against herpetic keratitis and systemic use (as on intravenous infusion at 15 mg/kg/day) against herpetic encephalitis (Whitley *et al.*, 1977, 1981). AraA has also been found to be efficacious in the systemic treatment of neonatal herpes (Whitley *et al.*, 1980) and severe mucocutaneous herpes simplex and varicella-zoster infections in immunosuppressed patients (Whitley *et al.*, 1976, 1982*a*, *b*, 1984).

In principle, the antiviral activity spectrum of the 'first-generation' antiherpes compounds should encompass all herpesviruses, including HSV-1, HSV-2, VZV, CMV and Epstein–Barr virus (EBV) and, indeed,

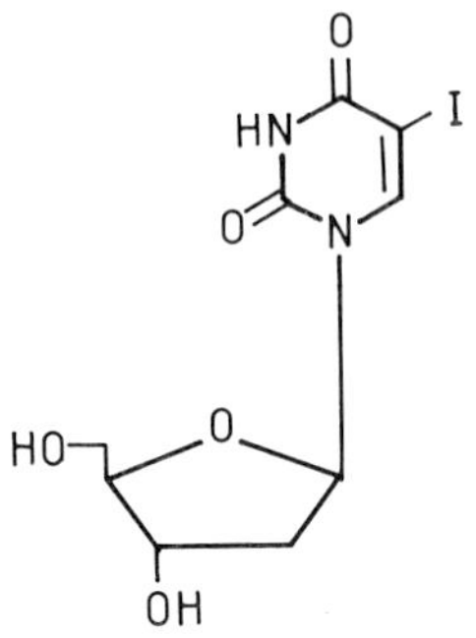

5-iodo-2'-deoxyuridine
(idoxuridine, IDU®, Stoxil®)

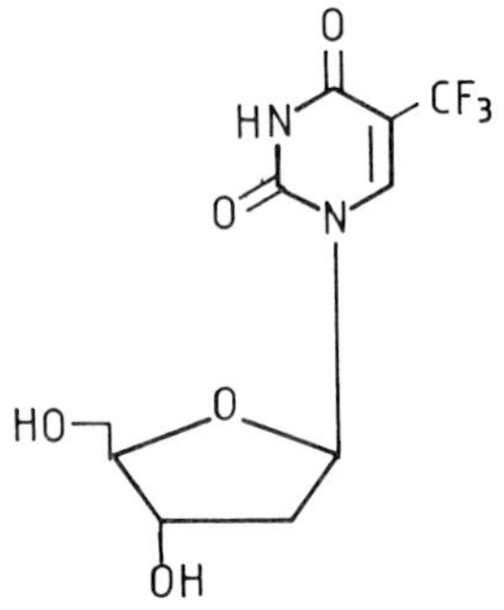

5-trifluoromethyl-2'-deoxyuridine
(trifluridine, trifluorothymidine, TFT, TFT-ophtiol®, Viroptic®)

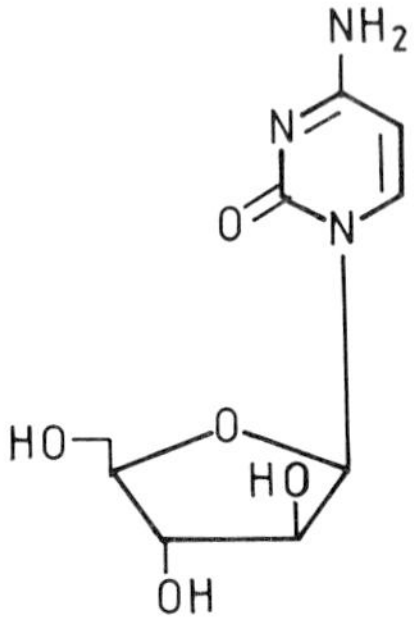

1-β-D-arabinofuranosylcytosine
(cytosine arabinoside, cytarabine, ara C, Cytosar®)

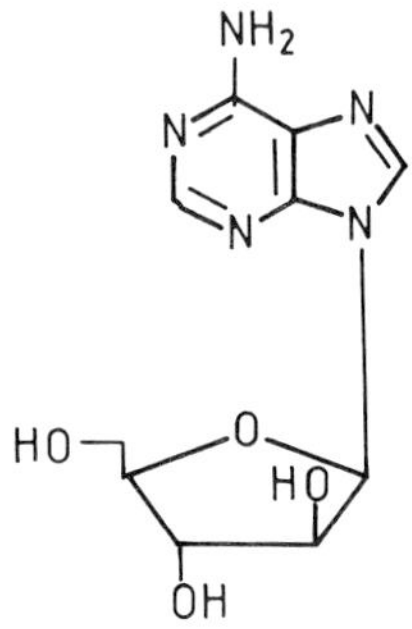

9-β-D-arabinofuranosyladenine
(adenine arabinoside, vidarabine, ara A, Vira-A®)

Fig. 5. 'First-generation' antiherpes compounds: IDU, TFT, araC and araA.

IDU, TFT, cytarabine (araC) and araA are effective inhibitors of HSV-1, HSV-2 and VZV replication (De Clercq *et al.*, 1980; Shigeta *et al.*, 1983). However, they exhibit little if any selectivity in their inhibitory effects on HSV or VZV replication, and TFT and araC are even negatively selective in that they interfere with normal cell metabolism at a concentration that is lower than that required for inhibition of virus replication. IDU, araC, araA and TFT are also effective against CMV (Sidwell *et al.*, 1970, 1972*a*; Wingard *et al.*, 1981) and the 50% inhibitory dose (ID_{50}) of TFT for CMV is extraordinarily low ($\sim 0{\cdot}003\ \mu g/ml$ for human CMV) (Wingard *et al.*, 1981, 1983). Whether TFT or the other drugs hold any promise for the treatment of CMV infections in humans is another matter. TFT as well as araC and IDU failed to protect mice against a lethal murine CMV infection (Kelsey *et al.*, 1976; Wingard *et al.*, 1981). Likewise, no apparent efficacy has been noted for araA in the treatment of CMV infection in renal transplant patients (Marker *et al.*, 1980).

2. Mechanism of action

The classical antiherpes compounds, IDU, TFT, araC and araA exhibit little or no selectivity in their antiviral action, because they are processed equally well by virus-infected and uninfected cells. IDU, TFT and araC are converted by pyrimidine nucleoside (and nucleotide) kinases, and araA by purine nucleoside (and nucleotide) kinases to their corresponding 5′-triphosphates. In this form, they may act either as an inhibitor or as a substrate of DNA polymerase. If they act as a substrate, they will be incorporated into DNA. As their 5′-triphosphates, the compounds may also act as allosteric inhibitors of a number of enzymes involved in nucleic acid biosynthesis, e.g. pyrimidine or purine nucleoside kinases, ribonucleotide reductase, deoxycytidylate deaminase etc.; and as its 5′-monophosphates, TFT may interact with deoxythymidylate (dTMP) synthetase. For IDU, however, the antiviral activity would depend primarily on its incorporation into DNA and the ensuing disturbance of the normal functioning of the DNA (Goz, 1978).

AraC and araA can also be incorporated into DNA, although the relationship between this incorporation and the antiviral action of the compounds is not straightforward: e.g. araA has a greater inhibitory effect on viral DNA synthesis than on cellular DNA synthesis (Shipman *et al.*, 1976), yet substantially more araA is incorporated into cellular DNA than into viral DNA (Pelling *et al.*, 1981). It is obvious that nucleoside analogues such as araA may also be directed at several other enzymatic reactions, including S-adenosylhomocysteine hydrolase, which makes it exceedingly difficult to sort out a single metabolic step as the target for their antiviral action.

3. In-vitro *interaction with the immune system*

In assays of both PHA-, ConA- or PWM-induced blastogenesis and HSV- and VZV-stimulated blastogenesis (Steele *et al.*, 1980) significant immunotoxicity has been noted for IDU at a concentration of 1·5 μg/ml, which is only tenfold higher than its minimal antiviral concentration (De Clercq *et al.*, 1980). The immuno- and myelotoxicity of TFT is even more impressive: this compound inhibits some lymphocyte functions (e.g. the mixed lymphocyte reaction and ConA-induced blastogenesis) (Wingard *et al.*, 1983) at a concentration of 0·03–0·04 μg/ml, which is tenfold lower than its minimal antiviral concentration (De Clercq *et al.*, 1980). At 10 μg/ml araC completely blocks lymphocyte proliferation, whether induced by mitogens or specific antigens (Steele *et al.*, 1980). Its ID_{50} for PHA-induced lymphocyte blastogenesis would be in the range of 0·01–0·02 μg/ml (Gray *et al.*, 1972). This, again, is lower than its minimal antiviral concentration (0·04 μg/ml) (De Clercq *et al.*, 1980).

AraA does not suppress the host cellular immune response at a concentration of 3 μg/ml (Steele *et al.*, 1975, 1980); however, it inhibits bone marrow progenitor cell proliferation at a concentration of 1 μg/ml (Wingard *et al.*, 1983). This concentration is lower than its minimal antiviral concentration (2–10 μg/ml) (De Clercq *et al.*, 1980). Of particular interest is the observation that araA is more toxic for bone marrow progenitor cells than for lymphocyte functions, whereas TFT inhibits lymphocyte functions more readily than haematopoietic precursor cell growth (Wingard *et al.*, 1983). Also, the varying ID_{50} values noted with araA from one assay to another, e.g. 120 μg/ml for the mixed lymphocyte reaction as compared with 1 μg/ml for bone marrow progenitor cell growth, indicates that no single *in-vitro* test suffices to predict the immunotoxic or myelotoxic potentials of the drugs.

4. In-vivo *interaction with the immune system*

AraC has been abandoned for clinical use as an antiviral agent, essentially because it was found to prolong rather than to shorten dissemination of herpes zoster in immunocompromised patients (Stevens *et al.*, 1973). At the dosage regimen used (100 mg/m^2/day for 3 days), araC had both immunosuppressive effects and haematologic toxicity. The patients most in danger from herpesvirus infection, those who could benefit most from effective antiviral chemotherapy, are hosts compromised by underlying disease leading to immunosuppression or requiring aggressive immunosuppressants. These patients are least able to sustain further immunosuppression or bone-marrow suppression. For reasons similar to those that terminated further clinical use of araC and, more specifically, for an unacceptable degree of bone-marrow suppression, IDU has also been abandoned as a systemic antiviral agent (Boston Interhospital Virus Study Group and NIAID-Sponsored Cooperative Antiviral Clinical Study, 1975). Notwithstanding its immuno- and myelosuppressive effects, IDU is still used routinely for topical treatment of herpetic keratitis and, in some countries, for topical treatment of mucocutaneous HSV and VZV infections.

Being equally if not more immuno- and myelotoxic as IDU, TFT has never been considered for systemic treatment of herpesvirus infections. Its clinical use is restricted to topical treatment of herpetic keratitis. The only member of the 'first-generation' antiherpes compounds that appears sufficiently safe for systemic use is araA. AraA is therapeutically effective in protecting immunosuppressed hosts (mice treated with antiserum to thymocytes) from an otherwise fatal vaccinia virus infection under conditions where araC and IDU do not show any protective effect (Worthington and Conliffe, 1977). Beneficial effects have been noted with araA in the systemic treatment of HSV and VZV infections in immunocompromised patients. In cancer patients with herpes zoster, it accelerates the healing process and the cessation of formation of new lesions concomitantly with an accelerated clearance of virus from the lesions (Whitley *et al.*, 1976, 1982*b*). In immunocompromised children with varicella, araA therapy reduces the risk of visceral complications (Whitley *et al.*, 1982*a*) and, as in adults, accelerates cessation of new vesicle formation; however, in order to accomplish these beneficial effects, treatment must start early in the course of infection, i.e. within 3 days after the appearance of rash. In children, araA can be administered at a dosage of 20 mg/kg/day (intravenously) for 5 days; in adults, toxic side effects such as nausea, vomiting, liver dysfunction, diarrhoea and neurologic disorders (pain, tremor, ataxia and seizures) preclude the use of araA at doses higher than 10 mg/kg/day.

AraA is of only limited benefit in the systemic treatment of mucocutaneous HSV infections in immunocompromised patients (Whitley *et al.*, 1984). It does not significantly alter the healing process as assessed by loss of virus from lesions, cessation of formation of new lesions or time to crusting. It may accelerate the resolution of pain but only in patients over 40 years of age. As already mentioned above, araA does not appear efficacious in the treatment of CMV infection in renal transplant patients, when given at the usual dose of 10 mg/kg/day for 5–7 days. In fact, four out of the nine renal transplant patients with CMV infection developed sudden irreversible neurologic deterioration during araA therapy (Marker *et al.*, 1980). This included tremors and myoclonus. In another patient, a 47-year-old woman with metastatic carcinoma of the breast, treated with araA for disseminated VZV infection, severe and ultimately fatal CNS disorders developed 48 h after completion of a 3-day course of araA (Van Etta *et al.*, 1981). Thus, toxic side effects, in particular to the CNS, that are normally not observed in immunocompetent patients treated with antiherpes drugs for an intercurrent herpesvirus infection, may occasionally occur in immunosuppressed patients. The role of araA in the pathogenesis of these neurologic disorders remains to be established.

D. 'Transition' Antiherpes Compounds

1. Antiviral spectrum

5′-Amino-5-iodo-2′,5′-dideoxyuridine (AIU), 5-ethyl-2′-deoxyuridine (EDU), 5-iodo-2′-deoxycytidine (IDC) and thymine arabinoside (araT) (Fig. 6) can

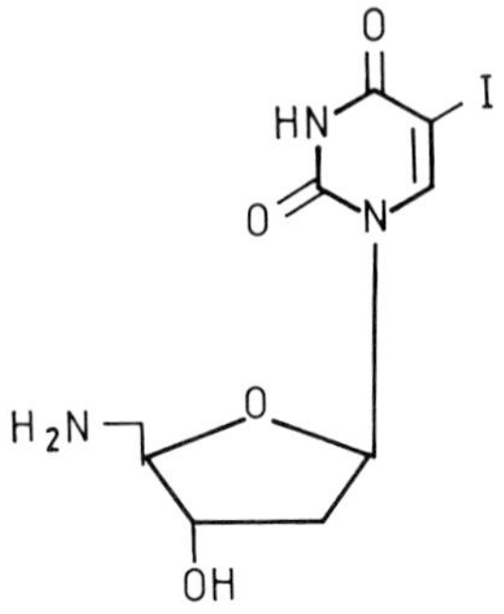

5'-amino-5-iodo-2',5'-dideoxyuridine (AIU)

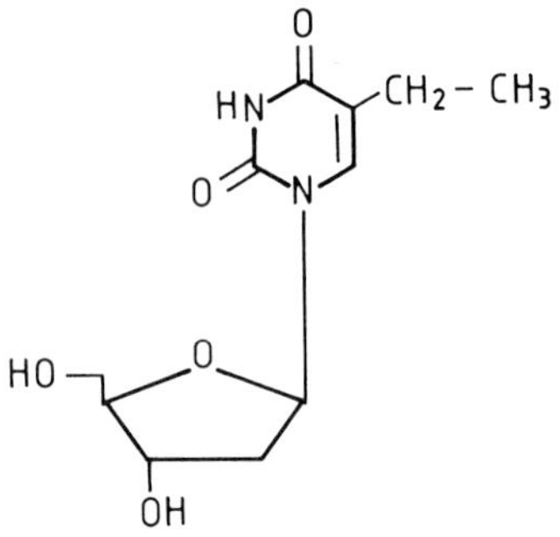

5-ethyl-2'-deoxyuridine (EDU, Aedurid®)

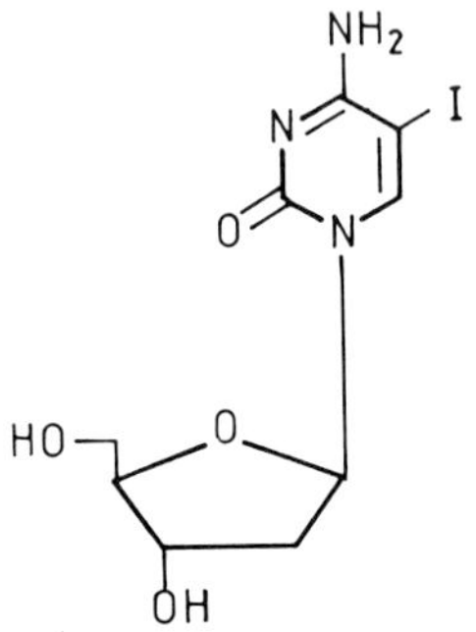

5-iodo-2'-deoxycytidine (IDC, Cébé-viran®, Cuterpes®)

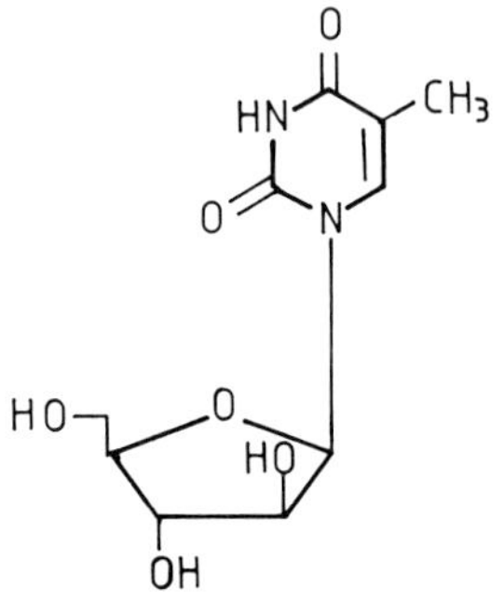

1-β-D-arabinofuranosylthymine (thymine arabinoside, ara T)

Fig. 6. 'Transition' antiherpes compounds: AIU, EDU, IDC and araT.

be considered as transition compounds between the first and second generation of antiherpes compounds. They are more selective in their antiherpes activity than are the classical antiherpes compounds, IDU, TFT, araC and araA, but for varying reasons, primarily because of insufficient potency (for AIU, see Sim *et al.*, 1981), they have not been pursued for clinical use. This notion does not take into account that EDU and IDC have been marketed (in F.R.G. and France, respectively) for topical treatment of herpetic keratitis (as 0·15% eyedrops) and herpetic skin lesions (IDC as a 1% ointment). The antiviral activity spectrum of AIU, IDU, IDC and araT is restricted mainly to HSV-1, HSV-2 and VZV (De Clercq *et al.*, 1980; Shigeta *et al.*, 1983). AraT is not inhibitory to CMV (Miller *et al.*, 1977) and there is no evidence that any of the other drugs would be effective against CMV. However, araT is an efficient inhibitor of EBV replication (Ooka and Calender, 1980; Ooka *et al.*, 1983).

2. *Mechanism of action*

The selectivity of AIU, EDU, IDC and araT as antiherpes agents is to a large extent dependent on a specific phosphorylation by the HSV- or VZV-induced deoxythymidine (dThd) kinase, which, because of its concomitant deoxycytidine (dCyd) kinase activity, can also be designated as a dThd(dCyd) kinase (e.g. see Dobersen *et al.*, 1976; Aswell *et al.*, 1977). Due to this specific phosphorylation, any further action of the compounds is essentially confined to the virus-infected cell. The virus-encoded dThd(dCyd) kinase would convert AIU successively to its 5′-mono- and 5′-diphosphate (Chen and Prusoff, 1979), and IDC, once converted to its 5′-monophosphate, may be deaminated to the corresponding dUMP analogue, IDUMP, by dCMP deaminase (Schildkraut *et al.*, 1975). Even the inhibitory effect of araT on EBV replication would depend on a specific phosphorylation by a newly induced dThd kinase (Ooka *et al.*, 1983).

In any case, the active forms of AIU, EDU, IDC and araT correspond to their final phosphorylation products, AIUTP, EDUTP, IDUTP and araTTP, respectively. In this form, they may interfere with the DNA polymerization reaction, as has been demonstrated for araTTP (Matsukage *et al.*, 1978). AraTTP inhibits cellular and viral DNA polymerases indiscriminately (Müller *et al.*, 1979). Its selectivity as an antiherpes agent would reside solely with a specific phosphorylation by the viral dThd(dCyd) kinase.

The 5′-triphosphates of AIU, EDU, IDC and araT may also serve as substrates for DNA polymerase and be incorporated into DNA. To the extent that the initial phosphorylation is restricted to the virus-infected cell, the subsequent incorporation into DNA would also be confined to the virus-infected cells, but within the infected cell the compound may be incorporated into both viral DNA and cellular DNA. The incorporation of AIU into DNA leads to the formation of phosphoramidate (P–N) bonds (Chen *et al.*, 1976), which are more prone to breakage than the usual phosphodiester linkages. However, the DNA breakage induced by the incorporation of AIU does not seem to be related to its antiviral activity (Fischer *et al.*, 1980).

3. In-vitro *interaction with the immune system*

EDU does not impair the growth of human lymphocytes at concentrations up to 100 μg/ml (Singh *et al.*, 1974), and like dThd, EDU restores proliferation of PHA-stimulated lymphocyte cultures placed under amethopterine block (Swierkowska *et al.*, 1973). However, araT depresses the proliferative response of hamster splenic lymphocytes to mitogens such as ConA and PWM, and these inhibitory effects are observed from a concentration of $\geqslant 5\ \mu g/ml$ (Barnett *et al.*, 1979). Apparently, mitogen-stimulated hamster splenic lymphocytes contain the necessary battery of kinases to convert araT to its active form (araTTP).

4. In-vivo *interaction with the immune system*

The immunosuppressive action of araT also extends to the situation *in vivo*. AraT inhibits the primary, but not the secondary, humoral immune response to *Brucella abortus* (a T-independent antigen) and sheep erythrocytes (a T-dependent antigen) (Barnett *et al.*, 1980). However, araT does not appear more immunosuppressive than dThd and, since only the primary humoral response is affected, the immunosuppression caused by araT might not be critical in immunocompromised patients (Barnett *et al.*, 1980), which is an important notion, if araT were ever to be considered for use in such patients.

Little is known about the interaction of EDU, IDU or AIU with the immune system *in vivo*. According to Davis *et al.* (1978), an uncompromised host defence mechanism may be required for manifestation of the full antiviral activity of EDU, since EDU did not prevent the final fatal outcome of an HSV-2 infection in mice immunosuppressed by irradiation, whereas in non-immunosuppressed mice infected with HSV-2 the mortality rate was significantly reduced upon EDU treatment. The EDU-treated animals surviving HSV-2 infection were resistant to rechallenge with the homologous virus, suggesting that EDU did not impair the ability of the mice to acquire an adequate immune response (Davis *et al.*, 1978).

E. 'Second-Generation' Antiherpes Compounds

1. *Antiviral spectrum*

The advent of the highly potent and selective antiherpes agents acyclovir (ACV, Fig. 7), bromovinyldeoxyuridine (BVDU, Fig. 8) and fluoroiodoaracytosine (FIAC, Fig. 9) has heralded a new era in antiviral chemotherapy. Of this second generation of antiherpes agents, only ACV has been licensed so far for clinical use, e.g. as a 3% eye ointment for topical treatment of herpetic keratitis, as a 5% ointment (in polyethylene glycol) for topical treatment of genital herpes, as an intravenous infusion at 15 mg/kg/day for systemic treatment of severe mucocutaneous HSV infections in immunocompromised patients, and as capsules (5×200 mg/day) for systemic treatment of genital herpes. As reviewed recently (De Clercq, 1984*a*), ACV may also be considered for the systemic

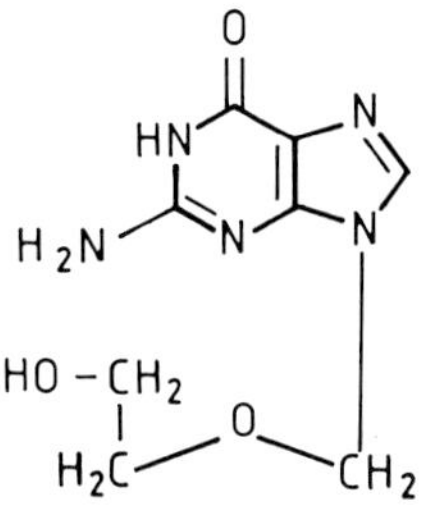

9-(2-hydroxyethoxymethyl) guanine (acycloguanosine, acyclovir, aciclovir, ACV, Zovirax ®)

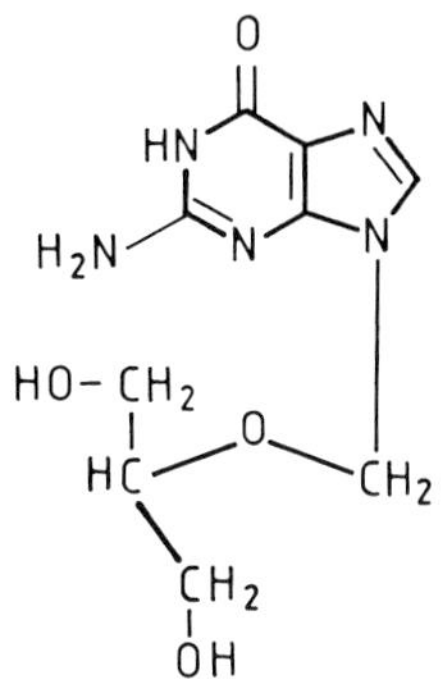

9-((2-hydroxy-1-hydroxymethyl) ethoxymethyl) guanine (dihydroxypropoxymethylguanine DHPG, BW-759, BIOLF-62, 2'-nor-2'-deoxyguanosine)

Fig. 7. 'Second-generation' antiherpes compounds: ACV and DHPG.

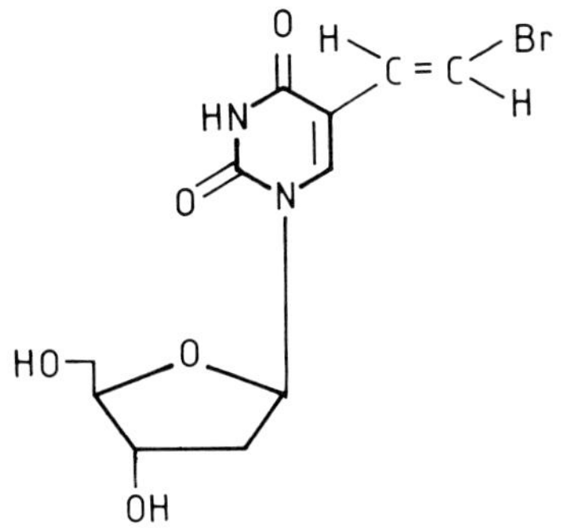

(E)-5-(2-bromovinyl)-2'-deoxyuridine (bromovinyldeoxyuridine, BVDU)

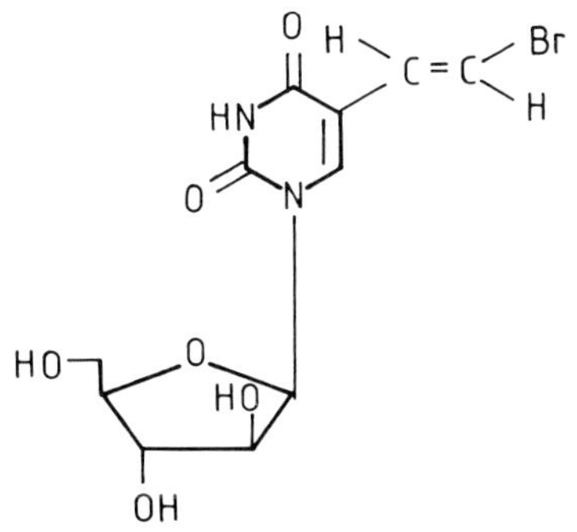

1-β-D-arabinofuranosyl-(E)-5-(2-bromovinyl) uracil (bromovinyluracil arabinoside, bromovinylarauracil, BVAU)

Fig. 8. 'Second-generation' antiherpes compounds: BVDU and BVAU.

therapy of VZV infections in both immunocompetent and immunocompromised patients and for the prophylaxis of recurrences of genital herpes and of HSV (and perhaps CMV) infections in bone-marrow transplant recipients. BVDU holds great promise for both topical and

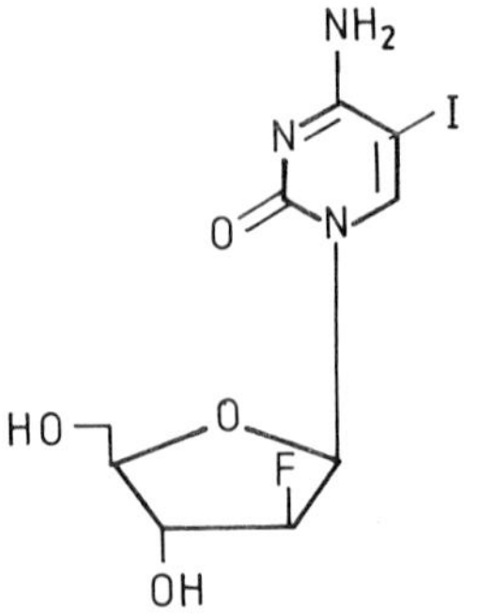

1-(2'-fluoro-2'-deoxy-β-D-
arabinofuranosyl-5-iodocytosine
(fluoroiodoaracytosine, FIAC)

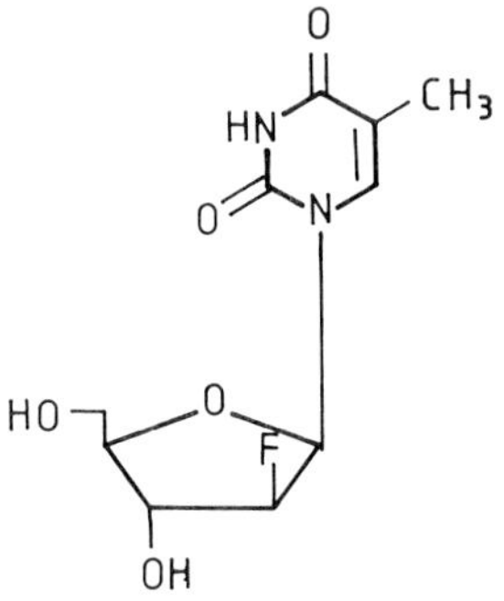

1-(2'-fluoro-2'-deoxy-β-D-
arabinofuranosyl-5-methyluracil
(fluoromethylarauracil, FMAU)

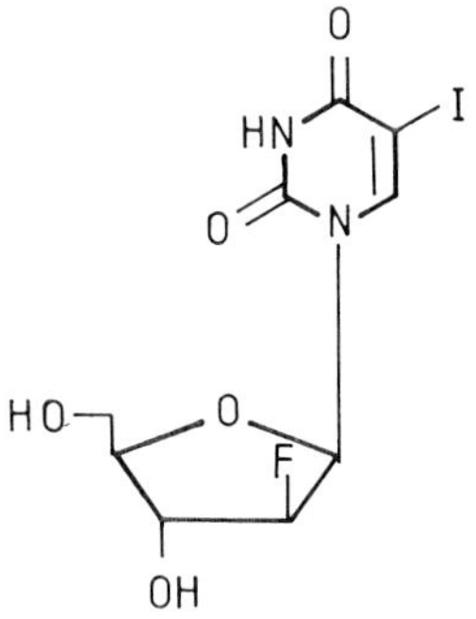

1-(2'-fluoro-2'-deoxy-β-D-
arabinofuranosyl-5-iodouracil
(fluoroiodoarauracil, FIAU)

Fig. 9. 'Second-generation' antiherpes compounds: FIAC, FMAU and FIAU.

systemic treatment of HSV-1 and VZV infections; in particular oral BVDU for the treatment of varicella-zoster in cancer patients, including children (Wildiers and De Clercq, 1984; Benoit *et al.*, 1984). FIAC has been found to be efficacious in the systemic (intravenous) treatment of VZV infections in immunocompromised patients (Young *et al.*, 1983).

The activity spectrum of ACV, BVDU and FIAC is primarily directed towards HSV-1, HSV-2 and VZV, although there are remarkable differences in the relative antiviral potencies of these drugs. For example, ACV and FIAC are equipotent against HSV-1 and HSV-2, but BVDU is significantly more inhibitory to HSV-1 than to HSV-2 [ID_{50}: 0·003–0·01 and 1–2 μg/ml, respectively (De Clercq *et al.*, 1979, 1980)]. On the other hand, BVDU is inhibitory to VZV in the concentration range of 0·001–0·01 μg/ml (Shigeta *et al.*, 1983), whereas ACV inhibits this virus only at a concentration of 1–10 μg/ml (Crumpacker *et al.*, 1979; Biron and Elion, 1980; Shigeta *et al.*, 1983). The differential susceptibility of VZV towards BVDU and ACV is also reflected by the marked difference in the efficacy of BVDU and ACV in the treatment of Simian varicella virus infection in monkeys, where ACV is only marginally effective at doses at which BVDU completely blocks all manifestations of the disease (Soike *et al.*, 1981*a*, *b*). FIAC and bromovinylarauracil (BVAU), a closely related analogue of BVDU (Fig. 8), are also active against VZV in the concentration range of 0·001–0·01 μg/ml (Lopez *et al.*, 1980; Machida *et al.*, 1982).

ACV and BVDU are rather weak inhibitors of CMV (Crumpacker *et al.*, 1979; De Clercq, 1984*c*). However, dihydroxypropoxymethylguanine (DHPG), a derivative of ACV (Fig. 7), is 10–100-fold more potent than ACV in inhibiting CMV replication in cell culture [ID_{50} in the range of 0·1–1 μg/ml (Cheng *et al.*, 1983; Field *et al.*, 1983; Mar *et al.*, 1983; Tocci *et al.*, 1984)]. FIAC and its congeners, fluoromethylarauracil (FMAU) and fluoroiodoarauracil (FIAU) (Fig. 9), are even more potent inhibitors than DHPG, since they inhibit CMV replication *in vitro* at a concentration of 0·01–0·1 μg/ml (Colacino and Lopez, 1983; Mar *et al.*, 1984). Based on these laboratory findings, it seems tempting to speculate on the potential clinical usefulness of DHPG, FIAC, FMAU or FIAU in the treatment of CMV infections in humans.

ACV (Colby *et al.*, 1980; Lin *et al.*, 1983, 1984), DHPG (Cheng *et al.*, 1983; Field *et al.*, 1983; Martin *et al.*, 1983; Lin *et al.*, 1984), BVDU (Lin *et al.*, 1983; Zhang *et al.*, 1984), FIAC (Lin *et al.*, 1983) and FMAU (Lin *et al.*, 1983) are all efficient inhibitors of EBV replication (at ID_{50} values varying between 0·01 and 10 μg/ml, depending on the compound and the parameters used to monitor EBV infection). BVDU, FIAC and FMAU can even be considered as irreversible inhibitors of EBV replication, since their inhibitory effects persist for up to 58 days after removal of the drugs (Lin *et al.*, 1983); the inhibitory effect of DHPG persists for more than 21 days (Lin *et al.*, 1984), whereas the inhibitory effect of ACV is readily reversed upon removal of the drug. The therapeutic implications of these findings, i.e. for the treatment of EBV-associated diseases, remain to be determined.

2. Mechanism of action

The prime target for the antiviral action of ACV, BVDU, FIAC [and their congeners DHPG, BVAU, FMAU and FIAU (Figs 7–9)] is the viral DNA, and their selectivity as antiviral agents is clearly attested by the markedly greater inhibition of viral DNA synthesis than of host cell DNA synthesis (Larsson and Öberg, 1981). All 'second-generation' antiherpes compounds share a common mechanism of action (De Clercq, 1984*b*), which can best be illustrated with BVDU as model. BVDU has a much greater affinity for the HSV- and VZV-encoded dThd kinase than for the corresponding cellular (cytosol) dThd kinase(s) (Cheng *et al.*, 1981), which explains why the compound is phosphorylated to a much greater extent in virus-infected cells than in uninfected cells (Descamps and De Clercq, 1981). The dThd kinase encoded by HSV-1 and VZV would convert BVDU successively to its 5′-monophosphate (BVDUMP) and 5′-diphosphate (BVDUDP), whereas the dThd kinase encoded by HSV-2 would convert BVDU only to BVDUMP (Descamps and De Clercq, 1981; Fyfe, 1982; Ayisi *et al.*, 1984). This difference in the phosphorylation pattern of BVDU in HSV-1- and HSV-2-infected cells may be related to its differential inhibitory effects on HSV-1 and HSV-2 replication (see above), since BVDU, once it has been trapped at the 5′-monophosphate stage, may be subject to degradation by dTMP synthetase to a number of inert metabolites (Barr *et al.*, 1983).

Upon further phosphorylation of BVDUDP (perhaps by cellular kinases) to BVDU 5′-triphosphate (BVDUTP), the drug may act in two ways:

(a) either as an inhibitor of DNA polymerase by direct competition with the natural substrate, dTTP, thereby inhibiting HSV DNA polymerase to a greater extent than the cellular DNA polymerases α, β and γ (Allaudeen *et al.*, 1981);
(b) or as an alternative substrate of the viral and cellular DNA polymerase, and thereby become incorporated into DNA (Allaudeen *et al.*, 1982). When used at supraoptimal concentrations (10 μg/ml), BVDU may be incorporated into both viral and host cell DNA of the virus-infected cell (Allaudeen *et al.*, 1982). However, at optimal concentrations (0·01–0·1 μg/ml), BVDU would be incorporated into viral DNA only (Mancini *et al.*, 1983). Furthermore, the amount of BVDU incorporated into HSV-1 DNA is directly proportional to the reduction in virus yield achieved with BVDU. As more BVDU is incorporated into HSV-1 DNA, the DNA becomes more unstable as ascertained by a dose-dependent increase in single-strand breaks. Whether this increased lability of the HSV-1 DNA is directly responsible for the antiviral effects of BVDU remains a matter of further study.

3. In-vitro *interaction with the immune system*

Of the compounds presented in Figs 7–9, only ACV and BVDU have been examined for their effects on lymphocyte functions. In contrast with the 'first-generation' antiherpes compounds (IDU, TFT, araC), the 'second-generation' antiherpes compounds exhibit little, if any, immunosuppressive activity. ACV does not depress the proliferative response of peripheral blood mononuclear cells to PHA or ConA at concentrations up to 6–11 μg/ml (Wingard *et al.*, 1983) or 20 μg/ml (Levin *et al.*, 1980). Its ID_{50} for the proliferation of human granulocyte-monocyte progenitor cells is approximately 40–80 μg/ml (McGuffin *et al.*, 1980; Parker *et al.*, 1982). Thus, ACV is immuno- or myelotoxic only at concentrations which are 100–1000-fold higher than its minimum inhibitory concentration for HSV-1 or HSV-2 replication. However, with respect to VZV, the safety margin of ACV is much smaller and does not exceed 1–10-fold.

BVDU is even less immunotoxic than ACV: it does not impair lymphocyte blastogenic responses at concentrations up to 60–150 μg/ml (Marmer *et al.*, 1982; Wingard *et al.*, 1983; Wittek *et al.*, 1983). Its ID_{50} for the growth of bone-marrow progenitor cells is 40 μg/ml according to Wingard *et al.* (1983) or 200 μg/ml according to Wittek *et al.* (1983). BVDU does not interfere with cell-mediated lympholysis, NK-cell activity or K-cell activity at a concentration of 100 μmol/l (33 μg/ml) (Wingard *et al.*, 1983). Based on a minimum antiviral concentration of 0·01 μg/ml for HSV-1 (De Clercq *et al.*, 1980) and 0·003 μg/ml for VZV (Shigeta *et al.*, 1983), and a minimum immuno- or myelotoxic concentration of 100 μg/ml (on average), the safety margin of BVDU could be estimated at about 10 000–30 000-fold. No other antiviral drug has ever been found to show such high selectivity index *in vitro*.

4. In-vivo *interaction with the immune system*

An intact immune system is not required for antiviral agents such as BVDU to exert their antiviral effects, since BVDU is fully protective against a lethal HSV-1 infection in athymic-nude (nu/nu) mice (De Clercq *et al.*, 1981). This contrasts with interferon, which did not alter progression of the HSV-1 infection in nu/nu mice when evaluated under the same conditions as BVDU. Also, when administered orally (at 7·5 mg/kg/day for 5 days) to immunocompromised (cancer) patients with herpes zoster infection, BVDU accomplished a prompt recovery from the zoster episode. In the majority of the patients progression of the VZV infection was arrested after 1 day of BVDU treatment (Wildiers and De Clercq, 1984). Similar beneficial effects were obtained with oral BVDU (at 15 mg/kg/day for 5 days) in leukaemic children suffering from an intercurrent varicella or zoster infection: all children responded rapidly to BVDU therapy and recovered completely without any complications (Benoit *et al.*, 1984).

ACV has been the subject of a number of studies in immunocompromised patients. A comprehensive trial of ACV in the therapy of acute herpes zoster in immunosuppressed patients (Balfour *et al.*, 1983*a*) demonstrated that ACV, when administered intravenously at 1500 mg/m^2/day for 7 days, prevented cutaneous or visceral dissemination of herpes zoster, but only if treatment was begun during the first 72 h after the onset of rash. Whether ACV would still be effective in patients with zoster of more than 3 days' duration, is uncertain (Fanelli and Sattler, 1984). In another study, conducted in immunosuppressed children with varicella, intravenous ACV treatment (at 1500 mg/m^2/day for 7 days) shortened the duration of viral shedding and prevented the development of visceral complications, but otherwise not much clinical benefit was noted (Prober *et al.*, 1982). In a small number of immunocompromised children with varicella, intravenous ACV treatment led to rapid recovery from the infection only if treatment was started before the third day of rash (Balfour, 1984). If treatment was started later, when there was already evidence of visceral varicella, the disease progressed despite ACV therapy and proved fatal in two out of four children (Balfour, 1984). This again makes it clear that if any beneficial effect were to be expected from ACV in the treatment of VZV infections in immunocompromised patients, treatment has to be started as soon as possible after onset of the disease.

ACV treatment (1500 mg/m^2/day, intravenously, for 5 days) does not seem to alter the humoral antibody response to VZV, as has been assessed in normal (immunocompetent) adults given ACV for acute herpes zoster (Bean *et al.*, 1982). The effect of ACV treatment on the cell-mediated immune response to VZV was not evaluated in this study.

While the effectiveness of ACV in the treatment of VZV infections is far from overwhelming, it appears more efficacious in the treatment of HSV infections. For instance, intravenous ACV treatment (at 750 mg/m^2/day for 7 days) significantly shortens the time to crusting, healing and therefore pain relief, concomitantly with a more rapid cessation of viral shedding, in kidney, heart or bone-marrow transplant recipients suffering from mucocutaneous HSV infections (Chou *et al.*, 1981; Mitchell *et al.*, 1981; Wade *et al.*, 1982). In addition, immunodeficient patients with recurrent mucocutaneous HSV infection responded favourably to intravenous ACV treatment, as monitored, for example, by the duration of viral shedding (Straus *et al.*, 1982). In these patients oral ACV treatment (at 15 mg/kg/day for up to 65 days) prevented recurrences of the HSV infection. Intravenous as well as oral ACV treatment would also be effective in the prophylaxis of recurrent HSV infections in bone-marrow transplant recipients (Saral *et al.*, 1981; Gluckman *et al.*, 1983*a*, *b*; Prentice, 1983) and patients with acute leukaemia receiving timed sequential chemotherapy (Saral *et al.*, 1983). According to Gluckman *et al.* (1983*a*, *b*), this prophylactic effect would even extend to CMV infections.

For the therapy of CMV infections in allograft (e.g. bone-marrow transplant) recipients, adequate treatment is still lacking. Balfour *et al.* (1982) have reported that intravenous ACV treatment (1500 mg/m^2/day for 7 days) may accelerate the rate of improvement and defervescence in immunocompromised patients (mainly renal transplant recipients) with various forms of CMV disease, but, in abeyance of a more uniform and extensive trial, the preliminary findings of Balfour *et al.* (1982) should not be considered as conclusive evidence for the effectiveness of ACV in the treatment of CMV infections. An attempt to treat CMV pneumonia in bone-marrow transplant recipients with high doses of ACV (up to 3000 mg/m^2/day) alone or in combination with human leucocyte interferon (up to 40×10^4 units/kg/day) proved unsucccessful (Wade *et al.*, 1983*a*; Meyers *et al.*, 1983*b*). Future attempts to treat CMV infections will undoubtedly be based on the use of DHPG or FIAC (FMAU, FIAU), either alone or combined with interferon.

The widespread use of antiviral agents such as ACV is clouded by the possible emergence of virus resistance to the drug. If such drug resistance were to occur, it should most likely arise in immunocompromised patients since they experience more severe recurrences more often than do immunocompetent patients and, therefore, require multiple drug treatment courses (Straus *et al.*, 1982). In fact, most of the ACV-resistant HSV mutants that have so far been isolated originated from immunodeficient or immunosuppressed patients who had received multiple courses of ACV (Burns *et al.*, 1982; Crumpacker *et al.*, 1982; Sibrack *et al.*, 1982; Wade *et al.*, 1983*b*). All these isolates were deficient in their ability to phosphorylate dThd and/or ACV, suggesting that they arose by a mutation in the dThd kinase locus. Alternatively, the drug-resistant mutant may have been present in the original virus population (Parris and Harrington, 1982) and selection of this variant may have occurred during drug therapy. Whatever mechanism (mutation and/or selection) the emergence of drug-resistant virus strains is based upon, it is not certain that they present a clinical problem, since ACV-resistant HSV-1 strains might be associated with diminished virulence (Sibrack *et al.*, 1982).

F. Interferon and Interferon Inducers

1. Antiviral spectrum

Interferon is not a purely antiviral agent; it has a variety of actions, including immunoregulatory (both immunoenhancing and immunosuppressive),

Table 2
Interferon and interferon inducers

1. *Interferon* (human interferon)[a]	
Type I:	HuIFN-α:α_1, α_2, α_3 etc.
	HuIFN-β:β_1
Type II:	HuIFN-γ
2. *Interferon inducers*	
Double-stranded RNAs: poly I:C (polyinosinic acid·polycytidylic acid), complexed with poly-L-lysine,[b] with or without carboxymethylcellulose	
Low-molecular-weight compounds: 5-halo-6-phenyl pyrimidinones,[c] e.g. ABPP (2-amino-5-bromo-6-phenyl-4-pyrimidinol)	

[a]De Clercq (1982).
[b]Krown *et al.* (1983).
[c]Stringfellow *et al.* (1980).

antitumour, antibacterial, antiprotozoal and antifungal properties (De Clercq, 1982). Theoretically, the antiviral activity spectrum of interferon encompasses all DNA and RNA viruses, but in practice interferon, and particularly HuIFN-α (Table 2), has been pursued only for certain virus infections. Interferon may have a beneficial effect in the therapy of papilloma virus infections (e.g. warts, laryngeal papilloma, condyloma acuminatum), adenovirus infections (e.g. epidemic adenovirus kerato-conjunctivitis), herpesvirus infections [e.g. herpetic keratitis (if combined with other antiviral agents), herpes zoster and varicella (in immuno-suppressed patients)] and chronic active hepatitis B. It may also be of value in the prophylaxis of acute respiratory tract virus infections (e.g. rhinovirus infections). Based on a reduction in virus shedding and diminution of nasal mucus production, HuIFN-α has shown efficacy when given as intranasal drops in the prophylaxis of rhinovirus infections (Scott *et al.*, 1982; Hayden and Gwaltney, 1983; Samo *et al.*, 1983). However, long-term intranasal administration of interferon may be associated with mucosal irritation, inflammation and ulceration and is therefore not a feasible strategy for the prophylaxis of respiratory viral infections (Hayden *et al.*, 1983*b*).

Since Greenberg *et al.* (1976) and Desmyter *et al.* (1976) reported that hepatitis B virus (HBV) infection may be sensitive to interferon (HuIFN-α and HuINF-β, respectively), interferon has also been considered for the treatment of chronic infection with HBV. However, the effectiveness of interferon treatment in patients with chronic HBV infection seems to be limited to a transient drop in serum Dane particle-associated DNA polymerase activity (Weimar *et al.*, 1980; Smith *et al.*, 1983). To achieve a permanent lack of HBV-associated DNA polymerase activity, it may be necessary to combine interferon with other antiviral agents (e.g. araA) (Scullard *et al.*, 1981*a*, *b*). Such a combination therapy may result in the loss of viral markers from serum and liver tissue and an improvement in symptoms, hepatic tests and histologic findings, but only in some of the patients. The response of chronic hepatitis B patients to HuIFN-α and araA treatment is far from uniform (Scullard *et al.*, 1981*b*) and some patients do not respond at all.

2. *Mechanism of action*

At the cellular level interferon exerts a myriad of effects which result in an enhancement of certain specialized cell functions, alterations of the outer cell plasma membrane and inhibition of cell division (De Clercq, 1982). At the molecular level, interferon shuts off protein synthesis. There are two pathways that lead to this inhibition of protein synthesis. First, interferon causes the induction of a protein kinase which phosphorylates and thereby inactivates eukaryotic initiation factor 2 (eIF-2). The initiation factor eIF-2 is required for the binding of methionyl-tRNA to 40S ribosomal subunits, an essential step in the initiation of protein synthesis. This step will not occur if eIF-2 is inactivated. Second, interferon causes the induction of a 2′–5′ oligoadenylate (2–5A) synthetase, which catalyses the formation of 2–5A from ATP, i.e. adenylate oligomers with 2′–5′ phosphodiester instead of the usual 3′–5′ phosphoediester linkages. These 2′–5′ adenylate oligomers then activate a preexisting endoribonuclease that breaks down RNAs, including rRNA and mRNA, which again results in an inhibition of protein synthesis. Both pathways are subject to additional control mechanisms, a phosphoprotein phosphatase that may dephosphorylate eIF-2 and a 2′–5′ phosphodiesterase that may degrade 2–5A. Furthermore, the exact role of the protein kinase and the 2–5A synthetase pathways in the establishment of the antiviral state of interferon is not very well defined.

3. In-vitro *interaction with the immune system*

In its interaction with the immune system, interferon stimulates some immune responses while obviating others: in general, it has an enhancing effect on T lymphocytes and a suppressive effect on B lymphocytes. Depending on the dose, interferon either enhances or inhibits the PFC response to T-cell-dependent antigens such as sheep red blood cells and T-cell-independent antigens such as *E. coli* lipopolysaccharide. Interferon stimulates IgE-mediated histamine release from human peripheral blood cells. It inhibits delayed-type hypersensitivity as well as the mixed lymphocyte reaction, but stimulates antibody-dependent cellular cytotoxicity (Zafra *et al.*, 1984). Interferon also enhances the phagocytic activity of macrophages, but inhibits the maturation of monocytes to macrophages. What has received most attention, however, is the stimulatory effect of interferon on natural killer (NK) cell activity (Vyakarnam, 1983). NK cells have spontaneous cytolytic activity towards tumour cells, virus-infected cells and some subpopulations of thymus cells, bone-marrow cells and macrophages (Herberman and Ortaldo, 1981), and their reactivity can be boosted further by interferon. Because NK cells have been implicated in the host defence against cancer and virus infections, it is plausible that the antiviral and antitumour effects of interferon are due at least in part to an augmented NK-cell activity. Interferon inducers [e.g. 2-amino-5-bromo-6-phenyl-4-pyrimidinol (ABPP)] may operate via an augmentation of NK-cell activity (Lotzova *et al.*, 1983), but these interferon inducers may also achieve their antiviral activity through mechanisms other than interferon induction or NK-cell augmentation.

4. In-vivo *interaction with the immune system*

From the complexity of effects that interferon can exert on the immune system it is obvious that, depending on a number of factors (dosage of interferon, time of administration, functional state of the immune system), interferon may either potentiate or suppress the host immune response or leave it unaffected. The beneficial effects of interferon treatment on some virus infections (e.g. chronic HBV infection) may be mediated through a stimulatory action on cell-mediated immunity (Dolen *et al.*, 1979). The inhibitory effects of interferon (HuIFN-α) on the progression (i.e. dissemination) of herpes zoster or varicella in immunosuppressed (cancer) patients (Merigan *et al.*, 1978, 1981; Arvin *et al.*, 1978, 1982) may be achieved through a direct antiviral action, independently from any interaction with the immune system. However, it does not exclude the possible contribution of an augmented NK-cell activity to the inhibitory effects of interferon on VZV infection in cancer patients, since the NK-cell activity of these patients is significantly increased upon interferon administration (Lotzova *et al.*, 1982).

Other observations suggest that interferon may require an intact immune system to exhibit an optimal antiviral activity. This is illustrated by the case of a 40-year-old female who developed a recurrent HSV infection while being treated with high doses of interferon (2×10^5 U/kg/day) for a metastatic breast cancer (Khan and Hill, 1980), and is further attested by the failure of interferon to alter the incidence of HSV infections in kidney transplant recipients (Weimar *et al.*, 1978; Cheeseman *et al.*, 1979). Neither is interferon effective in the prophylaxis or therapy of CMV infections in immunosuppressed patients (Weimar *et al.*, 1978; Cheeseman *et al.*, 1979; Meyers *et al.*, 1983*a*; Chou *et al.*, 1984). This failure may be related to the severely impaired immunoresponsiveness of the patients with CMV disease and their inability to react to the immunostimulatory activity of interferon. On the other hand, at the high-dose levels used in the latter two studies (5×10^7 U/day), HuIFN-α may act as an immunosuppressant and decrease several lymphocyte subpopulations, e.g. T (leu-1), suppressor T (leu-2), helper T (leu-3) and B cells (Smith *et al.*, 1983); and this immunosuppressive action may have counteracted any possible favourable effect that interferon could have had in the CMV patients.

G. Isoprinosine

1. Antiviral spectrum

Isoprinosine is a combination of the natural nucleoside inosine with the *p*-acetamidobenzoic acid salt of N,N-dimethylamino-2-propanol in a molar ratio of 1:3 (Fig. 10). Isoprinosine is principally an immunopotentiator. So are various other substances, e.g. transfer factor, thymosine, endotoxin, levamisole, Bacillus Calmette-Guérin, poly A·U (polyadenylic acid·polyuridylic acid), which are not discussed further in this chapter. In contrast with these other substances, isoprinosine has been pursued solely

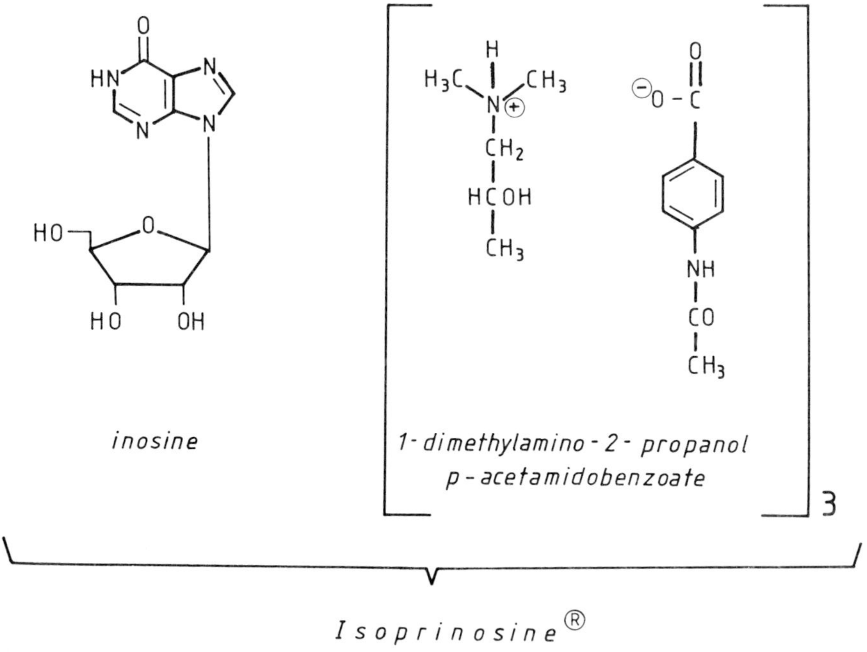

Fig. 10. Isoprinosine.

for its antiviral potentials. According to Gordon and Brown (1972), isoprinosine may be active against a wide variety of viruses, including influenza A, herpes simplex, polio and adeno, both *in vitro* and *in vivo* (mice). However, isoprinosine does not offer any protection from or alleviation of clinical illness associated with an influenza A virus infection in human volunteers (Longley *et al.*, 1973). Nor is there any evidence that the compound would be inhibitory to other viruses causing respiratory disease, such as rhinovirus infections, either *in vitro* (Muldoon *et al.*, 1972) or *in vivo* (humans) (Soto *et al.*, 1973; Pachuta *et al.*, 1974).

2. *Mechanism of action*

Very little is known about the mechanism by which isoprinosine exerts its putative antiviral effects. According to Gordon *et al.* (1974), the primary drug effect would be a modification in the physical or functional state of the host cell ribosomes which would then diminish their capacity to translate foreign (i.e. viral) mRNAs. No direct evidence has ever been provided for either a change in ribosome structure or reduced viral mRNA translation. Thus, the exact mode of action of isoprinosine remains unsettled.

3. In-vitro *interaction with the immune system*

Over a broad range of concentrations (0·2–250 μg/ml), isoprinosine augments the stimulatory effect of PHA on the proliferation of human peripheral blood lymphocytes (Hadden *et al.*, 1976). In the absence of PHA, isoprinosine does not stimulate lymphocyte proliferation. Hence, isoprinosine is not itself a mitogen nor an inducer of mitogenic factors. At a concentration range of 50–500 μg/ml it increases the percentage of active T-cell rosettes and yeast-phagocytosing cells; at a concentration range of 100–300 μg/ml it increases the number of non-adherent leucocytes; and at a concentration of 200–500 μg/ml it also increases the mixed lymphocyte reaction response (Wybran *et al.*, 1978). Thus, isoprinosine seems to activate both normal human T cells and monocytes and, possibly, also normal human neutrophils.

4. In-vivo *interaction with the immune system*

Human peripheral blood lymphocytes from apparently immunocompetent patients treated with isoprinosine exhibit a higher PHA reactivity than lymphocytes from placebo-treated patients (Bradshaw and Sumner, 1977), suggesting that the immunopotentiating effects of isoprinosine extend to the *in-vivo* situation. However, lymphocytes derived from immunosuppressed patients treated with isoprinosine for herpes zoster did not show an increased proliferative response to PHA or VZV as compared

Table 3
Immunosuppressive and myelosuppressive effects of antiherpes drugs *in vitro*

Parameter	ID$_{50}$ (μg/ml) IDU	TFT	AraC	AraA	ACV	BVDU	Reference
Mixed lymphocyte reaction		0·03		120		150	Wingard *et al.*, 1983
PHA-induced blastogenesis	< 1·5		≪10	> 3	160		Steele *et al.*, 1980
		2		5	6	100	Wingard *et al.*, 1983
						> 100	Wittek *et al.*, 1983
						60	Marmer *et al.*, 1982
					~ 20		Levin *et al.*, 1980
ConA-induced blastogenesis	< 1·5		≪10	> 3	84		Steele *et al.*, 1980
		0·04		2	11	90	Wingard *et al.*, 1983
						58	Marmer *et al.*, 1982
PWM-induced blastogenesis	< 1·5		≪10	> 3	200		Steele *et al.*, 1980
						84	Marmer *et al.*, 1982
HSV-stimulated blastogenesis	~ 1·5		≪10	> 3	> 20		Steele *et al.*, 1980
					~ 20		Levin *et al.*, 1980
VZV-stimulated blastogenesis	~ 1·5		≪10	> 3	< 20		Steele *et al.*, 1980
					~ 20		Levin *et al.*, 1980
						> 100	Wittek *et al.*, 1983
Cell-mediated lympholysis	0·08			> 50	> 20	> 33	Wingard *et al.*, 1983
NK-cell activity	> 30			> 25	> 20	> 33	Wingard *et al.*, 1983
K-cell activity	> 30			> 25	> 20	> 33	Wingard *et al.*, 1983
Growth of bone-marrow (granulocyte–monocyte) progenitor cells		0·4		1	> 20	40	Wingard *et al.*, 1983
						197	Wittek *et al.*, 1983
					~ 40		Parker *et al.*, 1982
					~ 80		McGuffin *et al.*, 1980

Table 4 Representative studies on the clinical efficacy of

Virus	Disease	Underlying disorder (majority of the patients)	Drug	Route of administration	Dosage
HSV	Mucocutaneous herpes simplex	Kidney transplant/cancer	AraA	i.v.	10 mg/kg/day
HSV	Mucocutaneous herpes simplex	Immunodeficiency	ACV	i.v. *p.o.*	15 mg/kg/day 15 mg/kg/day
HSV	Mucocutaneous herpes simplex	Kidney or bone-marrow transplant	ACV	i.v.	750 mg/m^2/day
HSV	Mucocutaneous herpes simplex	Heart transplant	ACV	i.v.	750 mg/m^2/day
HSV	Mucocutaneous herpes simplex	Bone-marrow transplant	ACV	i.v.	750 mg/m^2/day
HSV	Mucocutaneous herpes simplex	Bone-marrow transplant	ACV	i.v.	750 mg/m^2/day
HSV	Mucocutaneous herpes simplex	Acute leukaemia	ACV	i.v.	750 mg/m^2/day
HSV	Mucocutaneous herpes simplex	Bone-marrow transplant/ acute leukaemia	ACV	i.v.	10 mg/kg/day
HSV	Mucocutaneous herpes simplex	Bone-marrow transplant	ACV	*p.o.*	800 mg/day
VZV	Zoster (disseminated)	Cancer	AraC	i.v.	100 mg/m^2/day
VZV	Zoster (localized or disseminated)	Cancer	AraA	i.v.	10 mg/kg/day
VZV	Zoster (localized)	Cancer	AraA	i.v.	10 mg/kg/day
VZV	Varicella	Cancer	AraA	i.v.	20 mg/kg/day
VZV	Zoster (localized or disseminated)	Cancer	ACV	i.v.	1500 mg/m^2/day
VZV	Varicella	Cancer	ACV	i.v.	1500 mg/m^2/day
VZV	Varicella	Cancer	ACV	i.v.	1500 mg/m^2/day

antiherpes drugs in immunocompromised patients

Duration of treatment	Type of study	Therapeutic or prophylactic use	Principal clinical effect noted	Reference
7 days	DB	T	Accelerated relief of pain but only in older patients (>40 years)	Whitley *et al.* (1984)
5 days	O	T	Rapid healing	Straus *et al.* (1982)
up to 65 days	O	P	Prevention of recurrences	
7 days	DB	T	More rapid healing, relief of pain and cessation of new lesion formation	Mitchell *et al.* (1981)
7 days	DB	T	More rapid healing and relief of pain	Chou *et al.* (1981)
7 days	DB	T	More rapid healing and relief of pain	Wade *et al.* (1982)
18 days	DB	P	Prevention of the infection	Saral *et al.* (1981)
32 days	DB	P	Prevention of the infection	Saral *et al.* (1983)
throughout period of neutropenia	DB	P	Prevention of the infection	Prentice (1983)
44 days	DB	P	Prevention of the infection	Gluckman *et al.* (1983*a*, *b*)
3 days	DB	T	Dissemination prolonged	Stevens *et al.* (1973)
5 days	DB	T	More rapid cessation of new lesion formation	Whitley *et al.* (1976)
5 days	DB	T	More rapid healing, and lesser dissemination	Whitley *et al.* (1982*b*)
5 days	DB	T	More rapid cessation of new lesion formation and fewer visceral complications	Whitley *et al.* (1982*a*)
7 days	DB	T	Prevention of cutaneous and visceral dissemination	Balfour *et al.* (1983*a*, *b*)
7 days	DB	T	Fewer visceral complications	Prober *et al.* (1982)
7 days	O	T	Rapid recovery only if treatment started early	Balfour (1984)

(continued)

Table 4 (continued)

Virus	Disease	Underlying disorder (majority of the patients)	Drug	Route of administration	Dosage
VZV	Zoster (localized or disseminated)	Cancer	BVDU	*p.o.*	7.5 mg/kg/day
VZV	Varicella-zoster	Cancer	BVDU	*p.o.*	15 mg/kg/day
VZV	Zoster (localized or disseminated)	Cancer	FIAC	i.v.	$\geqslant 120$ mg/m^2/day
VZV	Zoster (localized)	Cancer	HuIFN-α	i.m.	$5 \cdot 1 \times 10^5$ U/kg/day
VZV	Varicella	Cancer	HuIFN-α	i.m.	$\leqslant 3 \cdot 5 \times 10^5$ U/kg/day
CMV	CMV pneumonia	Kidney transplant	AraA	i.v.	10 mg/kg/day
CMV	CMV pneumonia, hepatitis, retinitis, nephritis	Kidney transplant	ACV	i.v.	1500 mg/m^2/day
CMV	CMV pneumonia, hepatitis	Bone-marrow transplant	ACV	*p.o.*	800 mg/day
CMV	CMV pneumonia	Bone-marrow transplant	ACV	i.v.	up to 3600 mg/m^2/day
			ACV +	i.v.	up to 3000 mg/m^2/day
			HuIFN-α	i.m.	up to 4×10^5 U/kg/day
CMV HSV	CMV infection HSV infection	Kidney transplant	HuIFN-α	i.m.	3×10^6 U twice weekly
CMV HSV	CMV infection HSV infection	Kidney transplant	HuIFN-β	i.m.	3×10^6 U twice weekly
CMV Adenovirus	Pneumonia, esophagitis, nephritis	Bone-marrow transplant	HuIFN-α	i.m.	up to 10^6 U/kg/day
CMV	CMV retinitis	AIDS	HuIFN-α	i.m.	10^7 U/day up to $3 \cdot 6 \times 10^7$ U/day

Abbreviations: i.v., intravenously; i.m.; intramuscularly: *p.o.*, *per os*; O, open clinical study; DB, double-blind placebo-controlled study; T, therapeutic use; P, prophylactic use.

Table 4 (continued)

Duration of treatment	Type of study	Therapeutic or prophylactic use	Principal clinical effect noted	Reference
5 days	O	T	Rapid cessation of new lesion formation (within 1 day)	Wildiers and De Clercq (1984)
5 days	O	T	Rapid cessation of new lesion formation (within 1-3 days)	Benoit *et al.* (1984)
7 days	O	T	Stabilization of skin lesions within 2-3 days	Young *et al.* (1983)
5 days	DB	T	Prevention of cutaneous and visceral dissemination	Merigan *et al.*(1978)
2 days	DB	T	Modest effect on cutaneous dissemination	Merigan *et al.* (1981)
3-11 days	DB	T	More rapid cessation of new lesion formation	Arvin *et al.* (1982)
5-7 days	O+ DB	T	No apparent benefit	Marker *et al.* (1980)
7 days	DB	T	Tendency to improvement	Balfour *et al.* (1982)
44 days	DB	T	Prevention of the infection	Gluckman *et al.* (1983*a*, *b*)
4-32 days 1-27 days	O	T	No apparent benefit	Wade *et al.* (1983*a*); Meyers *et al.* (1983*b*)
6 weeks	DB	P	No prevention of the infection	Cheeseman *et al.* (1979)
3 months	DB	P	No prevention of the infection	Weimar *et al.* (1978)
7-14 days	O	T	No apparent benefit	Meyers *et al.* (1983*a*)
19-62 days	O	T	No apparent benefit	Chou *et al.* (1984)

with lymphocytes from placebo-treated patients (Feldman *et al.*, 1978). Neither did isoprinosine influence the course of the VZV infection in these patients. Although these findings do not justify the use of isoprinosine in the treatment of VZV infections in immunocompromised hosts, they do not preclude the possibility that in normal hosts with herpes zoster, the compound may have a more beneficial effect.

Of particular interest is the therapeutic potential that isoprinosine may offer in the treatment of subacute sclerosing pancephalitis (SSPE), a progressive and eventually fatal disease of the central nervous system in children or young adults, which is thought to be caused by a persistent measles-like virus infection in conjunction with a defective host immune response. Because of the immunopotentiating effects of isoprinosine and the hypothesized immune response defect in SSPE, isoprinosine has been administered to SSPE patients on numerous occasions (for representative studies, see Haddad and Risk, 1980; Jones *et al.*, 1982). The former study provides little support for any clinical efficacy of isoprinosine in SSPE; however, the latter does suggest that isoprinosine may prolong life in patients with SSPE. Thus, the therapeutic value of isoprinosine in the treatment of SSPE, or any other virus infection, remains a matter of conjecture.

IV. CONCLUSION

The most salient feature emerging from a review of the recent literature on the antiviral agents that are currently used in the clinic or being considered for clinical use is the paucity of data on their interaction with the immune system. Some antiviral agents have been investigated for their effects on some manifestations of cell-mediated immunity, but very few attempts have been made to determine the interaction of the antiviral agent with the cell-mediated immune response towards the virus for which it is used clinically. Yet it is imperative to know how the antiviral agent affects the immune response to the virus infection concerned. This would further help in delineating the optimal dose and time regimen and route(s) of administration of the compound. It is generally assumed that the antiviral compound would, if anything, depress the immune response, but, as exemplified by amantadine, ribavirin and interferon, antiviral agent may also augment immunoreactivity under well defined conditions. Again, it would be imperative to establish whether these immunostimulatory effects may be translated into a better therapeutic efficacy of the compound *in vivo*.

Most of the antiviral agents that have been developed in recent years are intended for the chemotherapy of herpesvirus infections, particularly those due to HSV and VZV. These herpesvirus infections are more prevalent than any other infections in immunocompromised patients. If the antiherpes compounds were to be used in immunosuppressed patients, they should not be harmful for the immune system, since immunocompromised patients are the least able to sustain additional immunosuppression. From Table 3 it is evident that the 'older' antiviral drugs IDU, TFT and araC are indeed immunosuppressive at therapeutically effective concentrations and therefore unsuitable for systemic treatment of herpesvirus infections. AraA is relatively non-toxic for the immune system, but yet more selective in their antiviral activity are ACV and especially BVDU, which does not impair the cell-mediated immune response unless it is used at a concentration that is 10^4-fold higher than its minimal antiviral concentration. Several aspects on the *in-vitro* and *in vivo* interactions with the immune system remain to be explored, viz. the effects of BVDU on the host immune response to those viruses (HSV and VZV) for which it offers the greatest therapeutic potential, and the effects of the newer antiviral compounds [i.e. FIAC (FMAU, FIAU) and DHPG] on the different parameters of the immune response.

Various antiherpes agents (e.g. araA, ACV, BVDU, FIAC and HuIFN-α) have been the subject of clinical trials in immunocompromised patients with either HSV, VZV or CMV infections (Table 4). Since these studies have not been conducted on a comparative base, it is difficult to assess the relative efficacy of the compounds. Yet, it appears well established that:

(1) araA has a modest beneficial effect in the treatment of VZV infections, which must be balanced, however, against the toxic side effects of the compound and the inconvenience of intravenous infusion of large volumes of fluid;
(2) ACV is clearly effective in the therapy and prophylaxis of HSV infections, but much less efficacious in the treatment of VZV infections and only so if treatment is started within 3 days after the onset of rash;
(3) for treatment of VZV infections, BVDU and FIAC offer greater potentials than either araA or ACV; BVDU has thereby the advantage that it can be administered orally which permits treatment on an outpatient base;
(4) HuIFN-α is also effective against VZV infections, but this effect is again far from overwhelming and has to be balanced against the discomfort (fever and other undesirable side effects) and costs of interferon therapy;
(5) neither araA nor ACV nor HuIFN-α offer any benefit in the treatment of CMV infections in immunocompromised patients. For

the treatment of such infections great expectations are now vested on the recently developed antiherpes compounds DHPG, FIAC (and its congeners FIAU and FMAU).

ACKNOWLEDGEMENT

I am most grateful to Christiane Callebaut for her invaluable help in the preparation of the typescript.

REFERENCES

Allaudeen, H. S., Kozarich, J. W., Bertino, J. R. and De Clercq, E. (1981). *Proc. Natl Acad. Sci. U.S.A.* **78**, 2698–2702.

Allaudeen, H. S., Chen, M. S., Lee, J. J., De Clercq, E. and Prusoff, W. H. (1982). *J. Biol. Chem.* **257**, 603–606.

Arvin, A. M., Feldman, S. and Merigan, T. C. (1978). *Antimicrob. Agents Chemother.* **13**, 605–607.

Arvin, A. M., Kushner, J. H., Feldman, S., Baehner, R. L., Hammond, D. and Merigan, T. C. (1982). *N. Engl. J. Med.* **306**, 761–765.

Aswell, J. F., Allen, G. P., Jamieson, A. T., Campbell, D. E. and Gentry, G. A. (1977). *Antimicrob. Agents Chemother.* **12**, 243–254.

Ayisi, N. K., De Clercq, E., Wall, R. A., Hughes, H. and Sacks, S. L. (1984). *Antimicrob. Agents Chemother.* **26**, 762–765.

Balfour, H. H., Jr. (1984). *J. Pediatr.* **104**, 134–136.

Balfour, H. H., Jr., Bean, B., Mitchell, C. D., Sachs, G. W., Boen, J. R. and Edelman, C. K. (1982). *Am. J. Med.* **73**(1A), 241–248.

Balfour, H. H., Jr., Bean, B., Laskin, O. L., Ambinder, R. F., Meyers, J. D., Wade, J. C., Zaia, J. A., Aeppli, D., Kirk, L. E., Segreti, A. C., Keeney, R. E. and the Burroughs Wellcome Collaborative Acyclovir Study Group (1983*a*). *N. Engl. J. Med.* **308**, 1448–1453.

Balfour, H. H., Jr., McMonigal, K. A. and Bean, B. (1983*b*). *J. Antimicrob. Chemother.* **12** (*Suppl. B*), 169–179.

Barnett, J. M., McGowan, J. J. and Gentry, G. A. (1979). *Infect. Immun.* **26**, 294–297.

Barnett, J. M., McGowan, J. J. and Gentry G. A. (1980). *Infect. Immun.* **28**, 160–162.

Barr, P. J., Oppenheimer, N. J. and Santi, D. V. (1983). *J. Biol. Chem.* **258**, 13627–13631.

Bean, B., Braun, C. and Balfour, H. H., Jr. (1982). *Lancet* **ii**, 118–121.

Benoit, Y., Laureys, G., Delbeke, M.-J. and De Clercq, E. (1985). *Eur. J. Pediatr.*, **143**, 198–202.

Biron, K. K. and Elion, G. B. (1980). *Antimicrob. Agents Chemother.* **18**, 443–447.

Bodey, G. P. (1975). *Cancer Treat. Rev.* **2**, 89–128.

Boston Interhospital Virus Study Group and the NIAID-Sponsored Cooperative Antiviral Clinical Study (1975). *N. Engl. J. Med.* **292**, 599–603.
Bradshaw, L. J. and Sumner, H. L. (1977). *Ann. N.Y. Acad. Sci.* **284**, 190–196.
Browne, M. J. (1978). *Antimicrob. Agents Chemother.* **15**, 747–753.
Bryson, Y. J., Monahan, C., Pollack, M. and Shields, W. D. (1980). *J. Infect. Dis.* **141**, 543–547.
Burns, W. H., Saral, R., Santos, G. W., Laskin, O. L., Lietman, P. S., McLaren, C. and Barry, D. W. (1982). *Lancet* **i**, 421–423.
Canonico, P. G., Jahrling, P. B. and Pannier, W. L. (1982). *Antiviral Res.* **2**, 331–337.
Cheeseman, S. H., Rubin, R. H., Stewart, J. A., Tolkoff-Rubin, N. E., Cosimi, A. B., Cantell, K., Gilbert, J., Winkle, S., Herrin, J. T., Black, P. H., Russell, P. S. and Hirsch, M. S. (1979). *N. Engl. J. Med.* **300**, 1345–1349.
Chen, M. S. and Prusoff, W. H. (1979). *J. Biol. Chem.* **254**, 10449–10452.
Chen, M. S., Ward, D. C. and Prusoff, W. H. (1976). *J. Biol. Chem.* **251**, 4833–4838.
Cheng, Y.-C., Dutschman, G., De Clercq, E., Jones, A. S., Rahim, S. G., Verhelst, G. and Walker, R. T. (1981). *Mol. Pharmacol.* **20**, 230–233.
Cheng, Y.-C., Huang, E.-S., Lin, J.-C., Mar, E.-C., Pagano, J. S., Dutschman, G. E. and Grill, S. P. (1983). *Proc. Natl Acad. Sci. U.S.A.* **80**, 2767–2770.
Chou, S., Gallagher, J. G. and Merigan, T. C. (1981). *Lancet* **i**, 1392–1394.
Chou, S., Dylewski, J. S., Gaynon, M. W., Egbert, P. R. and Merigan, T. C. (1984). *Antimicrob. Agents Chemother.* **25**, 25–28.
Colacino, J. M. and Lopez, C. (1983). *Antimicrob. Agents Chemother.* **24**, 505–508.
Colby, B. M., Shaw, J. E., Elion, G. B. and Pagano, J. S. (1980). *J. Virol.* **34**, 560–568.
Crumpacker, C. S., Schnipper, L. E., Zaia, J. A. and Levin, M. J. (1979). *Antimicrob. Agents Chemother.* **15**, 642–645.
Crumpacker, C. S., Schnipper, L. E., Marlowe, S. I., Kowalsky, P. N., Hershey, B. J. and Levin, M. J. (1982). *N. Engl. J. Med.* **306**, 343–346.
Davis, W. B., Oakes, J. E. and Taylor, J. A. (1978). *Antimicrob. Agents Chemother.* **14**, 743–748.
De Clercq, E. (1982). *In* "Virus Infections. Modern Concepts and Status" (Olson, L. C., ed.), pp. 87–138. Marcel Dekker, New York, Basel.
De Clercq, E. (1984*a*). *Eur. J. Clin. Microbiol.* **3**, 96–107.
De Clercq, E. (1984*b*). *Biochem. Pharmacol.* **33**, 2159–2169.
De Clercq, E. (1984*c*). *J. Antimicrob. Chemother.* **14** (*Suppl. A*), 85–95.
De Clercq, E, Descamps, J., De Somer, P., Barr, P. J., Jones, A. S. and Walker, R. T. (1979). *Proc. Natl Acad. Sci. USA* **76**, 2947–2951.
De Clercq, E., Descamps, J., Verhelst, G., Walker, R. T., Jones, A. S., Torrence, P. F. and Shugar, D. (1980). *J. Infect. Dis.* **141**, 563–574.
De Clercq, E., Zhang, Z.-X., Descamps, J. and Huygen, K. (1981). *J. Infect. Dis.* **143**, 846–852.
Descamps, J. and De Clercq, E. (1981). *J. Biol. Chem.* **256**, 5973–5976.

Desmyter, J., Ray, M. B., De Groote, J., Bradburne, A. F., Desmet, V. J., Edy, V. G., Billiau, A., De Somer, P. and Mortelmans, J. (1976). *Lancet* **ii**, 645-647.

Dobersen, M. J., Jerkofsky, M. and Greer, S. (1976). *J. Virol.* **20**, 478-486.

Dolen, J. G., Carter, W. A., Horoszewicz, J. S., Vladutiu, A. O., Leibowitz, A. I. and Nolan, J. P. (1979). *Am. J. Med.* **67**, 127-131.

Dolin, R., Reichman, R. C., Madore, H. P., Maynard, R., Linton, P. N. and Webber-Jones, J. (1982). *N. Engl. J. Med.* **307**, 580-584.

Drach, J. C., Thomas, M. A., Barnett, J. W., Smith, S. H. and Shipman, C., Jr. (1981). *Science* **212**, 549-551.

Eriksson, B., Helgstrand, E., Johansson, N. G., Larsson, A., Misiorny, A., Noren, J. O., Philipson, L., Stenberg, K., Stening, G., Stridh, S. and Öberg, B. (1977). *Antimicrob. Agents Chemother.* **11**, 946-951.

Fanelli, C. and Sattler, F. R. (1984). *N. Engl. J. Med.* **310**, 987.

Feldman, S., Hughes, W. T. and Kim, H. Y. (1973). *Am. J. Dis. Child.* **126**, 178-184.

Feldman, S., Hayes, F. A., Chaudhary, S. and Ossi, M. (1978). *Antimicrob. Agents Chemother.* **14**, 495-497.

Field, A. K., Davies, M. E., DeWitt, C., Perry, H. C., Liou, R., Germershausen, J., Karkas, J. D., Ashton, W. T., Johnston, D. B. R. and Tolman, R. L. (1983). *Proc. Natl Acad. Sci. U.S.A.* **80**, 4139-4143.

Fischer, P. H., Chen, M. S. and Prusoff, W. H. (1980). *Biochim. Biophys. Acta* **606**, 236-245.

Fyfe, J. A. (1982). *Mol. Pharmacol.* **21**, 432-437.

Gluckman, E., Lotsberg, J., Devergie, A., Zhao, X. M., Melo, R., Gomez-Morales, M., Mazeron, M. C. and Perol, Y. (1983*a*). *J. Antimicrob. Chemother.* **12** (*Suppl. B*), 161-167.

Gluckman, E., Lotsberg, J., Devergie, A., Zhao, X. M., Melo, R., Gomez-Morales, M., Nebout, T., Mazeron, M. C. & Perol, Y. (1983*b*). *Lancet* **ii**, 706-708.

Gordon, P. and Brown, E. R. (1972). *Can. J. Microbiol.* **18**, 1463-1470.

Gordon, P., Ronsen, B. and Brown, E. R. (1974). *Antimicrob. Agents Chemother.* **5**, 153-160.

Goz, B. (1978). *Pharmacol. Rev.* **29**, 249-272.

Gray, G. D., Nichol, F. R., Mickelson, M. M., Camiener, G. W., Gish, D. T., Kelly, R. C., Wechter, W. J., Moxley, T. E. and Neil, G. L. (1972). *Biochem. Pharmacol.* **21**, 465-475.

Greenberg, H. B., Pollard, R. B., Lutwick, L. I., Gregory, P. B., Robinson, W. S. and Merigan, T. C. (1976). *N. Engl. J. Med.* **295**, 517-522.

Haddad, F. S. and Risk, W. S. (1980). *Ann. Neurol.* **7**, 185-188.

Hadden, J. W., Hadden, E. M. and Coffey, R. G. (1976). *Infect. Immun.* **13**, 382-387.

Hall, C. B., McBride, J. T., Walsh, E. E., Bell, D. M., Gala, C. L., Hildreth, S., Ten Eyck, L. G. and Hall, W. J. (1983*a*). *N. Engl. J. Med.* **308**, 1443-1447.

Hall, C. B., Walsh, E. E., Hruska, J. F., Betts, R. F. and Hall, W. J. (1983*b*). *J. Am. Med. Assoc.* **249**, 2666-2670.

Hayden, F. G. and Gwaltney, J. M., Jr. (1983). *J. Infect. Dis.* **148**, 543–550.
Hayden, F. G., Hall, W. J., Douglas, R. G., Jr. and Speers, D. M. (1979). *Antimicrob. Agents Chemother.* **16**, 644–650.
Hayden, F. G., Hall, W. J. and Douglas, R. G., Jr. (1980). *J. Infect. Dis.* **141**, 535–542.
Hayden, F. G., Hoffman, H. E. and Spyker, D. A. (1983*a*). *Antimicrob. Agents Chemother.* **23**, 458–464.
Hayden, F. G., Mills, S. E. and Johns, M. E. (1983*b*). *J. Infect. Dis.* **148**, 914–921.
Herberman, R. B. and Ortaldo, J. R. (1981). *Science* **214**, 24–30.
Ho, M. (1977). *Arch. Virol.* **55**, 1–24.
Hruska, J. F., Bernstein, J. M., Douglas, R. G., Jr. and Hall, C. B. (1980). *Antimicrob. Agents Chemother.* **17**, 770–775.
Hruska, J. F., Morrow, P. E., Suffin, S. C. and Douglas, R. G., Jr. (1982). *Antimicrob. Agents Chemother.* **21**, 125–130.
Jackson, G. G. (1978). *J. Infect. Dis.* **138**, 567–568.
Jahrling, P. B., Hesse, R. A., Eddy, G. A., Johnson, K. M., Callis, R. T. and Stephen, E. L. (1980). *J. Infect. Dis.* **141**, 580–589.
Jolley, W. B., Call, T. W., Alvord, L. S. and Hinshaw, D. B. (1977). *Ann. N.Y. Acad. Sci.* **284**, 230–232.
Jones, C. E., Dyken, P. R., Huttenlocher, P. R., Jabbour, J. T. and Maxwell, K. W. (1982). *Lancet* **i**, 1034–1037.
Kelsey, D. K., Kern, E. R., Overall, J. C., Jr. and Glasgow, L. A. (1976). *Antimicrob. Agents Chemother.* **9**, 458–464.
Khan, A. and Hill, N. O. (1980). *Ann. Allergy* **44**, 289.
Klassen, L. W., Budman, D. R., Williams, G. W., Steinberg, A. D. and Gerber, N. L. (1977). *Science* **195**, 787–789.
Knight, V., Bloom, K., Wilson, S. Z. and Wilson, R. K. (1979). *Antimicrob. Agents Chemother.* **16**, 572–578.
Knight, V., McClung, H. W., Wilson, S. Z., Waters, B. K., Quarles, J. M., Cameron, R. W., Greggs, S. E., Zerwas, J. M. and Couch, R. B. (1981). *Lancet* **ii**, 945–949.
Koff, W. C. and Knight, V. (1979). *Proc. Soc. Exp. Biol. Med.* **160**, 246–253.
Krown, S. E., Friden, G. B., Khansur, T., Davies, M. E., Oettgen, H. F. and Field, A. K. (1983). *J. Interferon Res.* **3**, 281–290.
Larsson, A. and Öberg, B. (1981). *Antimicrob. Agents Chemother.* **19**, 927–929.
Levin, M. J., Leary, P. L. and Arbeit, R. D. (1980). *Antimicrob. Agents Chemother.* **17**, 947–953.
Lin, J.-C., Smith, M. C., Cheng, Y.-C. and Pagano, J. S. (1983). *Science* **221**, 578–579.
Lin, J.-C., Smith, M. C. and Pagano, J. S. (1984). *J. Virol.* **50**, 50–55.
Longley, S., Dunning, R. L. and Waldman, R. H. (1973). *Antimicrob. Agents Chemother.* **3**, 506–509.
Lopez, C., Watanabe, K. A. and Fox, J. J. (1980). *Antimicrob. Agents Chemother.* **17**, 803–806.
Lotzova, E., Savary, C. A., Gutterman, J. U. and Hersh, E. M. (1982). *Cancer Res.* **42**, 2480–2488.

Lotzova, E., Savary, C. A. and Stringfellow, D. A. (1983). *J. Immunol.* **130**, 965-969.

Machida, H., Kuninaka, A. and Yoshino, H. (1982). *Antimicrob. Agents Chemother.* **21**, 358-361.

Mancini, W. R., De Clercq, E. and Prusoff, W. H. (1983). *J. Biol. Chem.* **258**, 792-795.

Mar, E.-C., Cheng, Y.-C. and Huang, E.-S. (1983). *Antimicrob. Agents Chemother.* **24**, 518-521.

Mar, E.-C., Patel, P. C., Cheng, Y.-C., Fox, J. J., Watanabe, K. A. and Huang, E.-S. (1984). *J. Gen. Virol.* **65**, 47-53.

Mardiney, M. R., Jr. and Bredt, A. B. (1971). *Transplantation* **12**, 183-188.

Marker, S. C., Howard, R. J., Groth, K. E., Mastri, A. R., Simmons, R. L. and Balfour, H. H., Jr. (1980). *Arch. Intern. Med.* **140**, 1441-1444.

Marmer, D. J., Steele, R. W. and De Clercq, E. (1982). *In* "Current Chemotherapy and Immunotherapy" (Periti, P. and Grassi, G. G., eds), pp. 1065-1066. American Society for Microbiology, Washington, D. C.

Martin, J. C., Dvorak, C. A., Smee, D. F., Matthews, T. R. and Verheyden, J. P. H. (1983). *J. Med. Chem.* **26**, 759-761.

Matsukage, A., Ono, K., Ohashi, A., Takahashi, T., Nakayama, C. and Saneyoshi, M. (1978). *Cancer Res.* **38**, 3076-3079.

McClung, H. W., Knight, V., Gilbert, B. E., Wilson, S. Z., Quarles, J. M. and Divine, G. W. (1983). *J. Am. Med. Assoc.* **249**, 2671-2674.

McGuffin, R. W., Shiota, F. M. and Meyers, J. D. (1980). *Antimicrob. Agents Chemother.* **10**, 471-473.

Merigan, T. C., Rand, K. H., Pollard, R. B., Abdallah, P. S., Jordan, G. W. and Fried, R. P. (1978). *N. Engl. J. Med.* **298**, 981-987.

Merigan, T. C., Gallagher, J. G., Pollard, R. B. and Arvin, A. M. (1981). *Antimicrob. Agents Chemother.* **19**, 193-195.

Meyers, J. D., Day, L. M., Lum, L. G. and Sullivan, K. M. (1983*a*). *J. Infect. Dis.* **148**, 551-556.

Meyers, J. D., Wade, J. C., McGuffin, R. W., Springmeyer, S. C. and Thomas, E. D. (1983*b*). *J. Antimicrob. Chemother.* **12** (*Suppl. B*), 181-193.

Miller, R. L., Iltis, J. P. and Rapp, F. (1977). *J. Virol.* **23**, 679-684.

Mitchell, C. D., Bean, B., Gentry, S. R., Groth, K. E., Boen, J. R. and Balfour, H. H., Jr. (1981). *Lancet* **i**, 1389-1392.

Muldoon, R. L., Mezny, L. and Jackson, G. G. (1972). *Antimicrob. Agents Chemother.* **2**, 224-228.

Müller, W. E. G., Zahn, R. K., Arendes, J. and Falke, D. (1979). *J. Gen. Virol.* **43**, 261-271.

Ooka, T. and Calender, A. (1980). *Virology* **104**, 219-223.

Ooka, T., Calender, A., de Turenne, M. and Daillie, J. (1983). *J. Virol.* **46**, 187-195.

Oxford, J. S. (1984). *In* "Targets for the Design of Antiviral Agents" (De Clercq, E. and Walker, R. T., eds), pp. 159-176. NATO ASI Series A: Life Sciences Vol. 73. Plenum Press, New York.

Pachuta, D. M., Togo, Y., Hornick, R. B., Schwartz, A. R. and Tominaga, S. (1974). *Antimicrob. Agents Chemother.* **5**, 403-408.
Parker, L. M., Lipton, J. M., Binder, N., Crawford, E. L., Kudisch, M. and Levin, M. J. (1982). *Antimicrob. Agents Chemother.* **21**, 146-150.
Parris, D. S. and Harrington, J. E. (1982). *Antimicrob. Agents Chemother.* **22**, 71-77.
Peavy, D. L., Koff, W. C., Hyman, D. S. and Knight, V. (1980). *Infect. Immun.* **29**, 583-589.
Peavy, D. L., Powers, C. N. and Knight, V. (1981). *J. Immunol.* **126**, 861-864.
Pelling, J. C., Drach, J. C. and Shipman, C., Jr. (1981). *Virology* **109**, 323-335.
Pettersson, R. F., Hellström, P.-E., Penttinen, K., Pyhälä, R., Tokola, O., Vartio, T. and Visakorpi, R. (1980). *J. Infect. Dis.* **142**, 377-383.
Potter, C. W., Phair, J. P., Vodinelich, L., Fenton, R. and Jennings, R. (1976). *Nature* **259**, 496-497.
Powers, C. N., Peavy, D. L. and Knight, V. (1982). *Antimicrob. Agents Chemother.* **22**, 108-114.
Prentice, H. G. (1983). *J. Antimicrob. Chemother.* **12** (*Suppl. B*), 153-159.
Prober, C. G., Kirk, L. E. and Keeney, R. E. (1982). *J. Pediatr.* **101**, 622-625.
Richman, D. D., Yazaki, P. and Hostetler, K. Y. (1981). *Virology* **112**, 81-90.
Sabin, A. B. (1978). *J. Infect. Dis.* **138**, 557-566.
Samo, T. C., Greenberg, S. B., Couch, R. B., Quarles, J., Johnson, P. E., Hook, S. and Harmon, M. W. (1983). *J. Infect. Dis.* **148**, 535-542.
Saral, R., Burns, W. H., Laskin, O. L., Santos, G. W. and Lietman, P. S. (1981). *N. Engl. J. Med.* **305**, 63-67.
Saral, R., Ambinder, R. F., Burns, W. H., Angelopulos, C. M., Griffin, D. E., Burke, P. J. and Lietman, P. S. (1983). *Ann. Intern. Med.* **99**, 773-776.
Schildkraut, I., Cooper, G. M. and Greer, S. (1975). *Mol. Pharmacol.* **11**, 153-158.
Schimpff, S., Serpick, A., Stoler, B., Rumack, B., Mellin, H., Joseph, J. M. and Block, J. (1972). *Ann. Intern. Med.* **76**, 241-254.
Scholtissek, C. (1976). *Arch. Virol.* **50**, 349-352.
Scott, G. M., Phillpotts, R. J., Wallace, J., Gauci, C. L., Greiner, J. and Tyrrell, D. A. J. (1982). *Lancet* **ii**, 186-188.
Scullard, G. H., Andres, L. L., Greenberg, H. B., Smith, J. L., Sawhney, V. K., Neal, E. A., Mahal, A. S., Popper, H., Merigan, T. C., Robinson, W. S. and Gregory, P. B. (1981*a*). *Hepatology* **1**, 228-232.
Scullard, G. H., Pollard, R. B., Smith, J. L., Sacks, S. L., Gregory, P. B., Robinson, W. S. and Merigan, T. C. (1981*b*). *J. Infect. Dis.* **143**, 772-783.
Shannon, W. M. and Schabel, F. M., Jr. (1980). *Pharmacol. Ther.* **11**, 263-390.
Shigeta, S., Yokota, T., Iwabuchi, T., Baba, M., Konno, K., Ogata, M. and De Clercq, E. (1983). *J. Infect. Dis.* **147**, 576-584.
Shipman, C., Jr., Smith, S. H., Carlson, R. H. and Drach, J. C. (1976). *Antimicrob. Agents Chemother.* **9**, 120-127.
Sibrack, C. D., Gutman, L. T., Wilfert, C. M., McLaren, C., St. Clair, M. H., Keller, P. M. and Barry, D. W. (1982). *J. Infect. Dis.* **146**, 673-682.
Sidwell, R. W., Arnett, G. and Brockman, R. W. (1970). *Ann. N.Y. Acad. Sci.* **173**, 592-602.

Sidwell, R. W., Arnett, G. and Schabel, R. M. (1972*a*). *Chemotherapy* **17**, 259–282.
Sidwell, R. W., Huffman, J. H., Khare, G. P., Allen, L. B., Witkowski, J. T. and Robins, R. K. (1972*b*). *Science* **177**, 705–706.
Sidwell, R. W., Khare, G. P., Allen, L. B., Huffman, J. H., Witkowski, J. T., Simin, L. N. and Robins, R. K. (1975). *Chemotherapy* **21**, 205–220.
Sim, I. S., Stebbing, N. and Carey, N. H. (1981). *Antiviral Res.* **1**, 393–404.
Singh, S., Willers, I., Goedde, H. W. and Gauri, K. K. (1974). *Humangenetik* **24**, 135–139.
Skehel, J. J., Hay, A. J. and Armstrong, J. A. (1978). *J. Gen. Virol.* **38**, 97–110.
Smith, C. B., Charette, R. P., Fox, J. P., Cooney, M. K. and Hall, C. E. (1980). *J. Infect. Dis.* **141**, 548–554.
Smith, C. I., Weissberg, J., Bernhardt, L., Gregory, P. B., Robinson, W. S. and Merigan, T. C. (1983). *J. Infect. Dis.* **148**, 907–913.
Soike, K. F., Felsenfeld, A. D. and Gerone, P. J. (1981*a*). *Antimicrob. Agents Chemother.* **20**, 291–297.
Soike, K. F., Gibson, S. and Gerone, P. J. (1981*b*). *Antiviral Res.* **1**, 325–337.
Soto, A. J., Hall, T. S. and Reed, S. E. (1973). *Antimicrob. Agents Chemother.* **3**, 332–334.
Steele, R. W., Chapa, I. A., Vincent, M. M., Hensen, S. A. and Keeney, R. E. (1975). *Antimicrob. Agents Chemother.* **7**, 203–207.
Steele, R. W., Marmer, D. J. and Keeney, R. E. (1980). *Infect. Immun.* **28**, 957–962.
Stevens, D. A., Jordan, G. W., Waddell, T. F. and Merigan, T. C. (1973). *N. Engl. J. Med.* **289**, 873–878.
Straus, S. E., Smith, H. A., Brickman, C., de Miranda, P., McLaren, C. and Keeney, R. E. (1982). *Ann. Intern. Med.* **96**, 270–277.
Streeter, D. G., Witkowski, J. T., Khare, G. P., Sidwell, R. W., Bauer, R. J., Robins, R. K. and Simon, L. N. (1973). *Proc. Natl Acad. Sci. U.S.A.* **70**, 1174–1178.
Stringfellow, D. A., Vanderberg, H. C. and Weed, S. D. (1980). *J. Interferon Res.* **1**, 1–14.
Swierkowska, K. M., Jasinska, J. K. and Steffen, J. A. (1973). *Biochem. Pharmacol.* **22**, 85–93.
Taber, L. H., Knight, V., Gilbert, B. E., McClung, H. W., Wilson, S. Z., Norton, H. J., Thurson, J. M., Gordon, W. H., Atmar, R. L. and Schlaudt, W. R. (1983). *Pediatrics* **72**, 613–618.
Tocci, M. J., Livelli, T. J., Perry, H. C., Crumpacker, C. S. and Field, A. K. (1984). *Antimicrob. Agents Chemother.* **25**, 247–252.
Van Etta, L., Brown, J., Mastri, A. and Wilson, T. (1981). *J. Am. Med. Assoc.* **246**, 1703–1705.
Vyakarnam, A. (1983). *In* "Interferon and Cancer" (Sikora, K., ed.), pp. 53–63. Plenum Press, New York.
Wade, J. C., Newton, B., McLaren, C., Flournoy, N., Keeney, R. E. and Meyers, J. D. (1982). *Ann. Intern. Med.* **96**, 265–269.

Wade, J. C., McGuffin, R. W., Springmeyer, S. C., Newton, B., Singer, J. W. and Meyers, J. D. (1983*a*). *J. Infect. Dis.* **148**, 557-562.
Wade, J. C., McLaren, C. and Meyers, J. D. (1983*b*). *J. Infect. Dis.* **148**, 1077-1082.
Weimar, W., Schellekens, H., Lameijer, L. D. F., Masurel, N., Edy, V. G., Billiau, A. and De Somer, P. (1978). *Eur. J. Clin. Invest.* **8**, 255-258.
Weimar, W., Heijtink, R. A., Ten Kate, F. J. P., Schalm, S. W., Masurel, N., Schellekens, H. and Cantell, K. (1980). *Lancet* **i**, 336-338.
Whitley, R. J., Ch'ien, L. T., Dolin, R., Galasso, G. J., Alford, C. A., Jr. and the Collaborative Study Group (1976). *N. Engl. J. Med.* **294**, 1193-1199.
Whitley, R. J., Soong, S.-J., Dolin, R., Galasso, G. J., Ch'ien, L. T., Alford, C. A. and the Collaborative Study Group (1977). *N. Engl. J. Med.* **297**, 289-294.
Whitley, R. J., Nahmias, A. J., Soong, S.-J., Galasso, G. G., Fleming, C. L. and Alford, C. A. (1980). *Pediatrics* **66**, 495-501.
Whitley, R. J., Soong, S.-J., Hirsch, M. S., Karchmer, A. W., Dolin, R., Galasso, G., Dunnick, J. K., Alford, C. A. and the NIAID Collaborative Antiviral Study Group. (1981). *N. Engl. J. Med.* **304**, 313-318.
Whitley, R., Hilty, M., Haynes, R., Bryson, Y., Connor, J. D., Soong, S.-J., Alford, C. A. and the National Institute of Allergy and Infectious Diseases Collaborative Antiviral Study Group (1982*a*). *J. Pediatr.* **101**, 125-131.
Whitley, R., Soong, S.-J., Dolin, R., Betts, R., Linnemann, C., Jr., Alford, C. A., Jr. and the NIAID Collaborative Antiviral Study Group (1982*b*). *N. Engl. J. Med.* **307**, 971-975.
Whitley, R. J. Spruance, S., Hayden, F. G., Overall, J., Alford, C. A., Jr., Gwaltney, J. M., Soong, S.-J. and the NIAID Collaborative Antiviral Study Group (1984). *J. Infect. Dis.* **149**, 1-8.
Wildiers, J. and De Clercq, E. (1984). *Eur. J. Cancer Clin. Oncol.* **20**, 471-476.
Wingard, J. R., Stuart, R. K., Saral, R. and Burns, W. H. (1981). *Antimicrob. Agents Chemother.* **20**, 286-290.
Wingard, J. R., Hess, A. D., Stuart, R. K., Saral, R. and Burns, W. H. (1983). *Antimicrob. Agents Chemother.* **23**, 593-597.
Wittek, A. E., Cohen, P. S., Arvin, A. M., Smith, S. D., Koropchak, C. M. and De Clercq, E. (1983). *Antimicrob. Agents Chemother.* **24**, 803-806.
Worthington, M. and Conliffe, M. (1977). *J. Gen. Virol.* **36**, 329-333.
Wray, S. K., Gilbert, B. E. and Knight, V. (1985*a*). *Antiviral Res.* **5**, 39-48.
Wray, S. K., Gilbert, B. E., Noall, M. W. and Knight, V. (1985*b*). *Antiviral Res.* **5**, 29-37.
Wybran, J., Govaerts, A. and Appelboom, T. (1978). *J. Immunol.* **121**, 1184-1187.
Young, C. W., Schneider, R., Leyland-Jones, B., Armstrong, D., Tan, C. T. C., Lopez, C., Watanabe, K. A., Fox, J. J. and Philips, F. S. (1983). *Cancer Res.* **43**, 5006-5009.
Zafra, C., de la Fuente, M., Gaytan, F., Solana, R. and Pena, J. (1984). *Chemotherapy* **30**, 131-136.
Zhang, Z.-X., Liu, Y.-X., Hong-Shen, C., Allaudeen, H. S. and De Clercq, E. (1984). *J. Gen. Virol.* **65**, 37-46.

Chapter 3

Antibiotics and Antitumour Immunity

Kazimierz Roszkowski,[1] Waldemar Roszkowski,[1] Gerhard Pulverer[2] and Janusz Jeljaszewicz[3]

[1]*National Institute of Lung Diseases and Tuberculosis, Warsaw, Poland,* [2]*Institute of Hygiene, University of Cologne, Cologne, F.R.G. and* [3]*National Institute of Hygiene, Warsaw, Poland*

Bacterial infection is one of the most common complications encountered in the natural course and treatment of neoplastic disease. In about 60% of deaths of cancer patients, infections are a direct cause of death. Infections in malignancies result from suppression of the specific and non-specific host immunity initiated by the tumour itself and also by cytostatic antitumour treatment are depressed (Bodey *et al.*, 1966, 1975; Fainstein and Bodey, 1982). It is well known that during the development of malignancy some impairment of cellular reactivity may occur (Richards, 1980). Depression of immunity is considered an unfavourable prognosis; significant depression of humoral immunity is more often seen in advanced stages of cancer. It seems that lowering of antibody levels is rather dependent on progressing cachexia than on subtle immunoregulative abnormalities observed in less advanced stages of the disease (Stutman, 1975). Another incompletely investigated problem is the reactivity of phagocytic cells in cancer. Evidence exists that the number of monocytes and certain of their functions may increase in some kinds of malignancies (Bruckner *et al.*, 1982; Daunter *et al.*, 1982). This may lead to a depression of the specific immune reactivity (Twomey *et al.*, 1982). However, the correlation between suppression of the

Antimicrobial agents and immunity
ISBN 0-12-383830-4

immune reactivity and the antibacterial function of these cells is still not clear and it is not known whether an enhanced suppressive activity of monocytes is correlated to diminished antimicrobial properties.

Granulocytopenia is often observed during the natural course of several malignancies (Stutman, 1975). It is clear that cancer patients should be considered as immunocompromised hosts. The high incidence of bacterial complications in these patients leads to an extensive and sometimes long-lasting use of different antibiotics. Therefore the question arises as to whether and how antimicrobial antibiotics can influence the course of malignancy and antitumour chemotherapy, but there is a striking lack of information on these problems. Bossa *et al.* (1981) tested the activity of gentamicin and adriamycin in combination against eight strains of *Proteus mirabilis* using the celophane transfer technique. The same combination of antibiotics was examined for antitumour effects with application on Ehrlich ascites carcinoma in mice. They found evidence of some antagonism between these antibiotics as concerns the bactericidal activity. On the other hand, they observed a synergistic antitumour effect with adriamycin and gentamicin treatment: gentamicin alone did not affect the survival of tumour-bearing animals, but in combination with adriamycin resulted in an increase of the cure rate to 30%, as compared with 15% in mice treated with adriamycin alone. In these experiments the antimicrobial antibiotic was given only once after tumour implantation.

Jacobs *et al.* (1979) presented an opposite approach to the interaction between antimicrobial and antineoplastic antibiotics. These authors investigated the efficacy of 16 antibacterial drugs with activity against *Staphylococcus aureus* together with antineoplastic antibiotics. They observed that different combinations of these two groups of drugs may lead to synergistic or antagonistic antimicrobial effects, but they did not test the efficiency of such combinations in a tumour model.

Of particular interest are some observations of Ruben *et al.* (1973) concerning a rapid progression of small-cell lung cancer during therapy with rifampicin. This casuistic report points to a possible relation between rifampicin treatment and tumour progression, based on the fact that the discontinuation of antibiotic therapy led to the immediate inhibition of tumour growth. This clinical observation and the lack of other information on this problem led us to the study presented below. Obviously the problem of rifampicin has to be separated from similar questions concerning other antibiotics: antimycobacterial therapy has its own specificity, based on the fact that it takes an unusually long time, as compared with the treatment of other bacterial infections.

At first we tried to find out whether antimicrobial antibiotics influence experimental tumour growth or, when combined with an antitumour drug, if they influence the expected results of antitumour therapy. We used an experimental model of transplantable mouse sarcoma, metastasizing selectivity to the lungs. This tumour was isolated from a Balb/c mouse with spontaneous lung sarcoma and has been maintained more than 70 times in the same strain of animal. Subcutaneous implantation of 10^5 viable

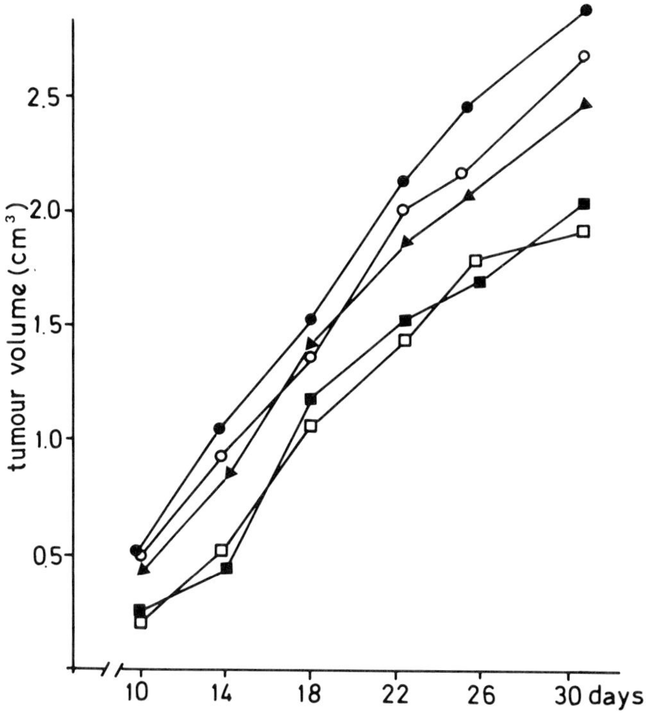

Fig. 1. L-1 Tumour growth in mice which were untreated (□——□) and treated with rifampicin for 3 days (■——■), 7 days (▲——▲), 10 days (○——○) and 14 days (●——●).

Table 1
Mean numbers of spontaneous lung metastases and mean survival time of tumour-bearing mice treated with rifampicin prior to tumour cell implantation

Time of treatment with with rifampicin (days)	Mean survival time (days)	Number of lung metastases (mean ± s.d.)
0 (control)	46	14·0±4·2
3	45	17·3±3·6
7	32[a]	24·1±4·9[a]
10	29[a]	27·1±5·0[a]
14	26[a]	32·0±6·2[a]

[a] $P<0{\cdot}05$.

tumour cells leads to the development of a solid sarcoma and to death of animals after approximately 35 days. On the day of death the mice usually have about 70 lung metastases. Metastases to other organs have never been observed. In order to investigate the effect of rifampicin on tumour growth, mice were treated for different periods of time (3–14 days) with this

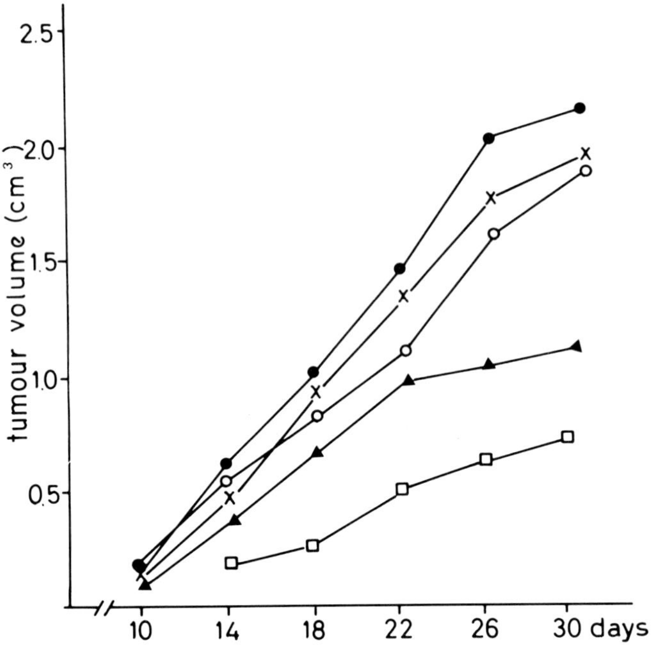

Fig. 2. L-1 Tumour growth in mice immunized with killed tumour cells and treated with rifampicin prior to tumour implantation: ●——●, Untreated and non-immunized controls; □——□, immunized; ▲——▲, immunized and treated with rifampicin for 7 days; X——X, immunized and treated with rifampicin for 10 days; ○——○, immunized and treated with rifampicin for 14 days.

Table 2
Mean numbers of lung metastases in mice treated with rifampicin prior to intravenous injection of tumour cells

Time of treatment with rifampicin (days)	Number of lung metastases (mean ± s.d.)	Metastases with diameter ⩾ 1 mm (%)
0	21·3±3·6	15
3	24·6±2·1	14
7	39·3±7·2[a]	36[a]
10	53·1±9·6[a]	47[a]
14	Uncountable[a]	—

[a] $P < 0{\cdot}05$.

antibiotic prior to tumour implantation. Treatment lasting longer than 7 days significantly enhanced tumour growth and shortened survival time of animals (Table 1, Fig. 1). It was interesting that the number of spontaneous metastases in lungs also increased (Table 2). This led to the question of whether increased numbers of metastases reflect a greater

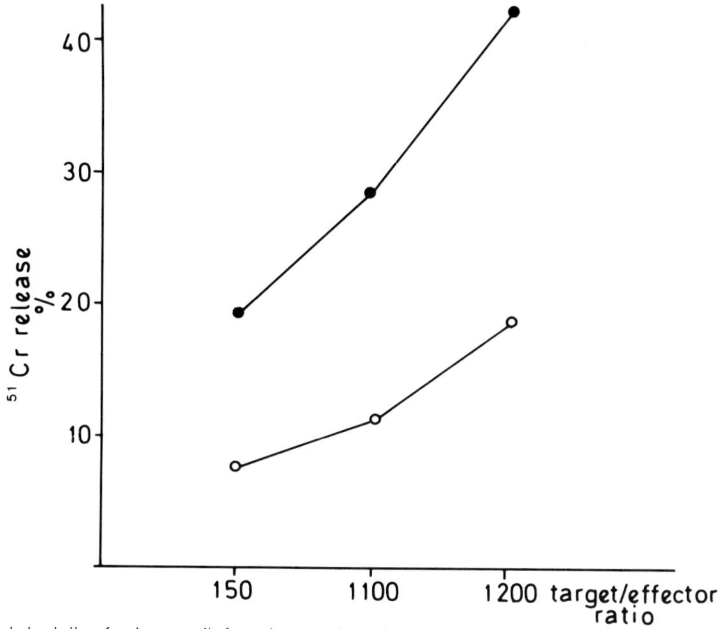

Fig. 3. Cytotoxicity of spleen cells from tumour-bearing mice directed towards syngeneic tumour cells: ●——●, untreated animals; ○——○, animals treated with rifampicin for 14 days.

Table 3
Mean numbers of spontaneous and artificial metastases in mice preimmunized with tumour cells and treated with rifampicin prior to tumour cell implantation

Experimental group	Number of spontaneous lung metastases (mean ± s.d.)	Number of lung colonies (mean ± s.d.)
Non-immunized controls	11·1±3·1	30·3±5·2
Tumour-preimmunized	1·3±1·1[a]	4·2±2·0[a]
Tumour-preimmunized +rifampicin 7 days	3·7±2·3[a]	10·8±7·6[a]
Tumour-preimmunized +rifampicin 10 days	7·7±2·8	21·3±4·1
Tumour-preimmunized +rifampicin 14 days	12·9±4·6	27·9±4·8

[a] $P<0 \cdot 05$ as compared with non-immunized controls.

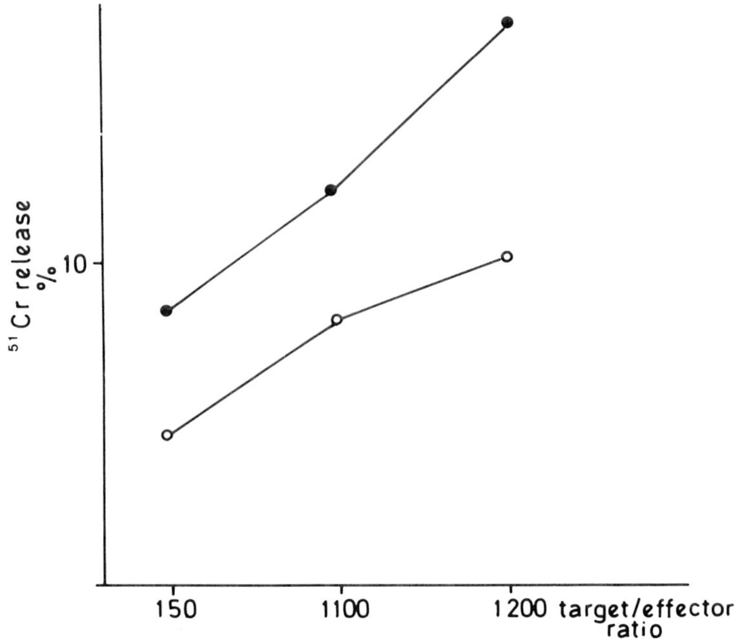

Fig. 4. Spontaneous cytotoxicity of spleen cells from healthy C3H mice directed towards YAC-1 cells: ●——●, untreated animals: ○——○, animals treated with rifampicin for 14 days.

Table 4
The effect of pretreatment with antibiotics on local sarcoma L-1 tumour growth and on the number of lung metastases[a]

	Tumour weight (g)		Number of lung metastases	
Antibiotic	mean ± s.d.	T/C (%)[b]	mean ± s.d.	T/C (%)[b]
Control	0·614 ± 0·107	100	44 ± 7	100
Cefotaxime	0·594 ± 0·096	97	48 ± 8	109
Clindamycin	0·648 ± 0·126	106	46 ± 6	105
Gentamicin	0·628 ± 0·129	102	49 ± 8	111
Mezlocillin	0·876 ± 0·127[a]	143	93 ± 14[c]	194
Piperacillin	0·748 ± 0·132	122	66 ± 10[c]	150

[a] Tumours were grafted after 10 days of antibiotic treatment; the mice were killed 14 days later.

[b] $\mathrm{T/C}\ (\%) = \dfrac{\text{mean value in antibiotic-treated Balb/c-mice}}{\text{mean value in untreated controls}} \times 100.$

[c] Difference statistically significant ($P < 0{\cdot}01$).

advancement of the primary tumour or a facilitation of settlement and development of circulating tumour cells. To resolve this problem, the lung colonies technique has been applied. It occurred that mice treated similarly with rifampicin developed higher numbers of lung colonies after intravenous administration of a suspension of tumour cells (Table 2). As rifampicin is known to affect several immune functions (Bellahsene and Forsgren, 1980), we investigated the possible involvement of immunological phenomena in the observed tumour-enhancing effect. In the following experiments, animals were immunized with killed L-1 tumour cells. This procedure resulted in a significant reduction of tumour growth, as compared with tumour growth in control mice (Fig. 2). Initiation of treatment with rifampicin after completing immunization and before implantation of live tumour cells resulted in total abrogation of the beneficial effects of immunization. This was also observed when the mean survival time, number of metastases and artificially induced lung colonies were examined (Table 3). The above results strongly suggest the participation of immune phenomena in the tumour-enhancing effects of rifampicin. It has also been shown that spleen lymphocytes from tumour-bearing and rifampicin-treated animals are significantly less cytotoxic for L-1 cells than are splenocytes from untreated controls (Fig. 3). Moreover, rifampicin seems to decrease natural-killer cell activity (Fig. 4). In this experiment YAC-1 cells were used as a non-specific target. Results obtained with rifampicin prompted the study of other antibiotics used in the treatment of bacterial infections. Taking into consideration the common dosage and duration of standard therapy with such antibiotics, the experimental period of treatment was established at 10 days and doses were calculated from typical therapeutic regimes. It was an arbitrarily chosen approach.

The antibiotics were applied before and after implantation of the tumour. The 10-day treatment of the animals resulted in a significant enhancement of tumour growth only in the group of mice injected with mezlocillin before tumour grafting (Table 4). The weight of 14-day-old tumours in mice pretreated with mezlocillin was approximately 40% higher than in controls. Other antibiotics used in this study had no effect on solid tumour growth. All the animals were treated similarly and were given a tumour cell suspension intravenously. It has been found that not only mezlocillin but also piperacillin enhanced the number of lung colonies. However, the enhancement was more pronounced for mezlocillin than for piperacillin.

In further experiments, the animals were treated with antibiotics after subcutaneous or intravenous implantation of sarcoma cells. In contrast to previous experiments, mezlocillin administered according to such a schedule possesses antitumour activity. In this case the solid tumours growing in mezlocillin-treated animals were 44% smaller than those in controls. Moreover, the mean survival of the treated animals was significantly prolonged. The other antibiotics studied had no effect on solid sarcoma growth (Table 5).

It is interesting that reduction of solid tumour size was not confirmed by lowering the number of lung colonies. Again, as in the case of the

Table 5
The influence of antibiotic treatment on early growth of sarcoma L-1 tumour[a]

	Tumour weight (g)		Survival time (days)	
Antibiotic	mean ± s.d.	T/C (%)[b]	mean ± s.d.	T/C (%)[b]
Control	0·553 ± 0·097	100	35 ± 6	100
Cefotaxime	0·475 ± 0·116	86	38 ± 7	109
Clindamycin	0·530 ± 0·104	96	34 ± 5	97
Gentamicin	0·616 ± 0·079	111	38 ± 5	109
Mezlocillin	0·314 ± 0·066[c]	56	58 ± 11[c]	166
Piperacillin	0·467 ± 0·101	84	40 ± 9	114

[a] Antibiotic treatment for a period of 10 days was started on the day of subcutaneous tumour grafting; tumour weight was evaluated 14 days later.

$$^{b}\mathrm{T/C}\ (\%) = \frac{\text{mean value in antibiotic-treated Balb/c-mice}}{\text{mean value in untreated controls}} \times 100.$$

[c] Difference statistically significant ($P < 0{\cdot}005$).

Table 6
The effect of antibiotic treatment on artificial metastatic spread[a]

	Total number of metastases	
Antibiotic	mean ± s.d.	T/C (%)[b]
Control	54 ± 11	100
Cefotaxime	49 ± 9	91
Clindamycin	61 ± 14	112
Gentamicin	47 ± 12	87
Mezlocillin	103 ± 19[c]	191
Piperacillin	80 ± 13[c]	148

[a] Antibiotic treatment for a period of 10 days was initiated on the day of tumour cell application; the number of lung colonies was evaluated 14 days later.

$$^{b}\mathrm{T/C}\ (\%) = \frac{\text{mean value in antibiotic-treated Balb/c-mice}}{\text{mean value in untreated controls}} \times 100.$$

[c] Difference statistically significant ($P < 0{\cdot}01$).

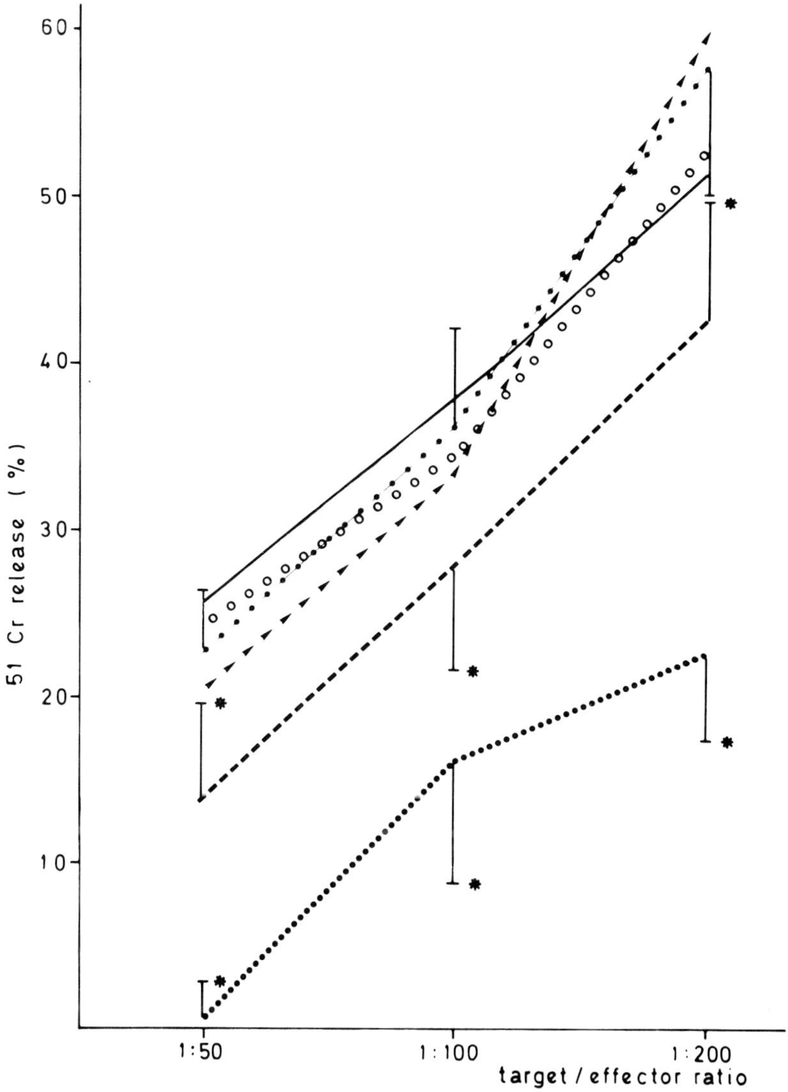

Fig. 5. Cytotoxicity of spleen cells from tumour-bearing mice directed toward syngeneic tumour cells. ●——●), Untreated animals; ——, cefotaxime treated animals; ► ►, clindamycin-treated animals; ○○○○, gentamicin-treated animals; ●●●●, mezlocillin-treated animals; – – –, piperacillin-treated animals.

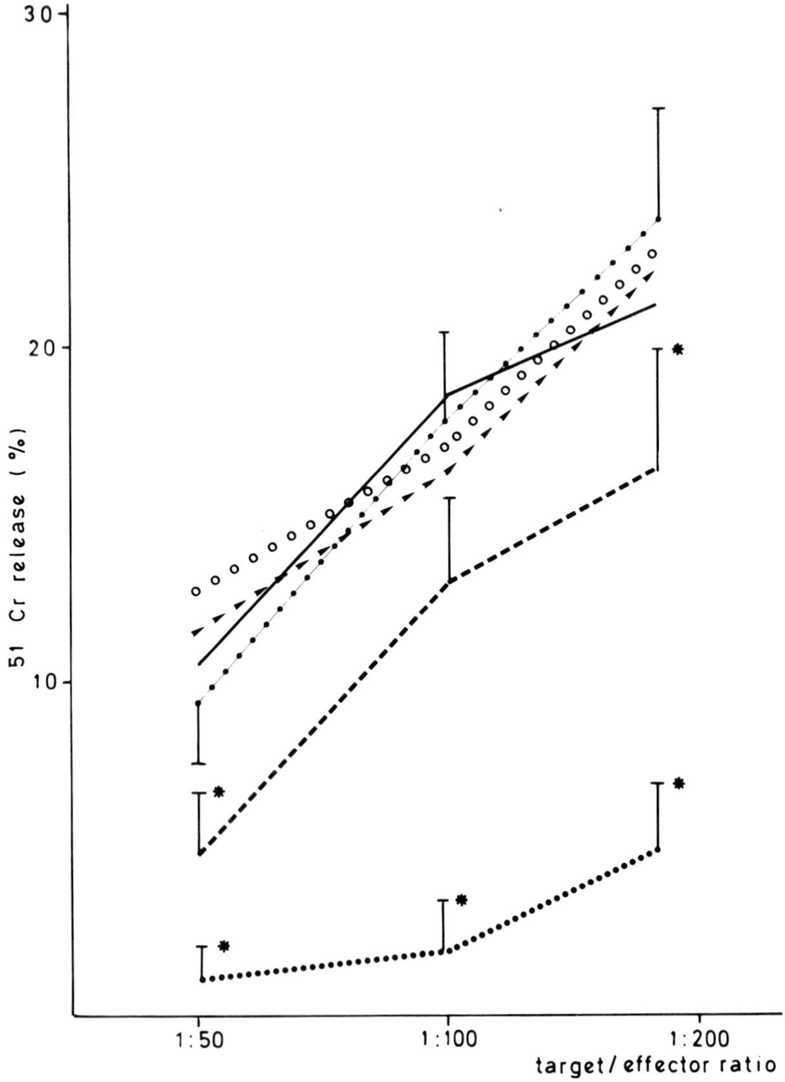

Fig. 6. Spontaneous cytotoxicity of spleen cells from healthy C3H mice directed toward YAC-1 cells. Untreated animals; ——, cefotaxime-treated animals; ► ►, clindamycin-treated animals; ○○○○, gentamicin-treated animals; ●●●●, mezlocillin-treated animals; - - -, piperacillin-treated animals.

mezlocillin-pretreated animals, the number of artificially induced metastases was higher than in controls (Table 6). The effect of mezlocillin on metastases seems to be unrelated to direct interaction of the drug with the tumour, as the tumour cells incubated *in vitro*, even in the presence of high concentrations of mezlocillin, exhibited similar cloning efficiency as those incubated without the drug (unpublished data).

These results indicate the existence of complex mechanisms responsible for facilitating tumour growth when animals were pretreated with mezlocillin, and for facilitating an antitumour effect when the drug was given after sarcoma cells implantation. Results of further experiments led us to the conclusion that involvement of the immune system may be the most probable explanation for tumour growth enhancement in mezlocillin-pretreated animals and a wider metastatic spread after pretreatment with mezlocillin and piperacillin. It was found that the specific

Table 7
The effect of different concentrations of antibiotics on the growth of mouse sarcoma L-1 tumour cells *in vitro*

Antibiotic concentration	Number of tumour cells at different times		
	0 h	48 h	72 h
Control	5×10^4	21×10^4	48×10^4
Cefotaxime			
30 μg/ml	5×10^4	21×10^4	48×10^4
60 μg/ml	5×10^4	21×10^4	47×10^4
90 μg/ml	5×10^4	20×10^4	46×10^4
Clindamycin			
10 μg/ml	5×10^4	19×10^4	46×10^4
20 μg/ml	5×10^4	19×10^4	45×10^4
30 μg/ml	5×10^4	19×10^4	44×10^4
Gentamicin			
6 μg/ml	5×10^4	18×10^4	44×10^4
12 μg/ml	5×10^4	19×10^4	44×10^4
18 μg/ml	5×10^4	18×10^4	43×10^4
Mezlocillin			
400 μg/ml	5×10^4	19×10^4	46×10^4
800 μg/ml	5×10^4	20×10^4	44×10^4
1200 μg/ml	5×10^4	17×10^4	40×10^4
Piperacillin			
100 μg/ml	5×10^4	21×10^4	46×10^4
200 μg/ml	5×10^4	19×10^4	46×10^4
300 μg/ml	5×10^4	18×10^4	45×10^4

cytotoxicity of spleen cells towards syngeneic tumour cells of mouse sarcoma L-1 is suppressed after 10 days of treatment with mezlocillin and piperacillin (Fig. 5). The natural cytotoxicity of spleen cells when using YAC-1 cells as target cells was also diminished after therapy with mezlocillin and piperacillin over 10 days (Fig. 6).

When investigating the mechanisms responsible for the antitumour effect of mezlocillin, two possibilities should be considered: mezlocillin may possess direct antitumour properties or it may influence tumour growth indirectly. A direct effect of the antibiotic seems to be the less probable in the light of results obtained from *in-vitro* studies. As shown in Table 7, even high concentrations of mezlocillin did not change the proliferative rate of sarcoma L-1 cells cultured *in vitro* in the presence of this drug. None of the antibiotics tested influenced the *in-vitro* growth of two human neoplastic cell lines: lung carcinoma E-14 and malignant melanoma MEW

Table 8
The effect of different concentrations of antibiotics on the growth of human lung cancer E-14 cells *in vitro*

Antibiotic concentration	Number of tumour cells at different times		
	0 h	48 h	72 h
Control	5×10^4	18×10^4	37×10^4
Cefotaxime			
30 μg/ml	5×10^4	17×10^4	35×10^4
60 μg/ml	5×10^4	17×10^4	36×10^4
90 μg/ml	5×10^4	16×10^4	34×10^4
Clindamycin			
10 μg/ml	5×10^4	17×10^4	36×10^4
20 μg/ml	5×10^4	18×10^4	36×10^4
30 μg/ml	5×10^4	17×10^4	36×10^4
Gentamicin			
6 μg/ml	5×10^4	17×10^4	36×10^4
12 μg/ml	5×10^4	16×10^4	35×10^4
18 μg/ml	5×10^4	16×10^4	34×10^4
Mezlocillin			
400 μg/ml	5×10^4	16×10^4	31×10^4
800 μg/ml	5×10^4	15×10^4	31×10^4
1200 μg/ml	5×10^4	15×10^4	31×10^4
Piperacillin			
100 μg/ml	5×10^4	17×10^4	35×10^4
200 μg/ml	5×10^4	16×10^4	34×10^4
300 μg/ml	5×10^4	16×10^4	34×10^4

(Tables 8, 9). These results allowed us to exclude the hypothesis of a direct cytotoxic activity of mezlocillin against L-1 cells. An additional argument against this hypothesis was found when investigating the dose–response relationship in mezlocillin treatment. When the drug was given in doses of 300 and 1000 mg/kg body weight, no difference in antitumour effectiveness was observed (Table 10). Mezlocillin administered at doses lower than 300 mg/kg body weight did not produce a significant reduction of tumour weight. However, the possibility of a direct antitumour activity of mezlocillin metabolites cannot be excluded, as this has not been studied. Therefore the pharmacokinetic properties of mezlocillin in mice were investigated. Evaluation of serum levels of the drug showed that mezlocillin is eliminated quickly from blood. Investigations of antibiotic elimination revealed that the drug reaches high and long-lasting concentrations in the intestinal tract (Fig. 7). This is in agreement with the results of

Table 9
The effect of different concentrations of antibiotics on the growth of human malignant melanoma MEW cells *in vitro*

Antibiotic concentration	Number of tumour cells at different times		
	0 h	48 h	72 h
Control	5×10^4	24×10^4	43×10^4
Cefotaxime			
30 μg/ml	5×10^4	24×10^4	43×10^4
60 μg/ml	5×10^4	24×10^4	42×10^4
90 μg/ml	5×10^4	24×10^4	42×10^4
Clindamycin			
10 μg/ml	5×10^4	23×10^4	42×10^4
20 μg/ml	5×10^4	23×10^4	41×10^4
30 μg/ml	5×10^4	23×10^4	42×10^4
Gentamicin			
6 μg/ml	5×10^4	23×10^4	42×10^4
12 μg/ml	5×10^4	22×10^4	42×10^4
18 μg/ml	5×10^4	22×10^4	41×10^4
Mezlocillin			
400 μg/ml	5×10^4	24×10^4	42×10^4
800 μg/ml	5×10^4	24×10^4	42×10^4
1200 μg/ml	5×10^4	24×10^4	41×10^4
Piperacillin			
100 μg/ml	5×10^4	24×10^4	43×10^4
200 μg/ml	5×10^4	24×10^4	42×10^4
300 μg/ml	5×10^4	23×10^4	42×10^4

Wiegersma *et al.* (1982) indicating mezlocillin as the antibiotic strongly suppressing colonization resistance of the digestive tract of mice. These observations led us to investigate the influence of mezlocillin and other antibiotics on the endogenous intestinal flora. After 10 days of antibiotic treatment, the endogenous intestinal bacterial flora was found to be

Table 10
The dose-response relationship in mezlocillin treatment of early sarcoma L-1 tumour[a]

Mezlocillin dose (mg/kg body weight)	Tumour weight (g)		Survival	
	mean ± s.d.	T/C (%)[b]	mean ± s.d.	T/C (%)[b]
Control	0·553 ± 0·097	100	35 ± 6	100
75	0·437 ± 0·047	79	44 ± 7	126
150	0·413 ± 0·042	74	48 ± 8	137
300	0·314 ± 0·066[c]	56	58 ± 8[c]	166
1000	0·285 ± 0·073[c]	51	62 ± 8[c]	177

[a] Mezlocillin treatment for 10 days was started on the day of subcutaneous tumour grafting; tumour weight was evaluated 14 days later.

[b] $T/C\ (\%) = \frac{\text{mean value in antibiotic-treated Balb/c-mice}}{\text{mean value in untreated controls}} \times 100.$

[c] Difference statistically significant ($P < 0{\cdot}01$).

Table 11
The influence of 10 days of antibiotic treatment on the endogenous intestinal flora and on tumour growth in Balb/c mice

Antibiotic used	Log no. of bacteria/1 g faeces (mean ± s.d.)			Relative caecal weight (mean ± s.d.)	Tumour weight (mg, mean ± s.d.)
	Enterobacteriaceae	*S. faecalis*	*S. viridans*		
Control	4·9 ± 0·9	5·5 ± 1·2	5·2 ± 1·6	2·7 ± 0·2	710 ± 149
Cefotazime	0·0 ± 0·0	6·2 ± 1·2	6·4 ± 1·8	2·9 ± 0·3	639 ± 127
Clindamycin	5·3 ± 1·1	5·7 ± 0·9	6·1 ± 1·9	3·0 ± 0·3	660 ± 136
Gentamicin	4·4 ± 0·8	6·1 ± 1·7	5·8 ± 1·3	2·5 ± 0·1	723 ± 142
Mezlocillin	0·0 ± 0·0	0·0 ± 0·0	0·0 ± 0·0	5·6 ± 0·7	350 ± 81
Piperacillin	3·5 ± 1·4	0·0 ± 0·0	0·0 ± 0·0	3·6 ± 0·4	611 ± 164

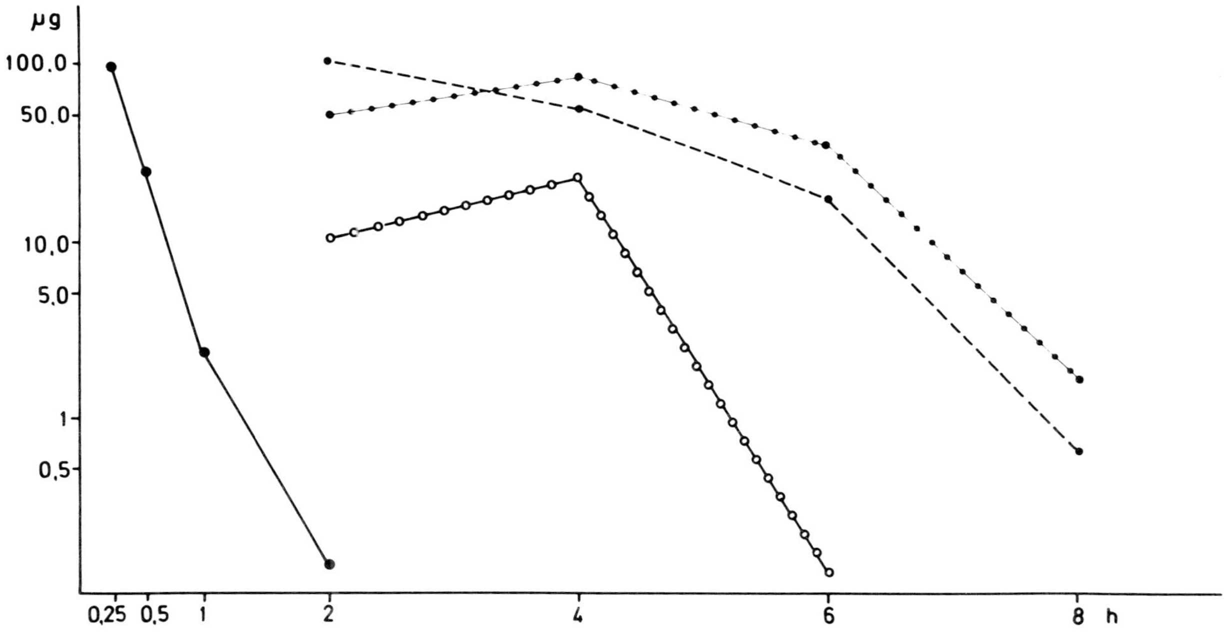

Fig. 7. Concentrations of mezlocillin in blood serum and in caecal content after systemic and oral administration of the antibiotic. ——, serum concentration after a single systemic administration of 150 mg/kg body weight; ----, caecal concentration after a single systemic administration of 150 mg/kg body weight; ○——○, caecal concentration after a single oral administration of 25 mg/kg body weight; — · — · —, caecal concentration after a single oral administration of 75 mg/kg body weight.

Table 12
The effect of mezlocillin on the endogenous intestinal flora and on tumour growth in Balb/c mice in relation to duration of treatment

Experimental group	Log no. of bacteria/1 g faeces (mean ± s.d.)			Relative caecal weight (mean ± s.d.)	Tumour weight (mg, mean ± s.d.)
	Enterobacteriaceae	*S. faecalis*	*S. viridans*		
Control	4·9±0·9	5·5±1·2	5·2±1·6	2·7±0·2	710±149
Mezlocillin					
10 days	0·0±0·0	0·0±0·0	0·0±0·0	5·6±0·7	350±81
7 days	0·0±0·0	0·0±0·0	0·0±0·0	5·4±0·8	381±94
3 days	0·0±0·0	0·0±0·0	0·0±0·0	3·5±0·3	320±118

modified with three out of five antibiotics tested (Table 11). However, the most potent influence was observed in the case of mezlocillin. This antibiotic produced a complete eradication of *Enterobacteriaceae* and streptococci. Cefotaxime treatment resulted in selective elimination of *Enterobacteriaceae*, whereas piperacillin influenced mainly Gram-positive bacteria. In the next experiment, the effect of mezlocillin on intestinal bacteria and on tumour growth was tested in relation to the duration of treatment. Even 3 days of treatment with mezlocillin produced the same effect on the flora and a similar reduction of tumour weight as compared with the effect of longer-lasting administration (Table 12). The caecal concentration of mezlocillin in mice after systemic administration is comparable to the concentration achieved after oral administration of the antibiotic at half of the systemically given dose (Fig. 7). As shown in Table 13, mezlocillin given orally in a dose of 150 mg/kg body weight completely eliminated aerobic intestinal flora, and was also accompanied by an inhibition of tumour growth. Knowing that orally applied mezlocillin is not absorbed at this dose, this observation strongly suggests that the antitumour activity of mezlocillin is related to the influence on the intestinal tract flora. However, the mechanisms of this phenomenon are not yet clear and need further investigation. It was observed that bacteria normally present in the intestinal tract can influence the proliferation of the intestinal epithelium (Abrams *et al.*, 1963) and can penetrate abdominal lymph nodes (Berg and Garlington, 1979). The relevance of this phenomenon is also unknown. One can speculate that the presence of the endogenous digestive tract flora may create a potent stimulus for the proliferation of normal untransformed cells, as was shown for plasma cells synthesizing IgA in the gut (Crabbe *et al.*, 1968). However, it is only a theoretical explanation

Table 13
Comparison of the effect of mezlocillin on the endogenous intestinal flora and on tumour growth after 3 days systemic or oral treatment

Route of administration and dose of mezlocillin	Log no. of bacteria/1 g faeces (mean ± s.d.)			Relative caecal weight (mean ± s.d.)	Tumour weight (mg, mean ± s.d.)
	Enterobacteriaceae	*S. faecalis*	*S. viridans*		
Control	4·3±0·7	5·1±1·3	4·6±0·8	2·4±0·2	854±173
300 mg/kg subcutaneously	0·0±0·0	0·0±0·0	0·0±0·0	4·6±0·6	432±106
150 mg/kg orally	0·0±0·0	0·0±0·0	0·0±0·0	5·2±0·8	331±68

Table 14
The effect of combined cytostatic and antibiotic treatment on an advanced sarcoma L-1 tumour[a]

	Tumour weight (g)		Survival time (days)	
Antibiotic	mean ± s.d.	T/C (%)[b]	mean ± s.d.	T/C (%)[b]
Control	3·64±0·87	—	33±5	—
Endoxan	0·49±0·12	100	61±14	100
Cefotaxime + endoxan	0·51±0·17	104	68±18	111
Clindamycin + endoxan	0·45±0·14	92	64±16	105
Gentamicin + endoxan	0·40±0·09	82	72±11	118
Mezlocillin + endoxan	0·18±0·05[c]	37	94±17[c]	154
Piperacillin + endoxan	0·35±0·09	71	76±13	125

[a] Endoxan was administered on days 10, 17 and 24; antibiotic treatment was initiated on day 17 after tumour grafting and lasted 10 days. Tumour weight was evaluated after 30 days after tumour grafting.

[b] $$\text{A+E (\%)} = \frac{\text{mean value in (antibiotic and endoxan)-treated Balb/c-mice}}{\text{mean value in (endoxan alone)-treated mice}} \times 100.$$

[c] Difference statistically significant ($P < 0{\cdot}01$).

and other possibilities have to be taken into consideration. It is interesting that intraperitoneal administration of non-pathogenic anaerobic bacteria to mezlocillin-treated mice can reverse the antitumour effect of the drug as well as the immunosuppression (unpublished data).

In further experiments we examined the effect of a combined cytostatic and antibiotic chemotherapy on an advanced sarcoma L-1 tumour. When administered to endoxan-treated Balb/c mice, mezlocillin produced a more pronounced reduction of tumour weight when compared with endoxan alone (Table 14). The mean survival time in animals treated with a combination of mezlocillin and endoxan was also significantly longer than in mice receiving endoxan alone. Of mice treated with this combination, 25% survived without any macroscopic signs of tumour. After 110 days these mice were killed and no tumour was found either macro- or microscopically. In none of the mice treated with endoxan alone was a complete response recorded. The remaining four antibiotics tested (cefotaxime, clindamycin, gentamicin and piperacillin) did not produce any significant effects on endoxan-treated animals.

The results presented above are based on an experimental tumour model which is different from human cancer. However, they may be of significance in clinical application. The results of clinical studies performed by the E.O.R.T.C. Gnotobiotic Project Group (1979) seem to be in agreement with our experimental observations. This group has found that non-Hodgkin's lymphoma patients with low numbers of different biotypes of *Enterobacteriaceae* species per faecal sample during remission induction chemotherapy survived significantly longer in comparison with patients with a higher number of various Gram-negative bacteria. This led the authors to the conclusion that elimination of Gram-negative flora may result in a decrease of the intestinal concentration of endotoxin which can be mitogenic for transformed human B cells (Ivanyi and Lehner, 1974). In our experiments, we have found that mezlocillin therapy affecting tumour growth was associated with a fall in the intestinal endotoxin level. The remaining four antibiotics examined did not influence the concentration of endotoxin in the intestinal tract. Even cefotaxime therapy, which resulted in a complete elimination of aerobic Gram-negative bacteria, did not significantly decrease the endotoxin concentration. This may be explained by the fact that besides aerobic Gram-negative bacteria, the anaerobic flora is a rich source of endotoxin and it was not affected by cefotaxime. Nevertheless, the role of endotoxin is only one of few possible explanations for the above phenomena. It is known that endotoxin possesses some antitumour properties (Kabir *et al.*, 1978). However, it is also known that endotoxin can stimulate B cells to proliferate, but this may be unique and limited only to such disorders as B-cell lymphoma. In the case of solid tumours, the above mechanism is much less probable. The results of this study strongly stress the need for clinical confirmation of the observed phenomena.

REFERENCES

Abrams, G. D., Bauer, H. and Sprinz, H. (1963). *Lab. Invest.* **12**, 335-364.

Bellahsene, A. and Forsgren, A. (1980). *Infection* **27**, 15-20.

Berg, R. D. and Garlington, A. W. (1979). *Infect. Immun.* **23**, 403-411.

Bodey, G. P., Bockley, M., Sath, Y. S. and Freireich, E. J. (1966). *Ann. Intern. Med.* **64**, 328-340.

Bodey, G. P., Hersh, E. M. and Valdivieso, M. (1975). *Postgrad. Med. J.* **58**, 67-74.

Bossa, R., Galatulas, I. and Perrone, G. (1981). *Chemotherapy* **27**, 350-353.

Bruckner, H. W., Lavin, P. T., Plaxe, S. C., Storch, J. A. and Livstone, E. M. (1982). *J. Am. Med. Assoc.* **247**, 1004-1006.

Crabbe, P. A., Bazin, H., Eyssen, H. and Heremans, J. F. (1968). *Int. Arch. Allergy* **34**, 362-375.

Daunter, B., Khoo, S. K. and Mackay, E. V. (1982). *Gynecol. Oncol.* **13**, 512-517.

E.O.R.T.C. Gnotobiotic Project Group writing Committee: van der Waaij, D., Went, F. and Gaus, W. (1979). *Zbl. Bakt. Suppl.* **7**, 345-356.

Fainstein, V. and Bodey, G. P. (1982). *In:* "Bacteria and Cancer" (Jeljaszewicz, J., Pulverer, G. and Roszkowski, W., eds), pp. 435-451. Academic Press, London.

Ivanyi, L. and Lehner, T. (1974). *Clin. Exp. Immunol.* **18**, 347-356.

Jacobs, J. Y., Michel, J. and Sacks, T. (1979). *Antimicrob. Agents Chemother.* **15**, 580-586.

Kabir, S., Rosenstreich, D. L. and Mergenhagen, S. E. (1978). *In:* "Bacterial Toxins and Cell Membranes" (Jeljaszewicz, J. and Wadström, T., eds), pp. 59-87. Academic Press, London.

Richards, V. (1980). *Prog. Exp. Tumor Res.* **25**, 1-60.

Ruben, F. L., Winkelstein, A., Fotadis, I. G. and Dessauer, P. (1973). *Lancet* **ii**, 978.

Stutman, O. (1975). *Adv. Cancer Res.* **22**, 261-422.

Twomey, J. J., Laughter, A. H., Rice, L. and Ford, R. J. (1982). *Blood* **60**, 316-322.

Wiegersma, N., Jansen, G. and van der Waaij, D. (1982). *J. Hyg. Camb.* **88**, 221-230.

Chapter 4

Immunomodulation by Antimicrobial Agents

Y. H. Thong
Department of Child Health, University of Queensland, Mater Children's Hospital, South Brisbane 4101, Australia

I. INTRODUCTION

Close encounters with microbial invaders occur throughout the lifetime of an individual. The outcome of each encounter is determined on one hand by the virulence and other intrinsic properties of the microbe and on the other by the integrity of the immune system. Under normal circumstances, most infections are asymptomatic, a minority are clinically apparent, while others may become chronic or persistent and a few even life-threatening.

The introduction of antimicrobial agents into clinical practice has changed the balance in favour of recovery from infection by susceptible microorganisms. However, there are many complications associated with antimicrobial chemotherapy, including allergy, idiosyncracy, toxicity, development of resistant strains, nosocomial and superinfections. The last three complications are particularly prone to develop in immunocompromised individuals receiving antimicrobial treatment, mainly because intact immunological responses are necessary for the complete elimination of invading microbes.

The interaction between antimicrobial agents and immunological responses has attracted increasing attention for a number of reasons. First, a better understanding of drug-host interactions may contribute to a

Antimicrobial agents and immunity
ISBN 0-12-383830-4

reduction in the problems of nosocomial and superinfections. Secondly, infections in immunocompromised patients are notoriously difficult to treat, and the selection of agents with immunostimulatory rather than immunosuppressive properties may aid in recovery from infection. Thirdly, newer and better immunosuppressive agents for control of transplant rejections and autoimmune diseases may be discovered; a case in point is the extremely useful drug cyclosporine, which was originally developed as an antibiotic. Fourthly, several antibiotics, such as actinomycin D and doxorubicin, are effective antitumour agents, and more may be forthcoming as research continues apace. Fifthly, although no effective immunostimulatory agents has joined the clinical armamentarium, this possibility is on the horizon, with antimicrobial agents such as levamisole, inosiplex and pyrimethamine at the forefront of these investigations. Finally, the molecular pharmacology of many antimicrobial agents are well understood, and those with immunomodulatory properties can be used as chemical probes for the study of immunoregulatory processes.

II. MOLECULAR PHARMACOLOGY OF ANTIMICROBIAL AGENTS

The ways in which antimicrobial agents affect microorganisms are many and varied, but five general mechanisms can be identified. These are (Sande and Mandell, 1980; Reynolds, 1982):

(1) disruption of bacterial cell wall synthesis,
(2) disruption of microbial cell membrane function,
(3) interference with microbial protein synthesis,
(4) interference with microbial nucleic acid synthesis,
(5) inhibition of microbial metabolic activity.

The 'magic bullet' concept of Paul Ehrlich defines the ideal antimicrobial agent as one that selectively poisons microbes with sparing of host tissues. However, in practice, the sparing of host tissue is relative rather than absolute, with the possible exception of the penicillins. This is because metabolic processes and structural components of mammalian and microbial cells may be somewhat identical, depending on the degree of evolutionary conservation.

Thus, the way in which antimicrobial agents interact with immune cells and tissues may be related to the way they interact with microbes, and knowledge of these processes offers an avenue to better appreciation of the immunomodulatory mechanism of the drugs. On the other hand, the manner of immunomodulation may be entirely unrelated to the drugs' antimicrobial activities, and represents a separate property of the drug itself.

A. Disruption of Bacterial Cell Wall Synthesis

The rigid framework of bacterial cell walls is made up of peptidoglycan. The biosynthesis of peptidoglycan takes place in three stages and involves approximately 30 bacterial enzymes; thus it is extremely vulnerable to disruption.

The β-lactam antibiotics—penicillins, cephalosporins, cephamycins—inhibit the transpeptidase enzyme, thus preventing the cross-linking of peptidoglycan strands (Waxman and Strominger, 1983). The antimicrobial spectrum of penicillin include Gram-positive bacteria, Gram-negative cocci, anaerobic bacteria, spirochaetes and actinomycetes. Ampicillin and its congeners are active against Gram-negative bacilli. The cephalosporins and cephamycins have even broader spectrums of activity.

Vancomycin, a complex glycopeptide, binds with high affinity to a precursor of peptidoglycan, thereby disrupting cell wall synthesis (Neito and Perkins, 1971). It is mainly used in the treatment of serious infections caused by staphylococci resistant to other agents.

Cycloserine competitively inhibits alanine racemase and dipeptidyl synthetase, in this way preventing the incorporation of peptidoglycan precursors (Hoeprich, 1963). It is used in the treatment of urinary infections caused by *Escherichia coli*.

Other precursors of peptidoglycan are mycolic acids, and isoniazid inhibits the elongation of 26-carbon fatty acids essential for their synthesis (Takayama *et al.*, 1972). This synthetic chemical is the primary drug for the chemotherapy to tuberculosis.

Since peptidoglycan is not a structural component of mammalian cells, any immunomodulation by drugs disrupting peptidoglycan biosynthesis is unlikely to be attributable to their pharmacological properties.

B. Disruption of Microbial Cell Membrane Function

The cell membrane is composed of a lipid bilayer with protein molecules interspersed. It separates the cell from its environment, and the cell organelles into discrete compartments within the cytoplasm. Among its many important functions are selective passage of ions and molecules, transmission of hormonal and other signals via receptors on its surface, and changes in shape and fluidity to allow for growth and movement. In short, its integrity is vital to the life processes of the cell.

Several antimicrobial agents act by causing damage to the microbial cell membrane. The polyene antibiotics—amphotericin B, nystatin—bind to the sterol moeity, especially ergosterol, and channels are formed through the membrane allowing the leakage of small molecules (Hamilton-Miller, 1974). They are very effective antifungal agents.

The polymyxins, polymyxin B and colistin (polymyxin E), interact avidly with phospholipids of the cell membrane to disrupt its structure (Brown and Wood, 1972). They are cationic detergents with a simple peptide configuration. They are used for the treatment of Gram-negative infections.

The highly substituted imidazole derivatives—clotrimazole, miconazole and ketoconazole—interfere with lipid biosynthesis, in particular the ergosterol moeity of the fungal cell membrane, leading to increased permeability (Van den Bossche *et al.*, 1978, 1979). They have broad-spectrum antifungal activity. Of the three, ketoconazole is the only one that is effective orally.

C. Interference with microbial protein synthesis

Proteins are assembled in ribosomes under the directions of messenger RNAs from individual amino acids carried by transfer RNAs. Proteins are vital to cellular processes either as enzymes or structural components.

Some of the most useful antimicrobial agents work by binding to ribosomes and inhibit protein synthesis. Chloramphenicol, erythromycin, lincomycin and clindamycin attach to the 30S ribosomal subunit, while spectinomycin, the tetracyclines and the aminoglycosides attach to the 50S subunit.

More specifically, chloramphenicol blocks the attachment of transfer RNA to the acceptor site, thereby suppressing peptide bond formation (Denslow and O'Brien, 1978). Erythromycin inhibits the late but not the early peptide bond formation; however, the exact mechanism is unknown (Mao and Wiegand, 1968). Lincomycin and clindamycin may inhibit the peptidyl synthetase enzyme (Wilson, 1977).

Like chloramphenicol, tetracyclines prevent the attachment of transfer RNA to the acceptor site, but at the 30S ribosomal unit and not the 50S subunit (Chopra and Howe, 1978). Spectinomycin affects translocation reactions between messenger RNA and the ribosome (Davies *et al.*, 1965). Aminoglycosides interfere with the initiation phase of protein synthesis as well as induce misreading of the messenger RNA code (Tai *et al.*, 1978).

In terms of therapeutic efficacy, the tetracyclines are broad-spectrum antibacterial agents, including many Gram-positive and Gram-negative bacteria, rickettsiae, mycoplasma, chlamydia, treponemes and amoebae. The spectrum of chloramphenicol is also very broad, and includes many Gram-positive and Gram-negative bacteria, as well as rickettsiae, chlamydia and mycoplasma. Erythromycin is mainly active against Gram-positive cocci, aerobic Gram-negative bacilli, mycoplasma, legionella and atypical mycobacteria. The aminoglycosides are useful in the treatment of Gram-negative bacterial infections and tuberculosis. Clindamycin is active against Gram-positive cocci, anaerobic bacteria, actinomycetes and toxoplasma. The polymyxins are useful mainly in the treatment of Gram-negative bacterial infections.

D. Interference with Microbial Nucleic Acid Synthesis

Some very useful antimicrobial agents disrupt microbial nucleic acid synthesis. Of these, rifampicin and other ansamycins are known to inhibit DNA-dependent RNA polymerase resulting in suppression of formation of RNA (Konno *et al.*, 1973). Their main use is in the treatment of tuberculosis.

The precise site of action of nalidixic acid is uncertain, but it appears to bind to a crucial protein involved with DNA synthesis (Brumfitt and Pursell, 1971). It is used mainly in urinary tract infections.

Chloroquine and other 4-aminoquinolines bind to DNA to inhibit the activity of DNA and RNA polymerases (Allison *et al.*, 1965). Mefloquine, the recently introduced 4-aminoquinoline derivative, does not seem to have this effect, and its antimalarial action may be related to the ability of 4-aminoquinolines to clump malarial pigment in erythrocytes, and indirectly disrupt amino-acid metabolism of the parasites (Fitch *et al.*, 1979).

Primaquine and other 8-aminoquinolines bind to DNA but do not inhibit DNA or RNA polymerases (Whichard *et al.*, 1968), so it may be that their antimalarial effects are mediated by active metabolites rather than the parent compounds.

Griseofulvin acts at a point later on in cell replication by disrupting the mitotic spindle as a result of its interaction with polymerized microtubules (Gull and Trinci, 1973). It is an effective antifungal drug.

Vidarabine (adenine arabinoside, ara A) is an adenosine analogue which inhibits DNA polymerase (Muller *et al.*, 1977). It has therapeutic efficacy against herpes simplex and herpes zoster infections.

The nitroimidazole derivatives such as metronidazole and tinidazole, bind to DNA and cause strand breakage and loss of its helical structure (Knight *et al.*, 1978). They are useful for therapy of infections caused by anaerobic bacteria and protozoa.

E. Inhibition of Microbial Metabolic Activity

There is a miscellaneous group of antimicrobial drugs which act by interfering with one aspect or another of microbial metabolic activity. Top of this list are the sulphonamides. They are structural analogues of P-aminobenzoic acid, an essential precursor for the biosynthesis of folic acid (Woods, 1962).

The synergistic combination of a sulphonamide—sulphamethoxazole—and trimethoprim acts by inhibition of two steps along the biosynthetic pathway for folic acid: sulphamethoxazole blocks the incorporation of P-aminobenzoic acid into folic acid, and trimethoprim suppresses the reduction of dihydrofolate to tetrahydrofolate (Hitchings and Burchall, 1965). As such, trimethoprim-sulphamethoxazole—also known as cotrimoxazole—has broad-spectrum antibacterial activity; in addition, it is effective against the protozoan parasite *pneumocystis carinii*. Pyrimethamine, an analogue of trimethoprim, is used in the treatment of malaria in combination with sulphadoxine, a sulphonamide analogue. On its own, it is used in the treatment of toxoplasmosis.

5-Fluorocytosine (flucytosine) is an antifungal agent which is enzymatically converted to fluorouracil, and subsequently metabolized to compounds which inhibit the enzyme thymidylate kinase (Santi and McHenry, 1972).

Quinine, an antimalarial isolated from chincona bark, is known as a general protoplasmic poison because of its propensity for interfering with a great variety of enzyme systems (Thompson and Werbel, 1972).

Pentamidine belongs to the diamidine group of drugs with antiprotozoal activity. It is useful in the treatment of Babesia and Pneumocystis infections. It acts by binding to the DNA of kinetoplast in trypanosomes and disrupt mitochondrial metabolism (Brack *et al.*, 1972).

Suramin is a polyanion which complexes strongly with proteins and inhibits a number of enzyme systems (Williamson and Macadam, 1965). It has activity against trypanosomes and filariae.

Arsenical compounds such as melarsoprol react with the sulphydryl groups of proteins and inhibit a number of enzyme systems, especially pyruvate kinase, a terminal enzyme of the glycolytic pathway (Flynn and Bowman, 1969). It is useful for therapy of the meningoencephalitic stage of trypanosomiasis.

Levamisole has broad-spectrum activity against nematode parasites. It has two primary actions: ganglionic stimulation leading to muscular paralysis, and inhibition of the enzyme fumarate reductase, but these effects cannot explain its well known immunomodulatory properties (Symoens and Rosenthal, 1977).

Thiabendazole is a substituted benzimidazole derivative with activity against gastrointestinal nematodes. It inhibits the enzyme fumarate reductase, but this may not be its main mechanism of action (Symposium, 1969). It has also been shown to interfere with microtubule functions (Davidse and Flach, 1978).

F. Antiviral Agents

The antiviral agents are a diverse group of substances which can act at different points in the infective cycle (Smith *et al.*, 1980). Some of them merely inactivate the virus. Others prevent its attachment, penetration or uncoating. Still others inhibit viron-associated enzymes, the translational processes of viral messenger RNA, the synthesis of viral DNA or the assembly process itself.

III. IMMUNOLOGICAL RESPONSES TO INFECTION

The immune system is complex, but four major constituents can be distinguished. These are the phagocytic cells, complement, B lymphocytes and T lymphocytes. They operate in concert during microbial invasion, but one or another component may take a more prominent role depending on the nature of the infection.

Thus, experimental data indicate that phagocytic cells are crucial in defence against pyogenic bacteria and fungi, and that these microorganisms are quite resistant to non-phagocytic immune mechanisms. This conclusion is substantiated by clinical observations of increased susceptibility to these types of infections in disorders of phagocytic function such as chronic granulomatous disease and Chediak–Higashi syndrome (Klebanoff and Clark, 1978; Nathan *et al.*, 1980).

Conversely, cell-mediated immune mechanisms involving T lymphocytes are preeminent in defence against viral and other intracellular pathogens, whereas B lymphocytes and the antibodies they secrete are particularly effective against toxin-producing microbes and certain viruses.

However, this is not to say that each constituent of the immune response functions in isolation from each other. On the contrary, the response to infection is a finely regulated and superbly orchestrated event, the elements of which are now beginning to be understood (Lachman and Peters, 1982; Stites *et al.*, 1982).

In infections caused by pyogenic bacteria, phagocytic cells of the polymorphonuclear neutrophil series arrive at the site of infection within 30 min (Dutcher *et al.*, 1981), and a delay of only 2 h results in a 10 000-fold increase in severity of the infection (Miles *et al.*, 1957). The process of phagocytosis is facilitated by antibody and complement acting as opsonins. Antibody is produced by B lymphocytes, and since recognition of many bacterial antigens is T-cell-dependent, this process is under the control of T lymphocytes. Antibodies not only act as opsonins, they also promote fusion of phagosomes and lysosomes. On their own, they can neutralize endotoxins and exotoxins and, in conjunction with complement, bring about bacteriolysis. A fuller account is presented by Lagrange and Closs (1979).

Phagocytic cells of the monocyte–macrophage series appear to play a pivotal role in resistance to infections caused by intracellular bacterial pathogens such as *Mycobacterium tuberculi* and *Salmonella typhi* (Daniel, 1980). On their own, however, they may be quite ineffectual; in fact, many of these bacteria are not just facultative but obligatory intracellular pathogens of monocytes and macrophages (Edelson, 1982). As a rule, mononuclear phagocytes acquire their propensity for killing these intracellular pathogens from T lymphocytes. This is mediated through biologically active molecules derived from activated T lymphocytes collectively known as lymphokines (Rocklin *et al.*, 1980). This aspect of cell-mediated immunity can be correlated with delayed-type hypersensitivity, a distinctive form of inflammatory reaction.

With regard to viral infections, the whole gamut of immunological responses is brought to bear on the microbial invader. Secretory antibody on mucosal surfaces and antibody and complement in tissue fluids have neutralizing actions on viruses (Sissons and Oldstone, 1980). Macrophages also have a role in presentation of viral antigen to T cells, as well as in transport, replication and destruction of viruses (Nathan *et al.*, 1980). Cytotoxic T cells lyse viral-infected cells and expose intracellular viruses to the lethal action of antibody, complement and macrophages (Zinkernagel and Doherty, 1979). Lymphokine-producing T cells release interferon which inhibits viral replication, and other soluble products such as macrophage inhibitory factor which recruit mononuclear phagocytes for defence. The phenomenon of antibody-dependent cell-mediated cytotoxicity has also been demonstrated in antiviral immunity (Pearson, 1978). Even more subtle mechanisms have been elucidated; for instance, in defence against Epstein–Barr Virus, a selective B-cell parasite, suppressor T cells are generated which reduce the number of B cells available to the virus (Tosato *et al.*, 1979).

Immunological mechanisms against systemic fungal infections are less well understood. Experimental findings indicate that circulating antibody has a minor role (Pearsall *et al.*, 1978). *In-vitro* studies have also shown that macrophages have difficulty in phagocytosing filamental forms of fungi, and that once phagocytosed, fungi have the capacity to multiply within the macrophage and eventually overwhelm the cell. Some experiments have shown macrophages to be capable of fungal killing (Peterson and Calderone, 1977), but the rate is always much slower in comparison with that of neutrophil polymorphs, which themselves are not very spectacular in *in-vitro* tests (Diamond *et al.*, 1972). However, clinical studies on neutropenic patients indicate that neutrophils have an important role in resistance to fungal infection (Lehrer and Cline, 1971). With regard to complement, studies in animals indicate that the alternative pathway and terminal components were more important than the classical pathway (Gelfand *et al.*, 1978). T cells have a central role in amplifying the immunological response to fungal infections but have no appreciable direct cytotoxic activity on their own (Beaman *et al.*, 1981). Their role is better defined in chronic mucocutaneous candiadiasis and the dermaphytoses than in the systemic mycoses (Gupta *et al.*, 1979). In any event, the principal effector cell in systemic mycoses appears to be the neutrophil leucocyte, which can adhere to fungal hyphae and damage them by direct contact (Diamond and Krzesicki, 1978).

The complexities of these immunological responses to parasitic infections have only been elucidated in recent years. Antibody against the surface glycoprotein appears to be the major defence mechanism against *Toxoplasma gondii* and *Trypanosoma cruzi*. However, their intracellular location shelters them from immune attack (Zinkernagel, 1979), and this strategy is successful even if the cell involved is the macrophage with parasiticidal capacity (Edelson, 1982), as the situation with *Leishmania* has shown (Chang and Dwyer, 1976). Antibody-mediated mechanisms are also important in defence against African trypanosomiasis, but the capacity of these parasites to change the antigenic composition of their surface glycoproteins renders them extremely elusive (Englund *et al.*, 1982). The malaria parasite combines the strategies of antigenic variation and intracellular location to evade host immunological responses, but this strategy is not entirely effective. Phagocytic cells (Wozencraft *et al.*, 1984), antibodies (Quin and Wyler, 1979) and T cells (Roberts and Weidanz, 1979) have been shown to kill the parasites. The strategy of camouflage is adopted by some metazoan parasites, such as schistosomes, which adopt host antigens and incorporate them on their own cell surfaces (Smithers and Terry, 1969). However, this is only one of several measures which include immunosuppression (Pelley *et al.*, 1976), rapid turnover of surface membrane (Wilson and Barnes, 1977) and inhibition of clotting mechanisms (Tsang *et al.*, 1977).

IV. IMMUNOLOGICAL CONSEQUENCES OF HOST-PATHOGEN INTERACTIONS

The most commonly seen phenomenon associated with parasitic infections is the induction by the parasites of a general state of non-specific immunosuppression (Bloom, 1979). This phenomenon is not confined to parasitic infections, but is also seen in viral (Ferrante *et al.*, 1980), fungal (Cox, 1979) and bacterial infections (Quie, 1983). It is now generally appreciated that host-pathogen interactions result in substantial modulation of immunological responses, and the straightforward action-reaction model is no longer adequate for description of the complex events (Thong, 1983).

Another immunological consequence of host–pathogen interaction is the development of autoimmune disease mediated by immune complexes or cytotoxic mechanisms. For instance, there is strong evidence that group A streptococci share a number of antigens with human tissues, and that this molecular mimicry is responsible for streptococcal-associated diseases such as rheumatic fever and acute glomerular nephritis (Yang *et al.*, 1977). Another example is seen in schistosomiasis where tissue damage is the result of intense inflammatory responses to egg antigens rather than to the adult worm (Tracy and Mahmoud, 1982).

Several important points need to be considered in the discussion of the complex relationships between host, infectious agent and antimicrobial drug. First, host response to infection is mediated by at least four major immunological mechanisms, one or another of which may be operative depending on the nature of the pathogen and the stage of the infection. Secondly, infectious agents have evolved tactics for circumventing immune attack. Thirdly, they have also developed effective methods for modulating host immune responses to their own advantage. Fourthly, host immune responses to infectious agents can elicit immunologically-mediated tissue injury. Finally, modulation of the immune response by antimicrobial agents should be viewed from the perspective of the above-mentioned interactions.

V. IMMUNOMODULATORY EFFECTS OF ANTIMICROBIAL DRUGS

A large volume of literature has accumulated on immunomodulation by antimicrobial drugs. This is best discussed in the context of the cell type or immunological component involved, but some degree of overlap cannot be avoided.

A. Phagocytic Cells

The two major phagocytic cells of the body, monocyte–macrophages and neutrophil polymorphonuclear leucocytes, are derived from the same precursor cells in the bone marrow. Monocytes released from the marrow remains in the circulation for about 3 days before moving into the tissues to mature into resident macrophages in organs such as the liver, spleen and lungs, where they can remain viable for more than 3 months (Nathan *et al.*, 1980; Adams *et al.*, 1981). On the other hand, neutrophils remain in the circulation for about 6 days, then leave the body via mucosal surfaces, never to return. There is a large marrow reserve of these cells and the marginating pool is 50% of the circulating cells. There are no comparable reserves for monocytes.

1. Adherence

Physiological changes during acute inflammation consist of capillary dilatation, leakage of fluid, adherence of leucocytes to vascular endothelium and their migration through the vessel wall into extravascular spaces (Klebanoff and Clark, 1978). Thus, adherence is the first step in the response of neutrophils and monocytes to infection, and is also the mechanism by which monocytes leave the circulation to become tissue macrophages. In spite of the importance of this modality, few studies have been reported on the influence of antimicrobial agents on neutrophil adherence, and only one on monocyte adherence. Odegaard and Lamvik (1976) reported that human monocyte adherence was unaffected by chloramphenicol even at high concentrations. Seklecki *et al.* (1978) studied five aminoglycosides and showed that they enhanced neutrophil adherence at therapeutic concentrations. Marmer *et al.* (1981) investigated the effects of ketoconazole, amphotericin B and amphotericin B methyl ester on several aspects of neutrophil function. For amphotericin B and its methyl ester, adherence was decreased at low drug concentrations, and increased at high drug concentrations. They had no explanation for this seemingly paradoxical effect. Ketoconazole was found to have no effect on all aspects of neutrophil function. Li Si-Ying *et al.* (1984) studied the effects of 24 antimicrobial agents on neutrophil adherence and found effects for six of them, and then only at supratherapeutic concentrations. Oxytetracycline and rifampicin enhanced adherence, polymyxin B, colistin, quinine and chloroquine suppressed adherence, while penicillin G, nafcillin, cephalothin, vancymycin, bacitracin, tetracycline, minocycline, doxycycline, chloramphenicol, erythromycin, lincomycin, neomycin, streptomycin, acetylspiramycin, 5-fluorocytosine, sulphioxaxole, tinidazole and primaquine had no effect even at high concentrations. Thus, the modality of adherence appears to be remarkably resistant to influence by antimicrobial drugs.

Gnarpe *et al.* (1984*a*, *b*) found that imipenem and ceftazidime, new β-lactam antibiotics, stimulated neutrophil adherence at therapeutic concentrations. King *et al.* (1983) showed that the antifilarial drug, diethylcarbamazine, stimulated eosinophil and neutrophil adherence.

2. Chemotaxis

Chemotaxis is the directed migration of phagocytic cells towards the site of infection by receptors on the cell membrane for complement C5a, bacterial peptides and other substances on receiving the appropriate signals (Snyderman and Goetzl, 1981). Many antimicrobial agents have been shown to influence this aspect of neutrophil function.

Agents which inhibit bacterial cell wall synthesis in general have little effect on neutrophil chemotaxis, and these include penicillin G, oxacillin and the cephalosporins (Forsgren and Schmeling, 1977; Esterly *et al.*, 1978; Forsgren *et al.*, 1978; Belsheim and Gnarpe, 1981). Nafcillin, a penicillinase-resistant penicillin, was found to be stimulatory at low concentrations but inhibitory at high concentrations (Majeski *et al.*, 1976). They later showed that cefoxitin but not cefamandole depressed neutrophil chemotaxis, although both were third-generation cephalosporins (Majeski *et al.*, 1978). Belsheim and Gnarpe (1981) studied eight β-lactam antibiotics and found no interference with chemotaxis. The polypeptide antibiotics—bacitracin, tyrocidin and gramicidin—were found to resemble bacterial peptides and act as chemostatic factors for neutrophils (Aswanikumar *et al.*, 1978).

As predicted, agents which disrupt cell membrane function have pronounced effects on neutrophil chemotaxis. Using the leading front method, Bjorksten *et al.* (1976) showed inhibition of chemotaxis by amphotericin B, but no inhibition by nystatin, griseofulvin and miconazole. Thong and Ness (1977) reported that both amphotericin B and miconazole inhibited neutrophil chemotaxis using the agarose method. Lohr and Snyderman (1980) showed that depression of neutrophil chemotaxis by amphotericin B was due to interference with binding to the chemotactic receptor. They also showed that nystatin suppressed chemotaxis to a lesser degree, while griseofulvin had no effect. Studies by Marmer *et al.* (1981) confirmed the suppressive effects of amphotericin B. They found no effect with ketoconazole. More recently, Rowan-Kelly *et al.* (1984) studied the effects of five imidazole derivatives on neutrophil chemotaxis. Metronidazole and tinidazole, which interfere with DNA synthesis in microbial systems, had no effect on neutrophil chemotaxis. The highly substituted imidazoles which disrupt cell membrane function, such as clotrimazole, miconazole and ketoconazole, were inhibitory at therapeutic concentrations. That Marmer *et al.* (1981) found no inhibitory effect by ketoconazole can be explained on methodological differences. Although both groups used the agarose method, Rowan-Kelly *et al.* (1984) incorporated the drug into the agar, so that a constant concentration of the drug is maintained in the chemotactic environment, whereas Marmer *et al.* (1981) did not. This procedure may be critical for some agents where actions are reversible.

Since protein synthesis is a requirement for chemotaxis to occur, it is not surprising that agents which inhibit protein synthesis also inhibit neutrophil chemotaxis. Martin *et al.* (1974) showed that tetracycline suppressed chemotaxis *in vitro*, and that serum obtained from patients taking tetracycline also inhibited control neutrophils. Forsgren and

Schmeling (1977) and Forsgren *et al.* (1978) found that tetracycline, lymecycline and doxycycline inhibited neutrophil chemotaxis. The study by Majeski and Alexander (1977) with eight tetracycline analogues suggested that the mechanism was interference with either chemotactic factor generation or binding to the chemotactic receptor on the neutrophil. However, Goodhart (1979) produced evidence to indicate that inhibition of neutrophil chemotaxis was due to chelation of intracellular cations by tetracyclines. The report by Esterly *et al.* (1978) identified not only tetracycline, but also erythromycin and clindamycin as inhibitors of neutrophil chemotaxis. Belsheim and Gnarpe (1981) found that doxycycline and lymecycline suppressed neutrophil chemotaxis *in vitro*. Belsheim *et al.* (1979*a*) found that neutrophils of patients treated with tetracyclines had defective chemotaxis *in vitro*. Gnarpe and Belsheim (1978) and Belsheim *et al.* (1979*b*) extended the findings by showing that neutrophils from tetracycline-treated patients had defective *in-vivo* chemotaxis, and this was confirmed by Elewiski *et al.* (1983) in a study using volunteers.

The effect of chloramphenicol on neutrophil chemotaxis is less clear. Majeski *et al.* (1976) found that chloramphenicol enhanced chemotaxis at low concentrations, while Forsgren and Schmeling (1977) and Forsgren *et al.* (1978) found the opposite. Admittedly, the first study used the Boyden Chamber while the second used the agarose technique, so the difference in results may be methodological. Comparative studies using several methods in order to resolve this problem have not yet been done.

With regard to the aminoglycosides, Goodhart (1977) examined the effects of gentamicin and amikacin on neutrophil chemotaxis and found no impairment. This finding confirms the work of Majeski *et al.* (1976). However, Seklecki *et al.* (1978) showed suppression of chemotaxis by all five aminoglycosides that they studied. This controversy may have been resolved by Khan *et al.* (1979) who showed that the vehicle of parenteral preparations of aminoglycosides was the active principle involved in the suppression of neutrophil chemotaxis, more so than the aminoglycosides themselves. A recent report by Belsheim and Gnarpe (1981) confirms that gentamicin and amikacin suppress neutrophil chemotaxis.

Of the agents that inhibit nucleic acid synthesis or metabolic activity, only a few have been studied with regard to neutrophil chemotaxis. Rifampicin was found by Forsgren and Schmeling (1977) and Forsgren *et al.* (1978) to be inhibitory; however, Gray *et al.* (1980) reported that, although it was inhibitory at low concentrations, it was stimulatory at high concentrations. They later showed that the drug was capable of blocking chemotactic receptors on neutrophils (Gray *et al.*, 1983). Sulphonamides were either not inhibitory (Forsgren and Schmeling, 1977; Esterly *et al.*, 1978; Forsgren *et al.*, 1978) or inhibitory only at high concentrations

(Majeski *et al.*, 1976). Neither metronidazole nor tinidazole were inhibitory at therapeutic concentrations (Rowan-Kelly *et al.*, 1984).

Levamisole was found to enhance neutrophil chemotaxis *in vitro* (Bourne *et al.*, 1974; Anderson *et al.*, 1976) as well as in humans receiving the drug (DeCree *et al.*, 1974; van Eygen *et al.*, 1976).

The benzimidazole derivative, nocodazole, has been shown to inhibit the movement and spreading of mouse peritoneal macrophages (Cheung and Terry, 1980).

3. Phagocytosis

The attachment of a particle to the phagocytic cell surface generates a signal which leads to the engulfment of the particle. Attachment is usually facilitated by antibody and complement C3b, but specific molecular sites on the particle surface are sometimes involved. Transmission of the phagocytic signal may be mediated by cyclic nucleotides. Repeated receptor–ligand binding takes place during the engulfment process, and the activity of certain esterase and protease enzymes are necessary for the process (Horowitz, 1982).

Using guinea-pig neutrophils, Downey and Pisano (1965) found that penicilin, chloramphenicol, streptomycin, neomycin and sulphanilamide had no effect on phagocytosis *in vitro*, whereas bacitracin and polymyxin B had inhibitory effects at high concentrations. According to Hoeprich and Martin (1970), phagocytosis of human neutrophils *in vitro* was not affected by tetracycline, polymyxin B and rifampicin at levels achievable during therapy with these drugs. Melby and Midtvedt (1977) investigated phagocytosis by rat polymorphonuclear leucocytes and showed that at high concentrations, oxytetracycline, doxycline, erythromycin, colistin, erythromycin and chloramphenicol depressed phagocytosis, but cephalothin, gentamicin and trimethoprim did not. They later showed that human neutrophil phagocytosis was impaired in the presence of high concentrations of cephalothin, chloramphenicol, colistin, erythromycin, gentamicin, oxytetracycline and trimethoprim (Melby and Midtvedt, 1980). Using human neutrophils, Chan and Belish (1978) reported that amphotericin B at concentrations of 1 μg/ml inhibited phagocytosis, while therapeutic concentrations of dicloxacillin, chloramphenicol and gentamicin were without effect.

Ohnishi *et al.* (1983, 1984) reported that a new semisynthetic cephalosporin, AC-1370, enhanced the phagocytic activity of macrophages, which in turn released factors which stimulated neutrophil phagocytosis.

The screening studies cited above suggest that tetracyclines may have inhibitory effects on phagocytosis, and this is confirmed by other reports. Inhibition of neutrophil phagocytosis *in vitro* was first observed by Munoz and Geister (1950). Subsequent experiments reported by Hoeprich and Martin (1970) and Forsgren and Gnarpe (1973) failed to confirm this. However, using more sensitive methods, Forsgren *et al.* (1974) and Gnarpe and Leslie (1974) showed suppression by tetracyclines at therapeutic concentrations. *In-vivo* experiments in rats and rabbits based on phagocytic clearance by macrophages of particles in the circulation support this view (Snell, 1960; Altura *et al.*, 1966).

That chloramphenicol has no influence on phagocytosis is confirmed by four reports (Downey and Pisano, 1965; Kaplan *et al.*, 1969; Odegaard and Lamvik, 1976; Chan and Belish, 1978). The aminoglycosides also have no effect on phagocytosis (Seklecki *et al.*, 1978; Ferrari *et al.*, 1980). Melsom and Seljelid (1974) found that the phagocytic activity of mouse macrophages was unaffected by rifamycin at high concentrations. Seneca and Peer (1966) reported that therapeutic concentrations of sulphadiazine enhanced phagocytosis, whereas higher levels of the drug depressed phagocytosis.

4. Metabolic and microbicidal activity

The process of phagocytosis is accompanied by a surge in oxidative metabolism via the hexose-monophosphate shunt. This results in the formation of reactive oxygen species with potent microbicidal activity. The contents of lysosomal and other granules in phagocytic cells are also microbicidal, and they are released into the phagosome on fusion (Root and Cohen, 1981). They are also released into the immediate environment and are not only microbicidal but immunoregulatory as well, for they contain chemotactic factors, leukotrienes and other biologically active molecules (Weissmann *et al.*, 1980).

Welch *et al.* (1981) studied the effects of 19 antimicrobial agents on neutrophil chemiluminescence, phagocytosis and killing. They found that at therapeutic concentrations, tetracycline, doxycycline and trimethoprim reduced both chemiluminescence and killing, while cephalothin only reduced killing. Fifteen agents had no effect: penicillin G, ampicillin, carbenicillin, cephalexin, cefazolin, cephaloridine, ceforanide, cefamandole, clindamycin, erythromycin, kanamycin, gentamicin, amikacin, sisomicin, sulphioxazole.

The antimicrobial agents with effects on these aspects of phagocytic cell function are primarily those with sites of action on cell membrane function, protein synthesis or microbial metabolism. In the case of amphotericin B, *in-vitro* studies by Bjorksten *et al.* (1976) showed suppression of chemiluminescence. Studies by Chunn *et al.* (1977) showed that even at the high concentration of 10 μg/ml, neutrophil oxidative metabolism was not affected. Lin *et al.* (1977) reported that a single peritoneal injection resulted in increased phagocytic and bactericidal activity of peritoneal macrophages. Marmer *et al.* (1981) studied the *in-vitro* effects of amphotericin B and ketoconazole in several aspects of neutrophil function. They found that amphotericin B depressed chemiluminescence and microbicidal function; ketoconazole depressed chemiluminescence but not microbicidal function. Ketoconazole and four other imidazole derivatives were investigated by Rowan-Kelly *et al.* (1984). Metronidazole and tinidazole had no effects on neutrophil function, clotrimazole inhibited chemotaxis only, while miconazole and ketoconazole suppressed bactericidal and fungicidal activity as well. The first two drugs inhibit DNA synthesis in microbial systems, while the last three disrupt cell membrane function, and the results appear to conform to this perspective. Another membrane-active agent, polymyxin B, has been shown to inhibit lysosomal enzyme release (Bannatyne *et al.*, 1977) but only high concentrations could it inhibit oxidative metabolism (Downey and Pisano, 1965).

Of the agents which inhibit protein synthesis, chloramphenicol and tetracycline received the most attention. Kaplan *et al.* (1969) noted that at very high concentrations chloramphenicol could suppress neutrophil oxidative metabolism and this was confirmed by McCurrach *et al.* (1970) and Lehrer (1973). Using cultured human macrophages, Odegaard and Lamvik (1976) found no effect of high concentrations on lysosomal digestion. With regard to tetracyclines, McCurrach *et al.* (1970) found no suppression of oxidative metabolism even at high concentrations, but Rubinstein and Pelet (1973) noted inhibition of nitro blue tetrazolium dye reduction, a phenomenon dependent on oxidative metabolism. The study by Seklecki *et al.* (1978) on aminoglycosides stated that these drugs had no effect on nitro blue tetrazolium dye reduction, and experiments by Ferrari *et al.* (1980) confirmed this but also showed that neutrophils treated with five aminoglycosides had impaired candidacidal activity. No effect of the macrolide antibiotics, erythromycin and rosamicin, on neutrophil chemiluminescence was observed (Martin *et al.*, 1980).

Other agents have also been studied briefly. Melsom and Seljelid (1974) observed that the cytotoxic effects of activated mouse peritoneal macrophages could be abrogated by low concentrations of rifampicin. Lehrer (1971) showed that the myeloperoxidase microbicidal system of phagocytic cells could be suppressed by sulphonamides at therapeutic concentrations. This was confirmed by Johnston *et al.* (1975), who also made the paradoxical observation that the microbicidal activity of neutrophils from patients with chronic granulomatous disease was enhanced by sulphioxaxole. Anderson *et al.* (1980) found no impairment of neutrophil functions except at high concentrations of trimethoprim–sulphamethoxaxole. The antiparasitic drug suramin interfered with the fusion between phagosome and lysosome in mouse peritoneal macrophages (D'Arcy Hart and Young, 1975).

B. The Complement System

The complement system consists of more than 20 serum proteins which interact with each other in a sequential manner reminiscent of that seen in blood coagulation (Fearon and Austen, 1980; Egwang and Befus, 1984). Activation of complement results in the generation of subcomponents with important functions in the inflammatory response. Antigen–antibody reactions activate complement through factors C1, C4 and C2 of the classical pathway. Microbial surfaces and endotoxins can activate complement via the alternative pathway through factors B, D and properdin. Both pathways converge at C3, which leads to completion of the sequence C5–C9 known as the membrane attack unit because of its capacity to lyse microbicidal and other cells. The subcomponents C3a, C4a and C5a induce mast cells, platelets and basophils to release vasoactive amines, enhance vascular permeability and stimulate contraction of smooth muscle, and are collectively known as anaphylotoxins. In addition, C5a is chemotactic for phagocytic cells and stimulates oxidative metabolism. The other cleavage products, C3b and C4b, interact with receptors on the membranes of phagocytic cells to promote phagocytosis.

Several studies have implicated antimicrobial agents with effects on complement function. Suramin is known to inhibit activation of the classical pathway and the whole complement sequence (Fong and Good, 1972; Eisen and Loveday, 1973), while activation of the alternative pathway can be suppressed by tetracycline, gentamicin and sulphonamides (Alexander, 1975).

Complement-mediated lysis of microbes is also subject to modification by antimicrobial agents. Traub and Sherris (1970) found that polymyxins enhanced lysis, but not ampicillin aminoglycosides. This effect of polymyxins was confirmed by Davis *et al.* (1971), Pruul and Reynolds (1972), Sud and Finegold (1975) and Fierer and Finley (1979). The effects of ampicillin are less substantiated, with Fierer and Finley (1979) confirming the work of Traub and Sherris (1970), Friedman and Warren (1976) finding that this agent enhances lysis, and Lorian and Atkinson (1979) claiming the opposite. These discrepancies can be attributed to methodological differences. The situation with tetracycline is more clear-cut; that is interfered with bacterial lysis was first reported by Waisbren and Brown (1964) and later confirmed by Forsgren and Gnarpe *in vitro* (1973), and in volunteers treated with the drug (Gnarpe and Belsheim, 1978). Chloramphenicol was also identified by Waisbren and Brown (1964) as another agent with possible suppressive effects on complement-mediated lysis. Other workers have published data to indicate that rifampicin can enhance lysis (Alexander *et al.*, 1980), and that penicillin (Yourtee *et al.*, 1980), cephalosporin, carbenicillin and aminoglycosides have no effect (Fierer and Finley, 1979).

C. Lymphocytes

Two major classes of lymphocytes, each with disparate functional capabilities, are present in the human body. B lymphocytes produce immunoglobulins and give rise to antibody-secreting plasma cells and memory cells. There are five isotypes of immunoglobulins; these are IgG, IgM, IgA, IgD and IgE; IgG has four subclasses and IgA has two. The specificity of antibody to antigen resides in the variability of amino-acid sequences in the variable regions of light and heavy chains of the immunoglobulin molecule (Leder, 1982).

T lymphocytes can be divided into two major functional categories. Regulatory T cells may be either helper or suppressor cells depending on whether they amplify or dampen the responses of other lymphocytes. Effector T cells mediate immunological reactions such as delayed-type hypersensitivity (DTH), graft rejection, tumour immunity and elimination of virus-infected cells by cytotoxic mechanisms (Reinherz and Schlossman, 1980). T lymphocytes are also secretory cells, and the soluble, biologically active molecules they produce include migration inhibitory factors affecting macrophages and neutrophils, chemotactic factors affecting macrophages, neutrophils, eosinophils and basophils, mitogenic factors affecting other lymphocytes, and lymphotoxins, interferon and growth inhibitory factors affecting diverse cell types (Rocklin *et al.*, 1980).

1. Penicillins and cephalosporins

In the presence of antigens or lectins and suitable culture conditions, lymphocytes undergo blast transformation and clonal proliferation. This response is generally regarded as an *in-vitro* correlate of immunity and has been used to evaluate the effects of antimicrobial agents.

In this regard, the penicillins are inert while some cephalosporins may be inhibitory. Dam and Malkinson (1975) reported that penicillin G had no effect on lymphocyte transformation. Forsgren and Banck (1978) and Banck and Forsgren (1979) found that benzylpenicillin, aminobenzylpenicillin, carboxybenzylpenicillin and cephazolin had no effect on lymphocyte proliferative responses. Likewise, Thong (1979) showed that penicillin G, methicillin, ampicillin, carbenicillin and cephalothin had no influence on mitogen-induced lymphocyte transformation when present in therapeutic concentrations of 10 μg/ml or less. In concentrations of 50 μg/ml, cephalothin, cephalexin and cephadrine suppressed responses to phytohaemagglutinin, while cephalexin, cephadrine and cefoxitin suppressed responses to pokeweed mitogen (Chaperon and Sanders, 1978). Moxalactam and cefuroxime, at concentrations of 25 and 50 μg/ml respectively, have also been reported to suppress mitogen-induced lymphocyte transformation (Manzella and Clark, 1983).

2. Polyene antibiotics

The polyene antibiotics, especially amphotericin B, have been the subject of extensive studies. The report by Hammarstrom and Smith (1976) that amphotericin B is antigenic for murine B lymphocytes has not been confirmed. Ferrante *et al.* (1979) and Walls and Kay (1982) showed that the drug suppressed murine lymphocyte transformation in the same concentrations used by the earlier workers. These later observations with murine lymphocytes would be in agreement with experiments using human lymphocytes. Tarnvik and Ansehn (1974) studied the effects of this drug on *in-vitro* lymphocyte proliferative responses to antigens, plant lectins and autologous cells and found dose-dependent inhibition. Using plant lectins, Thong and Rowan-Kelly (1978*a*, *b*) extended the studies to show that the inhibitory effects could be partially reversed by washing, and that the effects were quite pronounced even if the drug was added late in the experiments. These *in-vitro* effects on human lymphocytes were confirmed by Alford and Cartwright (1983).

The effects of amphotericin B *in vivo* depend on dosage schedule. Multiple doses of the drug over a period of time caused suppression of DTH but not antibody responses in mice (Ferrante *et al.*, 1979); DTH responses in tumour-bearing mice, already depressed, were further depressed by the drug (Ferrante and Thong, 1980). These findings were substantiated by Roselle and Kauffman (1980) in experiments using guinea pigs, where they reported suppression of cell-mediated immunity and lymphokine production.

In contrast, a simple injection of amphotericin B usually results in amplification of immunological responses. Thomas *et al.* (1973) treated mice with a single dose of the drug either 24 h before or 24 h after challenge with *Listeria monocytogenes*. Improved survival from the infection was observed in the group treated prior to challenge, while decreased survival occurred in the group treated after challenge. There was good correlation between these results and the number of viable bacteria in the liver and spleen of the animals. Medoff *et al.* (1974) showed that a combination of amphotericin B and an antitumour drug given 24 h prior to challenge of mice with a transplantable leukaemia resulted in improved survival. Amphotericin B given on the same day as the challenge was ineffective. Either of the drugs given alone did not influence survival rate. Moreover, mice that survived became immune to rechallenge with the leukaemia cells.

Ishikawa *et al.* (1975) reported enhancement of antibody synthesis *in vitro* by mouse splenic lymphocytes treated with amphotericin B. The studies by Blanke *et al.* (1977) indicated that the drug can stimulate B-cell responses to immunization with a hapten–protein complex and T-cell responses in graft-*vs*-host reactions. Shirley and Little (1979*a*, *b*) investigated the phenomenon further and reported augmentation of *in-vivo* contact sensitivity as well as *in-vitro* lymphocyte proliferative responses in mice treated *in vivo* with sensitizing agents and amphotericin B. They showed that the drug interacted with a subset of T cells with suppressor functions. A later report by Stewart *et al.* (1981) indicated that amphotericin B can activate monocytes and suppressor T cells in humans. The same group (Olds *et al.*, 1981) also showed that a single dose of the drug provided partial protection to mice challenged with *Schistosoma mansoni*, and that this protection may be due to activation of macrophages.

There are encouraging reports to suggest that amphotericin B may be a useful adjuvant in the chemotherapy of human malignancies (Presant *et al.*, 1977, 1980).

3. Griseofulvin

There is only one study on griseofulvin. This drug was reported to reduce the resistance of mice to challenge with *Listeria monocytogenes* (Mitchell *et al.*, 1973).

4. Nitroimidazoles

Tarnvik and Ansehn (1974) reported that clotrimazole suppressed lymphocyte transformation in the 4–10-μg/ml range. This was confirmed by the work of Gow *et al.* (1979).

Miconazole suppressed lymphocyte transformation in the 1–10-μg/ml range. The inhibition was reversible by washing. Delayed addition of the drug to lymphocyte cultures produced only slight inhibition (Thong and Rowan-Kelly, 1978). Experiments in mice demonstrated the capability of miconazole to suppress antibody production, skin-graft rejection and DTH (Thong and Ferrante, 1979*a*). In tumour-bearing mice, treatment with miconazole resulted in greater suppression of DTH than did the tumour-induced immunosuppression (Thong *et al.*, 1980).

Marshall *et al.* (1981) investigated the effects of ketoconazole on six patients with systemic fungal infections. In four patients, depressed levels of lymphocyte proliferative responses to T-cell mitogens were restored to normal after ketoconazole therapy. Serum containing 5 μg/ml of ketoconazole increased lymphocyte responses of five of six patients, but not those of lymphocytes from healthy individuals. However, the *in-vitro* effects of the drug at therapeutic concentrations are inhibitory rather than stimulatory (Alford and Cartwright, 1983; Buttke and Chapman, 1983).

Inhibition of DTH by metronidazole and misonidazole has been reported by Rockwell *et al.* (1983). Earlier, Grove *et al.* (1977) had shown that metronidazole was a potent suppressor of cell-mediated immunological responses.

5. Chloramphenicol

Ambrose and Coons (1963) first gave an indication that chloramphenicol has immunomodulatory properties. Using rabbit lymph nodes primed with antigen *in vivo*, they found that secondary antibody formation was inhibited by 5–50 μg/ml concentrations of chloramphenicol. Weisberger *et al.* (1964) studied the effects of chloramphenicol on antibody production and skin-graft rejection in rabbits, and showed that both were significantly suppressed by the drug and three of its analogues. These workers extended their studies to humans and reported the following year that normal oral doses suppressed tetanus antibody levels (Daniel *et al.*, 1965). DaMert and Sohnle (1979) showed suppression of lymphocyte transformation but not lymphokine production. Forsgren and Banck (1978) and Banck and Forsgren (1979) did not find that chloramphenicol inhibited lymphocyte transformation even at high concentrations, but Thong (1979) found suppression at concentrations of 10 μg/ml, and this may be related to the fact that Thong (1979) used pure chloramphenicol rather than chloramphenicol salts which require activation by tissue enzymes (Meissner and Smith, 1979).

Mice treated with chloramphenicol, or its analogue, thiamphenicol, produced less antibody *in vivo*. *In-vitro* spleen cell cultures from treated animals also produced less antibody than controls (Della Bella *et al.*, 1973). Thiamphenicol appears to have greater immunosuppressive activity than chloramphenicol. Both suppress mitogen-induced transformation of human lymphocyte at concentrations as low as 10 μg/ml (Ugazio *et al.*, 1974). Petruscu (1974) reported that thiamphenicol depressed antibody formation in mice, and this was confirmed by Vindel and Khoury (1974). It has been used as an immunosuppressive agent for the treatment of lupus nephritis (Richmond, 1979).

6. Tetracyclines

Inhibition of lymphocyte transformation by doxycycline was reported by Forsgren and Banck (1978) and Banck and Forsgren (1979). Thong and Ferrante (1979*b*) compared the effects of tetracycline, doxycycline and oxytetracycline on lectin-induced lymphocyte proliferation and observed that doxycycline was the most potent of the three analogues. They found that the inhibitory effect of doxycycline was completely reversible by washing, and that profound suppression occurred even when the drug was added 48 h after the initiation of lymphocyte culture. These findings were confirmed by Potts *et al.* (1983).

In an *in-vitro* study using human lymphocytes, it was shown that production of the lymphokine, migration inhibitory factor, was depressed in the presence of tetracycline at concentrations as low as 3 μg/ml (Ganguly *et al.*, 1983).

Thong and Ferrante (1980*a*) studied the effects of treatment of mice with four analogues of tetracycline. These analogues suppressed DTH but not antibody responses. The suppressive effects on DTH was most pronounced at the time of challenge with antigen.

7. Polymyxins

Thong (1979) observed inhibition of lymphocyte transformation by polymyxin B. Follow-up studies compared polymyxin B with colistin (polymyxin E) and found that colistin was a more potent inhibitor than polymyxin B (Ferrante *et al.*, 1982).

8. Aminoglycosides

In one report, gentamicin and kanamycin had no effects on lymphocyte transformation (Forsgren and Banck, 1978; Banck and Forsgren, 1979). In another study, gentamicin was also found to be without effect (Thong, 1979).

9. Rifampicin

Paunescu (1970) observed that rifampicin could inhibit antibody and DTH responses in rabbits and guinea pigs. Delayed rejection of skin grafts in rabbits treated by rifampicin was reported by Serrou *et al.* (1972). In guinea pigs, the drug was observed to suppress lymphocyte transformation and the tuberculin reaction (Grassi and Pozzi, 1972). Mice receiving rifampicin were found to be deficient in primary antibody responses (Bassi *et al.*, 1973). Working with guinea pings, Dajani *et al.* (1973) also found suppression of primary but not secondary antibody responses. Rats immunized with BCG were equally resistant to challenge with tubercle bacilli whether or not they received treatment with rifampicin and isoniazid in experiments using lymphocyte transfer (Lefford and McGregor, 1974). *In-vitro* production of antibody by mouse splenic lymphocytes was reported to be suppressed by rifamycin (Osoba, 1974). Kasik *et al.* (1976) studied six ansamycins, including rifampicin, and found inhibition of the tuberculin reaction in mice. However, Youmans *et al.* (1976) found that in spite of a reduction in DTH responses, mice receiving rifampicin had other intact responses such as granuloma formation and lymphokine production. In the first study of the effects of rifampicin on tumour immunity, Roszkowski *et al.* (1984) reported that tumour growth in mice was enhanced. They also reported that tumour resistance in preimmunized animals was abrogated after a 7-day or longer dosage schedule with rifampicin. Parallel experiments indicated a concomitant decline in the cytotoxic and natural killer cells of these animals.

Rifampicin is a potent immunosuppressive agent in humans as well. Moshkowitz *et al.* (1971) showed that local application reduced the inflammatory reaction to vaccination, but oral treatment did not. Mukerjee *et al.* (1973) showed that eight of 11 tuberculous patients became poorly responsive to the tuberculin test after receiving therapy with rifampicin for 2–6 months. Graber *et al.* (1973) found that patients treated with the drug responded poorly to immunization with two different antigens in terms of antibody production. Serrou (1974) reported that the drug suppressed human lymphocyte transformation and this was confirmed by Forsgren and Banck (1978) and Banck and Forsgren (1979). In the study by Litwin *et al.* (1974), a 2-week course of treatment reduced IgG antibodies but not DTH. A study reported by Ruben *et al.* (1974) showed suppression of several immunological parameters at 12–16 weeks after commencement of treatment with rifampicin, but not at 2 weeks. In another study, Gupta *et al.* (1975) noted reduction of T-cell rosettes in patients and volunteers treated with rifampicin; however, the levels of T-cell rosettes returned to normal 2 weeks after cessation of treatment. Goldstein *et al.* (1976) investigated 50 patients with tuberculosis, some of whom were receiving rifampicin. They found that lymphocyte transformation was depressed to phytohaemagglutinin, but not to pokeweed mitogen or concanavalin A. They also found that tuberculin responses were not impaired after 4–24 months of low-dose therapy.

10. Antimalarials

Hurvitz and Hirshhorn (1968) reported that chloroquine was a potent inhibitor of lymphocyte transformation. These findings were later extended to quinine (Gold and Ben-Efraim, 1978; Thong and Ferrante, 1978) and primaquine (Thong *et al.*, 1978). A later report by Gold *et al.* (1979) noted that quinine suppressed lymphocyte proliferative responses to autologous cells but not antibody formation by lymphocytes *in vitro*. The site of action of chloroquine appears to be the antigen-presenting macrophage (Lee *et* al., 1982; Ziegler and Unanue, 1982). *In-vivo* experiments with low dosages of quinine, chloroquine and primaquine showed that mice were not affected in their ability to mount DTH and antibody responses (Thong *et al.*, 1981).

The newly introduced antimalarial agent, mefloquine, also has inhibitory effects on lymphocyte transformation using human and mouse lymphocytes, as well as antibody production, but not DTH responses in mice (Thong *et al.*, 1979). The observation by Thong *et al.* (1979) of inhibition by mefloquine of human lymphocyte transformation induced by lectins was confirmed by Gilbreath *et al.* (1983*b*). These workers further showed that human lymphocyte responses to autologous cells were not impaired. The drug appears to affect both T and non-T lymphocytes. Serum obtained from volunteers and patients on low-dose mefloquine treatment did not suppress lymphocyte transformation.

11. Diaminopyrimidines

There was prolongation of skin-graft survival in mice treated with trimethoprim to the same degree as the standard immunosuppressive drug, azathioprine (Ghilchik *et al.*, 1970). Human lymphocyte transformation was also found to be suppressed by a combination of trimethoprim–sulphamethoxazole (Gaylarde and Sarkany, 1972), and the same combination suppressed booster antibody responses to tetanus immunization (Arvilommi *et al.*, 1972). However, Anderson *et al.* (1980) found suppression of *in-vitro* lymphocyte transformation only at high concentrations, while two out of three volunteers who ingested the drugs for 5 days had no depression of lymphocyte transformation. The third volunteer developed allergy to the drug and had impaired mitogen responsiveness.

In contrast, pyrimethamine was found to enhance both DTH and antibody responses in mice. The immunodeficiency of tumour-bearing mice was also reversed by high-dose pyrimethamine treatment (Thong and Ferrante, 1980*b*). Human lymphocyte transformation was also observed to be enhanced by pyrimethamine (Thong, 1979; Bygbjerg, 1981), but Gilbreath *et al.* (1983*a*) noted suppression instead. This discrepancy may be explained on the basis of methodological difficulties. Lymphocyte transformation is measured by incorporation of ^{3}H-thymidine. Since pyrimethamine is a folate antagonist, the lymphocyte cultures may be starved of folate, thereby leading to increased uptake of thymidine. This problem can be resolved by using less ambiguous methods of assessing lymphocyte transformation.

12. Pentamidine

Pentamidine was found to inhibit human lymphocyte transformation (Thong, 1979). Later experiments using mouse lymphocytes indicated that it has preferential suppressive effects on B cells. At low concentrations, only B cells were affected, whereas at high concentrations, both T and B lymphocytes were affected (Ferrante *et al.*, 1984).

13. Niridazole

Mahmoud and Warren (1974) observed that mice treated with niridazole and tartar emetic had impaired granuloma formation and DTH responses to schistosome egg antigens. In further experiments with mice, suppression of skin-graft rejection (Mahmoud *et al.*, 1975) but not antibody responses were noted (Pelley *et al.*, 1975).

In guinea pigs, Daniels *et al.* (1975*b*) found suppression of DTH by niridazole. Serum from niridazole-treated animals also suppressed lymphokine production. However, mixing of the drug with serum did not produce a similar effect, so they concluded that the immunosuppressive activity resided in a metabolite of the drug. They also found that suppression of lymphokine production depended on timing of niridazole administration. The suppression occurred only if niridazole was given before antigen, not after (Daniels *et al.*, 1975*a*).

Using the model of experimental allergic encephalitis, it was shown that niridazole ameliorated autoimmune tissue damage. Although no effects were seen on non-specific inflammation, antibody formation or lymphokine production, the drug prevented release of lymphokines by T cells (Bernard *et al.*, 1977). Studies in patients treated with niridazole confirm that it is a potent inhibitor of DTH (Webster *et al.*, 1975).

14. Levamisole

Renoux and Renoux (1972) and Chirigos *et al.* (1973) observed that levamisole treatment of mice resulted in a reduction of tumour progression and metastasis by an enhancement of antitumour immunity. However, Potter *et al.* (1974) found it to be ineffective in other tumour systems, and similar findings were made by Hopper *et al.* (1975). Trials in human cancer were also indeterminate. Tripodi *et al.* (1973) showed that the cutaneous allergy of cancer patients could be restored by levamisole, while Ramot *et al.* (1976) showed restoration of E-rosette levels in Hodgkin's disease. Reports of improved survival (Amery, 1975, 1976) in patients with lung cancer were contradicted by another study of increased deaths from cardiopulmonary arrests of unknown cause (Anthony *et al.*, 1979). A randomized double-blind controlled trial in 203 patients with malignant melanoma showed no benefit except in those with Stage I disease (Spitler and Sagebiel, 1980). Thus, the variable results in cancer therapy may be due to the degree of tumour burden.

Studies on the mechanisms of immunomodulation by levamisole suggest that it may mimic some of the actions of thymic hormones. It augments mitogen-induced lymphocyte transformation (Hadden *et al.*, 1975), enhances skin reactivity to DTH antigens (Pabst and Crawford, 1975), restores azathioprine sensitivity to spleen cells of adult thymectomized mice (Van Ginckel and Holbecke, 1976), retards development of antinuclear antibodies in NZB/w mice (Russell, 1976), stimulates maturation of human null cells to rosette-forming lymphocytes (Rosenthal *et al.*, 1976; Thomas *et al.*, 1976), potentiates DTH and skin-graft rejection, but not antibody responses in mice (Renoux *et al.*, 1976), induces the expression of thymic antigens in splenic lymphocytes of nude mice (Renoux and Renoux, 1977), depresses the level of autologous rosette-forming cells in the spleen of nude mice (van Wauwe and van Nijen, 1977), and enhances DNA synthesis and lymphokine production in T cells (Kazura *et al.*, 1979).

Studies by Whitcomb *et al.* (1976) and Pike *et al.* (1977) indicate that levamisole may act by facilitating participation of monocytes in cell-mediated immune responses. The active principle appears to be a metabolite of the drug (Van Ginckel and De Brabander, 1979). Besides cancer, levamisole has been used in the experimental therapy of a large number of clinical conditions, but its acceptance has been limited by a number of undesirable side-effects, the most serious of which are neutropenia and agranulocytosis (El-Ghobarey *et al.*, 1978). However, it has been used with safety in children by Van Eygen *et al.* (1976); in a double-blind trial on 70 children with recurrent upper respiratory infections, treatment over 6 months reduced the frequency and severity of the infections.

15. Benzimidazoles

This group of anthelminthic agents has interesting effects on immune responses. One analogue has been shown to enhance antibody formation (Warren *et al.*, 1979) and others have modulating effects on lymphocyte reactivity (Holden *et al.*, 1980; Colot and Mickshe, 1982; Durand and Olive, 1982). Thiabendazole was reported by Hewlett *et al.* (1981) to suppress DTH responses *in vivo*, confirming and extending previous studies that it is a potent immunosuppressive agent (Campbell, 1971), but at odds with reports that it may have immunopotentiating properties (Lundy and Lovett, 1976; Lovett and Lundy, 1977). These conflicting data may be due to differences in dosage schedule, as seen in studies with amphotericin B (Ferrante *et al.*, 1979), or they may be the result of selective inhibition of suppressor cells, as seen in the cyclophosphamide model (Braciale and Parish, 1980).

16. Diethylcarbamazine

This antifilarial agent has been shown to affect antibody synthesis in patients (Grove, 1981; Piessens *et al.*, 1981). Another interesting effect is its ability to inhibit leukotriene synthesis (Mathews and Murphy, 1982).

Its immunosuppressive properties have been foreshadowed by previous authors (Muller, 1971; Thevathason and Litt, 1971; Sharma *et al.*, 1979).

17. Nifurtimox

Lelchuk *et al.* (1977) observed that immunological alterations occurred in patients with Chagas disease receiving treatment with nifurtimox, and *in vitro* inhibition of leucocyte migration was also abrogated. In animal experiments, it was shown that the *in-vitro* and *in-vivo* reactivity of guinea pigs to tuberculin was inhibited by the drug.

18. Antiviral agents

Steele *et al.* (1980) reported that cytosine arabinoside and idoxuridine suppressed lymphocyte functions, but adenine arabinoside and acyclovir did not. Wingard *et al.* (1983) screened five antiviral agents for their effects on lymphocyte transformation, mixed lymphocyte reaction and lymphocyte cytotoxicity. Acyclovir and bromovinyldeoxyuridine were the least suppressive, vidarabine and trifluorothymide were most suppressive, while (S)-9-(2,3-dihydropropyl) adenine was intermediate.

Vidarabine was studied by Steele *et al.* (1975, 1977). They found that concentrations of vidarabine as high as 3 μg/ml did not inhibit lymphocyte transformation to lectins and viral antigens. Parallel experiments showed suppression by cytosine arabinoside, a related drug. They also examined immunological responses of four patients with herpes simplex encephalitis receiving vidarabine, and found no suppression of lymphocyte transformation or lymphotoxicity. They later studied a further 13 treated and two untreated patients, and reported that immunological reactivity was not affected by the drug.

Wingard *et al.* (1983) and Wittek *et al.* (1983) showed that the new antiviral agent, bromovinyldeoxyuridine had minimal inhibitory effects on lymphocyte functions *in vitro*.

Bennett *et al.* (1982) compared the effects of two antiviral agents in mice. They found that 5′-amino-5′-deoxythymidine, a new compound, had no effect, while 5-iodo-2′-deoxyuridine was immunosuppressive.

Gordon *et al.* (1974) observed that isoprinosine (inosiplex, methiosprinol) had antiviral properties, but that some of its efficacy may be immunological in origin. Hadden *et al.* (1976, 1977) reported that this drug was capable of augmenting lectin-induced lymphocyte transformation, both in mouse and human cells, and that this effect was not mediated by cyclic nucleotides. It also increases the percentage of active T-cell rosettes (Friedman *et al.*, 1980). Bradshaw and Summer (1977) showed that inosiplex enhanced lymphotoxin production in patients with herpes simplex infection. Patients with subacute sclerosing panencephalitis improved after prolonged treatment (Huttenlocher and Mattson, 1979). It restores DTH reactions in patients with herpes zoster (Laude *et al.*, 1980).

Ribavirin has been shown to suppress antibody formation in mice (Suganuma and Ishida, 1973) and skin-graft rejection in rabbits (Jolley *et al.*, 1977) when high dosages were used. Schofield *et al.* (1975) reported that ferrets treated with ribavirin (virazole) had impaired serum and secretory antibody response. Potter *et al.* (1976) also showed that high-dose ribavirin treatment of guinea pigs resulted in abrogation of antibody synthesis but not cell-mediated immunity. However, in the mouse model, relatively high doses of ribavirin did not interfere with antibody formation or interferon production (Huffman *et al.*, 1977). *In-vitro* experiments indicate that this drug is capable of suppressing lymphocyte proliferative responses and antibody formation (Peavy *et al.*, 1980, 1981), and that suppressor T-cell populations are affected at low concentrations, while B cells are also affected at high concentrations (Powers *et al.*, 1982).

VI. CONCLUSIONS

In the preceding paragraphs, a large number of studies have been condensed into a small number of pages. It is appropriate at this stage to examine the pertinence of this kaleidoscope of observations to the clinical situation and determine the avenues for future research.

A. Clinical Relevance

From the immunological standpoint, there is little doubt that the tripartite interactions between microbe, immune system and antimicrobial agent have tremendous implications on clinical practice. Allergy to antimicrobial agents constitutes a major proportion of the problem of drug allergy encountered in medical practice (Parker, 1982). Much remains to be learned about the mechanisms of IgE regulation in relation to drug allergy, but some general understanding of the process has emerged in recent years (Katz, 1982). Non-IgE mechanisms are also important in drug allergy; antibody-mediated thrombocytopenia and haemolytic anaemia has followed administration of penicillins, tetracyclines, aminoglycosides, isoniazid, rifampicin and antimalarial agents (Conley, 1981).

That many antimicrobial agents have immunosuppressive effects is also well documented. The antimalarial drugs, such as chloroquine and quinine, have long been used in the treatment of autoimmune diseases (Lanham and Hughes, 1982). Antibiotics such as actinomycin D and doxorubicin are established anticancer agents (Umezawa, 1983). Another antibiotic, cyclosporine, is now the mainstay of many organ transplantation programmes (White and Calne, 1982). Thiamphenicol, the analogue of chloramphenicol that has enjoyed wide usage in Europe as an antimicrobial agent, has been used successfully as an immunosuppressive agent in lupus nephritis (Richmond, 1979). Many other commonly used antimicrobial agents surveyed in this review have been shown to affect one or more modalities of the immune response. It would be prudent at this stage to consider these findings in the choice of an antimicrobial agent, especially in patients with therapeutic immunosuppression for cancer and organ transplantation (Chang *et al.*, 1976), autoimmune diseases (Cohen, 1983), malnutrition (Gross and Newberne, 1980) and other debilitating illnesses. In this regard, recent editorials have advised caution in the use of antimicrobials, particularly for prolonged periods in immunosuppressed patients (Finch, 1980; Hauser and Remington, 1982).

Paradoxically, some antimicrobials achieve some of their beneficial effects in the treatment of infections because of their immunosuppressive properties. A case in point is the use of niridazole in the treatment of schistosomiasis, where the drug is able to reduce the inflammatory response to egg antigens (Mahmoud and Warren, 1974; Mahmoud *et al.*, 1975). Another example is ribavirin, a new antiviral agent whose efficacy is partly due to suppression of viral-induced immunopathology (Powers *et al.*, 1982).

Conversely, antimicrobials with immunopotentiating properties such as levamisole (Symoens and Rosenthal, 1977), pyrimethamine (Thong *et al.*, 1979) or AC-1370 (Ohnishi *et al.*, 1983) may be helpful to patients with borderline immunocompetence.

Another aspect of antimicrobial therapy not covered in this review is the well documented observation, summarized by McDonald *et al.* (1981), that even a brief exposure to antibiotics render some bacteria more susceptible to phagocytic destruction. The implications are that the current prescriptive practice of frequent dosing to sustain high blood levels of antibiotics may not be necessary for the treatment of many infections. Thus, as more is learned about how antimicrobial agents modulate immune responses, simplistic views will be abandoned in favour of more rational approaches to prescriptive practice.

B. Future Research

The topic under discussion in this chapter lies at the confluence of three active fields of enquiry. It is an interdisciplinary area of research that will benefit from developments in pharmacology, immunology and microbiology. In these last few paragraphs, new and old information will be related to these developments to arrive at some directions for future research.

A much clearer picture has emerged about penicillin-binding proteins in relation to the mechanism of action of β-lactam antibiotics (Waxman and Strominger, 1983), and about sterol specificity and phospholipid complexes with regard to the mechanism of action of antifungal agents (Medoff *et al.*, 1983). The systematic approach adopted in the design of antiviral agents has produced a number of drugs with actions at several points in the virus–host cell cycle (Smith *et al.*, 1980). The interferons, naturally occurring antiviral substances, have been shown to have remarkable immunomodulatory effects (Heron *et al.*, 1983). These complexities of drug action would certainly lend themselves to investigation of immunomodulatory properties.

However, the immunomodulatory effects of some antimicrobial agents may not be related to their actions on microorganisms. For example, the aminoglycosides inhibit protein synthesis in microbial cells, but their effects on the immune system may be related to their extrapharmacological effects on cell membrane polyphosphoinositide metabolism (Schacht, 1976), or energy metabolism of mammalian tissues (Tachibana *et al.*, 1976). Chloramphenicol also inhibits protein synthesis in microbial cells, but its effects on mammalian cells are on mitochondria rather than ribosomes (Yunis, 1973). It suppresses bone marrow by the same mechanism, yet, paradoxically, it can induce neutrophil maturation in patients with chronic neutropenia (Adams and Pearson, 1983). Although some of the immunomodulating effects of polymyxin antibiotics may be attributed to their effects on cell membranes (Brown and Wood, 1972), others may be a direct result of their capacity to cause degranulation and release of histamine from mast cells (Tizard and Holmes, 1974). The known action of chloroquine and its analogues on malaria parasites is by binding to DNA (Allison *et al.*, 1965), but its immunomodulatory effects have been localized to inhibition of phospholipase A_2, a key enzyme in the pathway of prostaglandin and leukotriene synthesis (Flower, 1974; Dise *et al.*, 1982). These arachidonic acid metabolites are not only important in inflammation, they are also key factors in the regulation of lymphocyte function (Hirata *et al.*, 1980; Namiuchi *et al.*, 1984).

It can be appreciated from the preceding paragraph that inflammatory processes (Larsen and Henson, 1983) are an integral part of immunological responses. The study of this aspect of immunomodulation by antimicrobial agents is much neglected and needs early rectification.

The effects of antimicrobial agents on the immune system must be understood in terms of the interactions between the complement system (Reid and Porter, 1981), phagocytic cells (Daniel, 1980; Nathan *et al.*, 1980) and the various lymphocyte subpopulations which make up the immunologic network. The capacity of these lymphocyte subpopulations to respond to other cells, biologically active molecules and antigens is governed by genes of the major histocompatibility complex (Klein and Nagy, 1982). The immunologic network is also regulated by feedback loops involving T cells (Gree *et al.*, 1983), T–B cell interactions (Singer and Hodes, 1983), immunoglobulin synthesis (Wall and Kuehl, 1983) and idiotypic antibodies (Rajewski and Takemori, 1983). Because of the complexity of the immunologic network, antimicrobial agents can affect the immune system at various levels, on multiple sites and by varied mechanisms. Some attempts have been made, particularly in connection with amphotericin B, levamisole, niridazole and a few other agents, to dissect out these effects so that they can be understood with some clarity. There are also valuable studies employing antimicrobial agents as chemical probes in order to understand better the intricacies of immunological interactions, as seen in the reports by Lee *et al.* (1982) and Ziegler and Unanue (1982) with chloroquine.

C. Concluding Remarks

Pathogenic microbes and the immune system have evolved alongside each other for millions of years. Each new invasive or evasive tactic would be met by the invention of a novel defence strategy and, in time, the relationship between the protagonists became closely intermeshed. This complex relationship is now beginning to be understood (Thong, 1983). The process generally involves alteration of immune response by microbial products or biological adaptations (Bloom, 1979; Cox, 1979; Ferrante *et al.*, 1980; Peterson and Quie, 1981). Alteration of host immune responses can also lead to the development of autoimmune or inflammatory diseases (Yang *et al.*, 1977; Tracy and Mahmoud, 1982). Thus the effects of antimicrobial agents on the immune system need to be understood in the context of immunological events during the course of an ongoing infection. Carefully designed experiments in humans and whole animals along these lines would contribute greatly to knowledge about the intricate relationships discussed in this chapter. Much can be achieved if immunological testing is included in the standard development protocol for new antimicrobial and anticancer agents by the pharmaceutical industry.

ACKNOWLEDGEMENTS

The author's work cited herein was supported in part by grants from the National Health and Medical Research Council of Australia, and the Mayne, Henker and Adams Bequest Funds of the University of Queensland.

My dear friend and former colleague in Adelaide, Dr Antonio Ferrante, participated in many of these studies. I am indebted to Ms Erlene Chun for careful typing of the manuscript and Miss Barbara Ryan for excellent library assistance.

REFERENCES

Adams, D. O., Edelson, P. J. and Koren, H. S. (eds) (1981). "Methods for Studying Mononuclear Phagocytes." Academic Press, London.

Adams, G. R. and Pearson, H. A. (1983). *N. Engl. J. Med.* **309**, 1039–1041.

Alexander, J. W. (1975). *Bull. N. Y. Acad. Sci.* **51**, 1039–1045.

Alexander, J. W., Cobbs, C. G. and Curtiss, R. (1980). *Infect. Immun.* **28**, 923–926.

Alford, R. H. and Cartwright, B. B. (1983). *Antimicrob. Agents Chemother.* **24**, 575–578.

Allison, J. L., O'Brien, R. C. and Hahn, F. E. (1965). *Science* **149**, 1111–1113.

Altura, B. M., Hershey, S. G., Ali, M. and Thaw, C. (1966). *J. Reticuloendothel. Soc.* **3**, 447–457.

Ambrose, C. T. and Coons, A. H. (1963). *J. Exp. Med.* **117**, 1075–1088.

Amery, W. K. (1975). *Br. Med. J.* **iii**, 461–463.

Amery, W. K. (1976). *Ann. N. Y. Acad. Sci.* **277**, 260–268.

Anderson, R., Glover, A., Koornhof, H. J. and Rabson, A. R. (1976). *J. Immunol.* **117**, 428–432.

Anderson, R., Grabow, G., Oosthuizer, R., Theron, A. and Van Rensburg, A. J. (1980). *Antimicrob. Agents Chemother.* **17**, 322–326.

Anthony, H. M., Mearns, A. J., Mason, M. K., Scott, D. G., Moghissi, K., Deverall, P. B., Rozycki, Z. J. and Watson, D. A. (1979). *Thorax* **34**, 4–12.

Arvilommi, H., Vuori, M. and Salmi, A. (1972). *Br. Med. J.* **2**, 761–762.

Aswanikumar, S., Schiffman, E., Corcoran, B. A., Pert, C. B., Morrell, J. L. and Gross, E. (1978). *Biochem. Biophys. Res. Commun.* **80**, 464–471.

Banck, G. and Forsgren, A. (1979). *Antimicrob. Agents Chemother.* **16**, 554–560.

Bannatyne, R. M., Harnett, N. M., Lee, K. Y. and Biggar, W. D. (1977). *J. Infect. Dis.* **136**, 469–474.

Bassi, L., Di Bernardino, L., Arioli, V., Silvestri, G. and Cherie Ligniere, E. L. (1973). *J. Infect. Dis.* **128**, 736–744.

Beaman, L., Benjamini, E., Pappagianis, D. (1981). *Infect Immun.* **34** 347–353.

Belsheim, J. A., Gnarpe, G. H. (1981). *Acta Pathol. Microbiol. Scand. Sect. C* **89**, 217–221.

Belsheim, J., Gnarpe, H. and Persson, S. (1979*a*). *Scand. J. Infect. Dis.* **11**, 141–145.

Belsheim, J. Gnarpe, H. and Lofberg, J. (1979*b*). *Scand. J. Infect. Dis.* **11**, 289–290.

Bennett, J. A., Savoca, P. E., Lin, P. S. and Prusoff, W. H. (1982). *Int. J. Immunopharmacol.* **4**, 559–566.

Bernard, C. C. A., Leydon, J. and Mackay, I. R. (1977). *Int. Arch. Allergy Clin. Immunol.* **53**, 555–559.

Bjorksten, B., Ray, C. and Quie, P. G. (1976). *Infect. Immun.* **14**, 315-317.
Blanke, T. J., Little, J. R., Shirley, S. F. and Lynch, R. G. (1977). *Cell. Immunol.* **33**, 180-190.
Bloom, B. R. (1979). *Nature* **279**, 21-26.
Bourne, H. R., Lichtenstein, L. M. and Melmon, K. L. (1974). *Science* **184**, 19-28.
Braciale, V. L. and Parish, C. R. (1980). *Cell. Immunol.* **51**, 1-12.
Brack, C., Delain, E. and Riou, G. (1972). *Proc. Natl. Acad. Sci. U.S.A.* **69**, 1642-1646.
Bradshaw, L. J. and Summer, H. L. (1977). *Ann. N.Y. Acad. Sci.* **284**, 190-196.
Brown, M. R. W. and Wood, S. M. (1972). *J. Pharm. Pharmacol.* **24**, 215-228.
Brumfitt, W. and Pursell, R. (1971). *Postgrad. Med. J.* **47**, 16-18.
Buttke, T. M. and Chapman, S. W. (1983). *Antimicrob. Agents Chemother.* **24**, 478-485.
Bygbjerg, I. C. (1981). *Acta Pathol. Microbiol. Scand. Sect. C* **89**, 111-113.
Campbell, W. C. (1971). *J. Am. Med. Assoc.* **216**, 2143-2145.
Chan, C. K. and Belish, E. (1978). *Canad. J. Microbiol.* **24**, 363-364.
Chang, H. Y, Rodriguez, V., Narboni, G., Bodey, G. P., Luna, M. A. and Freireich, E. J. (1976). *Medicine* **55**, 259-268.
Chang, K. P. and Dwyer, D. M. (1976). *Science* **193**, 678-680.
Chaperon, E. A. and Sanders, W. E., Jr. (1978). *Infect. Immun.* **19**, 378-384.
Cheung, H. T. and Terry, D. S. (1980). *Cell Biol. Int. Rep.* **4**, 1125-1129.
Chirigos, M. A., Pearson, J. W. and Pryor, J. (1973). *Cancer Res.* **33**, 2615-2618.
Chopra, I. and Howe, T. G. B. (1978). *Microbiol. Rev.* **42**, 707-724.
Chunn, C. J., Starr, P. R. and Gilbert, D. N. (1977). *Antimicrob. Agents Chemother.* **12**, 226-230.
Cohen, J. (1983). *J. R. Soc. Med.* **76**, 508-513.
Colot, M. and Micksche, M. (1982). *J. Immunopharmacol.* **4**, 367-376.
Conley, C. L. (1981). *Johns Hopkins Med. J.* **149**, 101-109.
Cox, R. A. (1979). *Am. Rev. Resp. Dis.* **120**, 143-149.
Dajani, B. M., Kasik, J. E. and Thompson, J. (1973). *Antimicrob. Agents Chemother.* **3**, 451-455.
Dam, W. C. and Malkinson, F. D. (1975). *Experientia* **31** 375-376.
DaMert, G. J. and Sohnle, P. G. (1979). *J. Infect Dis.* **139**, 220-224.
Daniel, T. M. (1980). *Clin. Chest Med.* **1** 189-201.
Daniel, T. M., Suhrland, L. G. and Weisberger, A. S. (1965). *N. Engl. J. Med.* **273**, 367-369.
Daniels, J. C., Fajardo, I. and David, J. R. (1975*a*). *Proc. Natl. Acad. Sci.* **72**, 4569-4572.
Daniels, J. C., Warren, K. S. and David, J. R. (1975*b*). *J. Immunol.* **115**, 1414-1421.
D'Arcy Hart, P. and Young, M. R. (1975). *Nature* **256**, 47-49.
Davidse, L. C. and Flach, W. (1978). *Biochem. Biophys. Acta.* **543**, 82-85.
Davies, D. R. Metzger, H. (1983). *Ann. Rev. Immunol.* **1**, 87-118.
Davies, J., Anderson, P. and Davis, B. D. (1965). *Science* **149**, 1096-1098.
Davis, A. T., Brunning, R. C., Jr. and Quie, P. G. (1971). *N. Engl. J. Med.* **285**, 789-790.

DeCree, J., Verhaegen, H., DeCock, M., Vanheule, R., Brugmans, J. and Schuermans, V. (1974). *Lancet* **ii**, 294-295.
Della Bella, D., Petrescu, D., Marca, G. and Veronese, M. (1973). *Exp. Chemother.* **18**, 99-111.
Denslow, N. D. and O'Brien, T. W. (1978). *Eur. J. Biochem.* **91**, 441-448.
Diamond, R. D. and Krzesicki, R. (1978). *J. Clin. Invest.* **61**, 360-369.
Diamond, R. D., Root, R. K. and Bennett, J. E. (1972). *J. Infect. Dis.* **125**, 367-376.
Dise, C. A., Burch, J. W. and Goodman, D. B. P. (1982). *J. Biol. Chem.* **257**, 4701-4704.
Downey, R. J. and Pisano, J. C. (1965). *J. Reticuloendothel. Soc.* **2**, 75-88.
Durand, R. E. and Olive, P. L. (1982). *J. Histochem. Cytochem.* **30**, 111-116.
Dutcher, J. P., Schiffer, C. A. and Johnston, G. S. (1981). *N. Engl. J. Med.* **304**, 486-489.
Edelson, P. J. (1982). *Rev. Infect. Dis.* **4**, 125-135.
Egwang, T. G. and Befus, A. D. (1984). *Immunology* **51**, 207-224.
Eisen, V. and Loveday, C. (1973). *Br. J. Pharmacol.* **49**, 678-687.
Elewiski, B. E., Lamb, B. A. J., Sams, M., Jr. and Gammon, W. R. (1983). *J. Am. Acad. Dermatol.* **8**, 807-812.
El-Ghobarey, A. F., Mavrikakis, M. E., MacLeod, M., Reynolds, P. M. G., Capell, H. A., Spencer, D. G., Balint, G., Mathieu, J. P., MacAllister, T., Cooney, A. and Dick, W. C. (1978). *Quart. J. Med.* **47**, 385-400.
Englund, P. T., Bajduk, S. L. and Marini, J. C. (1982). *Ann. Rev. Biochem.* **51**, 695-726.
Esterly, N. B., Furey, N. L. and Flanagan, L. E. (1978). *J. Invest. Dermatol.* **70**, 51.
Fearon, D. T. and Austen, K. F. (1980). *N. Engl. J. Med.* **303**, 259-266.
Ferrante, A. and Thong, Y. H. (1980). *Int. J. Immunopharmacol.* **1**, 299-301.
Ferrante, A., Rowan-Kelly, B. and Thong, Y. H. (1979). *Clin. Exp. Immunol.* **38**, 70-76.
Ferrante, A., O'Keefe, D. E. and Thong, Y. H. (1980). *Med. Microbiol. Immunol.* **168**, 227-233.
Ferrante, A., Rowan-Kelly, B. and Thong, Y. H. (1982). *Int. Arch. Allergy Appl. Immunol.* **69**, 279-281.
Ferrante, A., Secker, L. K. and Thong, Y. H. (1985). *Int. J. Immunopharmacol.* **7**, 281-285.
Ferrari, F. A., Pagani, A., Marconi, M., Stefanoni, R. and Siccardi, A. G. (1980). *Antimicrob. Agents Chemother.* **17**, 87-88.
Fierer, J. and Finley, F. (1979). *J. Infect. Dis.* **140**, 581-589.
Finch, G. D. (1980). *J. Antimicrob. Chemother.* **6**, 691-694.
Fitch, C. D., Chan, R. L. and Chevli, R. (1979). *Antimicrob. Agents Chemother.* **15**, 258-262.
Flower, R. J. (1974). *Pharmacol. Rev.* **26**, 33-45.
Flynn, I. W. and Bowman, I. B. R. (1969). *Trans. R. Soc. Trop. Med. Hyg.* **63**, 121-122.

Fong, J. S. C. and Good, R. A. (1972). *Clin. Exp. Immunol.* **10**, 127–138.
Forsgren, A. and Banck, G. (1978). *Infection* **6**, 91–97.
Forsgren, A. and Gnarpe H. (1973). *Nature New Biol.* **244**, 82–83.
Forsgren, A. and Schmeling, D. (1977). *Antimicrob. Agents Chemother.* **11**, 580–584.
Forsgren, A., Schmeling, D. and Quie, P. G. (1974). *J. Infect. Dis.* **130**, 412–415.
Forsgren, A., Schmeling, D. and Banck, G. (1978). *Infection* **6**, 102–106.
Friedman, H. and Warren, G. H. (1976). *Proc. Soc. Exp. Biol. Med.* **153**, 301–304.
Friedman, H., Cole, R. and Morin, A. (1980). *Int. J. Immunopharmacol.* **2**, 153–164.
Ganguly, R., Pennock, D. and Kluge, R. M. (1983). *J. Infect. Dis.* **148**, 611.
Gaylarde, P. M. and Sarkany, I. (1972). *Br. Med. J.* **3**, 144–146.
Gelfand, J. A., Hurley, D. L., Fauci, A. S. and Frank, M. M. (1978). *J. Infect. Dis.* **138**, 9–16.
Ghilchik, M. W., Morris, A. S. and Reeves, D. S. (1970). *Nature* **227**, 393–394.
Gilbreath, M. J. Groves, J., Pavanand, K., Phisphumvithi, P. (1983*a*). *Trans. R. Soc. Trop. Med. Hyg.* **77**, 743–747.
Gilbreath, M. J., Kongchavoen, S., Wimonnrattrawatee, T., Phisphumvithi, P., Pavanand, K. (1983*b*). *Trans. Roy. Soc. Trop. Med. Hyg.* **77**, 767–770.
Gnarpe, H. and Belsheim, J. (1978). *Microbios* **22**, 45–59.
Gnarpe, H. and Leslie, D. (1974). *Microbios* **10A**, 127–138.
Gnarpe, H., Belsheim, J., Blomquist, C. and Lundback, A. (1984*a*). *Antimicrob. Agents Chemother.* **25**, 179–181.
Gnarpe, H., Belsheim, J., Blomquist, C. and Svensson, A. (1984*b*). *J. Antimicrob. Chemother.* **13**, 369–375.
Gold, E. F. and Ben-Efraim, S. (1978). *Int. Arch. Allergy Appl. Immunol.* **57**, 177–182.
Gold, E. F., Ophir, R. and Ben-Efraim, S. (1979). *Int. Arch. Allergy Appl. Immunol.* **58**, 447–452.
Goldstein, R. A., Ang, U. H., Foellmar, J. W. and Janicki, B. W. (1976). *Am. Rev. Resp. Dis.* **113**, 197–202.
Goodhart, G. L. (1977). *Antimicrob. Agents Chemother.* **12**, 540–542.
Goodhart, G. L. (1979). *J. Reticuloendothel. Soc.* **25**, 545–554.
Gordon, B., Ronsen, P. and Brown, E. R. (1974). *Antimicrob. Agents Chemother.* **5**, 153–160.
Gow, P. J., Corrigall, V. and Panayi, G. S. (1979). *Agents Actions* **9**, 543–548.
Graber, C. D., Jebaily, J., Galphin, R. L. and Doering, E. (1973). *Am. Rev. Resp. Dis.* **107**, 713–717.
Grassi, G. G. and Pozzi, E. (1972). *J. Infect. Dis.* **126**, 542–544.
Gray, G. D., Knight, K. A. and Talley, C. A. (1980). *Fed. Proc.* **39**, 878.
Gray, G. D., Smith, C. W., Hollers, J. C., Chenoweth, D. E., Fiegel, V. D. and Nelson, R. D. (1983). *Antimicrob. Agents Chemother.* **24**, 777–783.
Gree, D. R., Flood, P. M. and Gershon, R. K. (1983). *Ann. Rev. Immunol.* **1**, 439–464.
Gross, R. L. and Newberne, P. M. (1980). *Physiol. Rev.* **60**, 188–302.
Grove, D. I. (1981). *Southeast Asian J. Trop. Med. Pub. Health* **12**, 487–491.

Grove, D. I. and Warren, K. S. (1976). *Ann. Trop. Med. Parasitol.* **70**, 449-453.
Grove, D. I., Mahmoud, A. A. F. and Warren, K. S. (1977). *Int. Arch. Allergy Appl. Immunol.* **54**, 422-427.
Gull, K. and Trinci, A. P. J. (1973). *Nature* **244**, 292-294.
Gupta, S., Grieco, M. H. and Siegel, I. (1975). *Ann. Intern. Med.* **82**, 484-488.
Gupta, S., Kirkpatrick, C. H. and Good, R. A. (1979). *Clin. Immunol. Immunopathol.* **14**, 86-95.
Hadden, J. W., Coffey, R. G., Hadden, E. M., Lopes-Corrales, E. and Sunshine, G. H. (1975). *Cell. Immunol.* **20**, 98-103.
Hadden, J. W., Hadden, E. M. and Coffey, R. G. (1976). *Infect. Immun.* **13**, 382-387.
Hadden, J. W., Lopez, C., O'Reilly, R. J. and Hadden, E. M. (1977). *Ann. Ny. Acad. Sci.* **284**, 139-152.
Hamilton-Miller, J. M. T. (1974). *Adv. Appl. Microbiol.* **17**, 109-134.
Hammarstrom, L. and Smith, E. (1976). *Scand. J. Immunol.* **5**, 37-43.
Hauser, W. P., Jr. and Remington, J. S. (1982). *Am. J. Med.* **72**, 711-716.
Heron, I., Hokland, M. and Berg, K. (1983). *J. Interferon Res.* **3**, 231-239.
Hewlett, E. L., Hamid, D. Y., Ruffier, J. and Mahmoud, A. A. F. (1981). *Immunopharmacology* **3**, 325-332.
Hirata, F., Toyoshima, S., Axelrod, J. and Waxdal, M. J. (1980). *Proc. Natl Acad. Sci. U.S.A.* **77**, 862-865.
Hitchings, G. H. and Burchell, J. J. (1965). *Adv. Enzymol.* **27**, 417-468.
Hoeprich, P. D. (1963). *Ann. Intern. Med.* **112**, 405-414.
Hoeprich, P. D. and Martin, C. H. (1970). *Clin. Pharmacol. Therap.* **11**, 418-422.
Holden, H. E., Crider, P. A. and Wahrenberg, M. G. (1980). *Environ. Mutagen.* **2**, 67-73.
Hopper, D. G., Pimm, M. V. and Baldwin, R. W. (1975). *Lancet* **i**, 574-575.
Horowitz, M. A. (1982). *Rev. Infect. Dis.* **4**, 104-123.
Huffman, J. H., Anderson, M. A., Allen, L. B. and Sidwell, R. W. (1977). *J. Antimicrob. Chemother.* **3**, 79-85.
Hurvitz, D. and Hirshhorn, K. (1968). *N. Engl. J. Med.* **273**, 23-26.
Huttenlocher, P. R. and Mattson, R. H. (1979). *Neurology* **29**, 763-771.
Ishikawa, H., Narimatsu, H. and Saito, K. (1975). *Cell Immunol.* **17**, 300-305.
Johnston, R. B., Jr, Wilfert, C. M., Buckley, R. H., Webb, L. S., DeChatelet, L. R. and McCall, C. E. (1975). *Lancet* **i**, 824-827.
Jolley, W. B., Call, T. W., Alvord, L. S. and Hinshaw, D. B. (1977). *Ann. N.Y. Acad. Sci* **284**, 230-232.
Jordan, W. M., Bodey, G. P., Rodriguez, V., Ketchel, S. J. and Henney, J. (1979). *Antimicrob. Agents Chemother.* **16**, 792-797.
Kaplan, S. S., Perillie, P. E. and Finch, S. C. (1969). *Proc. Soc. Exp. Biol. Med.* **130**, 839-843.
Kasik, J. E., Monick, M. and Thompson, J. S. (1976). *Antimicrob. Agents Chemother.* **8**, 470-473.
Katz, D. H. (1982). *Prog. Allergy* **32**, 105-160.
Kazura, J. W., Negendahk, M., Guerry, D. and Schreiber, A. D. (1979). *Clin. Exp. Immunol.* **35**, 258-268.

Khan, A. J., Evans, H. E., Glass, L., Khan, P., Chang, C. T. and Nair, S. R. (1979). *J. Lab. Clin. Med.* **93**, 295–300.

King, C. H., Green, B. M. and Spagnuolo, P. J. (1983). *Antimicrob. Agents Chemother.* **24**, 453–456.

Klebanoff, S. J. and Clark, R. A. (1978). "The Neutrophil: Function in Clinical Disorders." North Holland, Amsterdam.

Klein, J. and Nagy, Z. A. (1982). *Adv. Cancer Res.* **37**, 233–317.

Knight, R. C., Skolimovski, I. M. and Edwards, D. I. (1978). *Biochem. Pharmacol.* **27**, 1089–2093.

Konno, K., Dizumo, K. and Oka, S. (1973). *Am. Rev. Resp. Dis.* **107**, 1006–1012.

Lachman, P. J. and Peters, D. K. (1982). "Clinical Aspects of Immunology", 4th edn. Blackwell, Oxford.

Lagrange, P. H. and Closs, O. (1979). *Scand. J. Immunol.* **10**, 285–290.

Lanham, J. G. and Hughes, G. R. (1982). *Clin. Rheum. Dis.* **8**, 279–298.

Larsen, G. L. and Henson, P. M. (1983). *Ann. Rev. Immunol.* **1**, 335–359.

Laude, J., Le Sound, B., Rancurel, G., Doumere, S. and Moulias, R. (1980). *Int. J. Immunopharmacol.* **2**, 195.

Leder, O. (1982). *Scient. Am.* **246**, 102–111.

Lee, K. C., Wong, M. and Spitzer, D. (1982). *Transplantation* **34**, 150–153.

Lefford, M. J. and McGregor, D. D. (1974). *J. Infect. Dis.* **129**, 473–476.

Lehrer, R. I. (1971). *J. Clin. Invest.* **50**, 2498–2505.

Lehrer, R. I. (1973). *J. Infect. Dis.* **127**, 40–48.

Lehrer, R. I. and Cline, M. J. (1971). *Cancer* **27**, 1211–1217.

Lelchuk, R., Cardoni, R. L. and Levis, S. (1977). *Clin. Exp. Immunol.* **30**, 469–473.

Lin, H., Medoff, G. and Kobayashi, G. S. (1977). *Antimicrob. Agents Chemother.* **11**, 154–159.

Li Si-Ying, Seow, W. K. and Thong, Y. H. (1985). *Int. Arch. Allergy Appl. Immunol.* **76**, 151–155.

Litwin, A., Brooks, S. M. and Claew, F. (1974). *Chest* **65**, 548–551.

Lohr, K. M. and Snyderman, R. (1982). *J. Immunol.* **129**, 1594–1599.

Lorian, V. and Atkinson, B. (1979). *Rev. Infect. Dis.* **1**, 797–806.

Lovett, E. J. and Lundy, J. (1977). *Transplantation* **24**, 93–97.

Lundy, J. and Lovett, E. J. (1976). *Surg. Forum* **27**, 132–134.

Macario, A. J. L. and DeMacario, E. C. (1978). *Clin. Exp. Immunol.* **31**, 282–290.

Mahmoud, A. A. F. and Warren, K. S. (1974). *J. Immunol.* **112**, 222–228.

Mahmoud, A. A. F., Mandel, M. A., Warren, K. A. and Webster, L. T., Jr. (1975). *J. Immunol.* **114**, 279–286.

Majeski, J. A. and Alexander, J. W. (1977). *J. Lab. Clin. Med.* **90**, 259–265.

Majeski, J. A., McClellan, M. A. and Alexander, J. W. (1976). *Amer. Surg.* **42**, 785–788.

Majeski, J. A., Morris, M. J. and Alexander, J. W. (1978). *J. Antibiot.* **41**, 1059–1062.

Manzella, J. P. and Clark, J. K. (1983). *Antimicrob. Agents Chemother.* **23**, 360–363.

Mao, J. C. H. and Wiegand, R. G. (1968). *Biochim. Biophys. Acta* **157**, 404–413.

Marmer, D. J., Fields, B. T., France, G. L. and Steele, R. W. (1981). *Antimicrob. Agents Chemother.* **20**, 660–665.
Marshall, G. D., Wilson, J. B., Mader, J. T. and Reinarz, J. A. (1981). AFCR Meeting, New Orleans, Louisiana, January 15–17.
Martin, R. R., Warr, G. A., Couch, R. B., Yeager, H. and Knight, V. (1974). *J. Infect. Dis.* **129**, 110–116.
Martin, R. R., Futuan, M., Greenberg, S. B., Wallace, R. J., Jr. and Wilson, S. Z. (1980). *J. Med.* **11**, 39–48.
Mathews, W. R. and Murphy, R. C. (1982). *Biochem. Pharmacol.* **31**, 2129–2132.
McCurrach, P. H., Park, J. K. and Perry, W. L. M. (1970). *Br. J. Pharmacol.* **38**, 608–615.
McDonald, P. J., Wetherall, B. L. and Pruul, H. (1981). *Rev. Infect. Dis.* **3**, 38–44.
Medoff, G., Valeriote, F., Lynch, R. G., Schlessinger, D. and Kobayashi, G. S. (1974). *Cancer Res.* **34**, 974–978.
Medoff, G., Brajtburg, J. and Kobayashi, G. S. (1983). *Ann. Rev. Pharmacol. Toxicol.* **23**, 303–330.
Meissner, H. C. and Smith, A. L. (1979). *Pediatrics* **64**, 348–356.
Melby, K. and Midtvedt, T. (1977). *Scand. J. Infect. Dis.* **9**, 9–12.
Melby, K. and Midtvedt, T. (1980). *Acta Pathol. Microbiol. Scand. Sect. B.* **88**, 103–106.
Melsom, H. and Seljelid, R. (1974). *Exp. Cell Res.* **86**, 415–419.
Miles, A. Z., Miles, E. M. and Burke, J. (1957). *Br. J. Exp. Pathol.* **38**, 79–96.
Mitchell, F., Yamamoto, R. S. and Weisberger, J. H. (1973). *Proc. Soc. Exp. Biol. Med* **143**, 165–167.
Moshkowitz, A., Goldblum, N. and Heller, G. (1971). *Nature* **229**, 422–424.
Mukerjee, P., Schuldt, S. and Kasik, J. E. (1973). *Antimicrob. Agents Chemother.* **4**, 607–611.
Muller, R. (1971). *Trans. R. Soc. Trop. Hyg.* **65**, 843–844.
Muller, W. E. G., Zahn, R. K., Bittlingmaier, K. and Falks, D. (1977). *Ann. N.Y. Acad. Sci.* **284**, 34–48.
Munoz, J. and Geister, R. (1950). *Proc. Soc. Exp. Biol. Med.* **75**, 367–371.
Namiuchi, S., Kumagai, S., Imura, H., Suginoshita, T., Hattori, T. and Hirata, F. (1984). *J. Immunol.* **132**, 1456–1460.
Nathan, C. F., Murray, H. W. and Cohn, Z. A. (1980). *N. Engl. J. Med.* **303**, 622–626.
Neito, M. and Perkins, H. R. (1971). *Biochem. J.* **124**, 845–852.
Nilsson, B. S. (1971). *Lancet* **ii**, 374.
Odegaard, A. and Lamvik, J. (1976). *Acta Path. Microbiol. Scand.* **84**, 37–44.
Ohnishi, H., Kosozume, H., Inaba, H., Okura, M., Mochizuki, H., Suzuki, Y. and Fujii, R. (1983). *Antimicrob. Agents Chemother.* **23**, 874–880.
Ohnishi, H., Inaba, H., Mochizuki, H. and Kosozume, H. (1984). *Antimicrob. Agents Chemother.* **25**, 88–92.
Olds, G. R., Stewart, S. J. and Ellner, J. J. (1981). *J. Immunol.* **126**, 1667–1670.
Osoba, D. (1974). *J. Immunol.* **112**, 844–848.

Pabst, H. F. and Crawford, J. (1975). *Clin. Exp. Immunol.* **21**, 468-473.
Parker, C. W. (1982). *Pharmacol. Rev.* **34**, 85-104.
Paunescu, E. (1970). *Nature* **228**, 1188-1190.
Pearsall, N. A., Adams, B. L. and Bunni, R. (1978). *J. Immunol.* **120**, 1176-1180.
Pearson, G. R. (1978). *Curr. Top. Microbiol. Immunol.* **80**, 65-96.
Peavy, D. L., Koff, V. C., Hyman, D. H. and Knight, V. (1980). *Infect. Immun.* **29**, 583-589.
Peavy, D. L., Powers, C. N. and Knight, V. (1981). *J. Immunol.* **126**, 861-864.
Pelley, R. P., Pelley, R. J., Stavitsky, A. B., Mahmoud, A. A. F. and Warren, K. S. (1975). *J. Immunol.* **15**, 1477-1482.
Pelley, R. P., Ruffier, J. J. and Warren, K. S. (1976). *Infect. Immun.* **13**, 1176-1183.
Peterson, E. M. and Calderone, R. A. (1977). *Infect. Immun.* **15**, 910-915.
Peterson, P. K. and Quie, P. G. (1981). *Ann. Rev. Med.* **32**, 29-43.
Petruscu, D. (1974). *Postgrad. Med. J.* **50** (Supple. 5), 97-104.
Piessens, W. F., Ratiwayanto, S., Piessens, P. W., Tuti, S. and Dennis, D. T. (1981). *Acta Tropica* **38**, 227-234.
Pike, M. C., Daniels, C. A. and Snyderman, R. (1977). *Cell Immunol.* **32**, 234-238.
Pious, D. A. and Hawley, P. (1972). *Pediatr. Res.* **6**, 687-692.
Plewig, G. and Schopf, E. (1975). *J. Invest. Dermatol.* **65**, 532-536.
Potter, C. W., Carr, I., Jennings, R., Rees, R. C. McGinty, F. and Richardson, W. M. (1974). *Nature* **249**, 267-269.
Potter, C. W., Phair, J. P., Vodelinich, L., Fenton, R. and Jennings, R. (1976). *Nature* **259**, 496-497.
Potts, R. C. Hassan, H. A. A., Brown, R. A., MacConnachie, A., Gibbs, J. H., Robertson, A. J. and Beck, J. S. (1983). *Clin. Exp. Immunol.* **53**, 458-464.
Powers, C. N., Peavy, D. L. and Knight, v. (1982). *Antimicrob. Agents Chemother.* **22**, 108-114.
Presant, C. A., Klahr, C. and Santaia, R. (1977). *Ann. Intern. Med.* **86**, 47-53.
Presant, C. A. Hiblinger, S. H. and Klahr, C. (1980). *Cancer* **45**, 6-12.
Pruul, H. and Reynolds, P. L. (1972). *Infect. Immun.* **6**, 709-717.
Quie, P. G. (1983). *J. Infect. Dis.* **148**, 189-193.
Quin, T. C. and Wyler, P. J. (1979). *J. Clin. Invest.* **63**, 1187-1194.
Rajewski, K. and Takemori, T. (1983). *Ann. Rev. Immunol.* **1**, 569-607.
Ramot, B., Binilaminov, M., Shoham, C. H., and Rosenthal, E. (1976). *N. Engl. J. Med.* **294**, 809-811.
Reid, K. B. M. and Porter, R. R. (1981). *Ann. Rev. Biochem.* **50**, 433-464.
Reinherz, E. L. and Schlossman, S. F. (1980). *N. Engl. J. Med.* **303**, 370-373.
Renoux, G. and Renoux, M. (1972). *Nature New Biol.* **240**, 218.
Renoux, G. and Renoux, M. (1977). *J. Exp. Med.* **145**, 466-473.
Renoux, G., Renoux, M., Teller, M. N., McMahon, S. M. and Guillaumin, J.-M. (1976). *Clin. Exp. Immunol.* **25**, 188-296.
Reynolds, J. E. F. (1982). "Martindale: The Extra Pharmacopoeia." Pharmaceutical Press, London.
Richmond, D. E. (1979). *Aust. N.Z. J. Med.* **9**, 670-675.
Roberts, D. W. and Weidanz, N. P. (1979). *Am. J. Trop. Med. Hyg.* **28**, 1-3.

Rocklin, R. E., Bendtzen, K. and Greineder, D. (1980). *Adv. Immunol.* **29**, 55–136.
Rockwell, S., Irvin, C. G. and Neaderland, M. B. (1983). *Int. J. Radiat. Oncol. Biol. Phys.* **9**, 701–706.
Root, R. K. and Cohen, M. S. (1981). *Rev. Infect. Dis.* **3**, 565–598.
Roselle, G. A. and Kauffman, C. A. (1980). *Clin. Exp. Immunol.* **40**, 186–192.
Rosenthal, M., Trabert, U. and Muller, W. (1976). *Clin. Exp. Immunol.* **25**, 493–499.
Roszkowski, W., Lipenska, R., Roszkowski, K., Jeljaszewicz, J. and Pulverer, G. (1984). *Med. Microbiol. Immunol.* **172**, 197–205.
Rowan-Kelly, B., Ferrante, A., and Thong, Y. H. (1984). *Int. J. Immunopharmacol.* **6**, 389–393.
Ruben, F. L., Winkelstein, A. and Fotiadis, I. G. (1974). *Antimicrob. Agents Chemother.* **5**, 383–387.
Rubinstein, A. and Pelet, B. (1973). *Lancet* **i**, 382.
Russell, A. S. (1974). *J. Rheumatol.* **3**, 380–384.
Sande, M. A. and Mandell, G. L. (1980). *Chemotherapy for microbial disease. In* "Goodman and Gilman's: The Principles of Therapeutics" (Gilman, A. G., Goodman, L. S., Gilman, A., eds) Macmillan, New York.
Santi, D. V. & McHenry, C. S. (1972). *Proc. Natl. Acad. Sci. U.S.A.* **69**, 1855–1857.
Schacht, J. (1976). *J. Accoust. Soc. Am.* **59**, 940–944.
Schofield, K. P., Potter, C. W., Edey, D., Jennings, R. and Oxford, J. S. (1975). *J. Antimicrob. Chemother.* **1**, (*Suppl.*), 63–69.
Seklecki, M. M., Quintilliani, R. and Maderazo, E. G. (1978). *Antimicrob. Agents Chemother.* **13**, 552–554.
Seneca, H. and Peer, P. (1966). *J. Am. Geriatr. Soc.* **14**, 187–199.
Serrou, B. (1974). *Lancet* **ii**, 172.
Serrou, B., Solassol, C., Joyeux, H., Pujol, H. and Romien, C. (1972). *Transplantation* **14**, 654–655.
Sharma, V. P., Bathore, H. S. and Sharma, M. M. (1979). *Am. J. Trop. Med. Hyg.* **28**, 658–660.
Shirley, S. F. and Little, J. R. (1979*a*). *J. Immunol.* **123**, 2878–2882.
Shirley, S. F. and Little, J. R. (1979*b*). *J. Immunol.* **123**, 2883–2889.
Singer, A. and Hodes, R. J. (1983). *Ann. Rev. Immunol.* 211–242.
Sissons, J. G. P. and Oldstone, M. B. A. (1980). *Adv. Immunol.* **29**, 209–260.
Smith, R. A., Sidwell, R. W. and Robins, R. K. (1980). *Ann. Rev. Pharmacol. Toxicol.* **20**, 259–284.
Smithers, S. R. and Terry, R. J. (1969). *Adv. Parasit.* **71**, 41–93.
Snell, J. F. (1960). *Ann. N.Y. Acad. Sci.* **88**, 56–77.
Snyderman, R. and Goetzl, E. J. (1981). *Science* **213**, 830–837.
Spitler, L. E. and Sagebiel, R. (1980). *N. Engl. J. Med.* **303**, 1143–1147.
Steele, R. W., Chapa, I. A., Vincent, M. M., Hensen, S. A. and Keeney, R. E. (1975). *Antimicrob. Agents Chemother.* **7**, 203–207.
Steele, R. W., Keeney, R. E., Brown, J. III and Young, E. J. (1977). *J. Infect. Dis.* **135**, 593–599.

Steele, R. W., Marmer, D. J. and Keeney, K. E. (1980). *Infect. Immun.* **28**, 957-962.
Stewart, S. J., Spagnulo, P. J. and Ellner, J. J. (1981). *J. Immunol.* **127**, 135-139
Stites, D. P., Stobo, J. D., Fudenberg, H. H. and Wells, J. V. (1982). "Basic and Clinical Pharmacology", 4th edn. Lange, Los Altos.
Sud, I. J. and Finegold, D. S. (1975). *Antimicrob. Agents Chemother.* **8**, 34-39.
Suganuma, T. and Ishida, N. (1973). *Tohoku J. Exp. Med.* **110**, 405-406.
Symoens, J. and Rosenthal, M. (1977). *J. Reticuloendothel Soc.* **21**, 175-221.
Symposium (1969). *Tex. Rep. Biol. Med.* **27**, 533-708.
Tachibana, M., Mizukoshi, O. and Kuriyama, K. (1976). *Biochem. Pharmacol.* **25**, 2297-2301.
Tai, P. C., Wallace, B. J. and Davis, B. D. (1978). *Proc. Natl Acad. Sci. U.S.A.* **75**, 275-279.
Takayama, K., Wang, L. and David, H. L. (1972). *Antimicrob. Agents Chemother.* **2**, 29-35.
Tarnvik, A. and Ansehn, S. (1974). *Antimicrob. Agents Chemother.* **6**, 529-533.
Thevathason, O. I. and Litt, M. (1971). *Clin. Exp. Immunol.* **9**, 657-660.
Thomas, H. C., Freni, M., Sanchez-Tapias, J., DeVilliers, D., Jain, S. and Sherlock, S. (1976).*Clin. Exp. Immunol.* **26**, 222-228.
Thomas, M. Z., Medoff, G. and Kobayashi, G. S. (1973). *J. Infect. Dis.* **127**, 373-377.
Thompson, P. E. and Werbel, L. M. (1972). "Antimalarial Agents: Chemistry and Pharmacology." Academic Press, New York.
Thong, Y. H. (1979). The immunopharmacology of antimicrobial drugs. M.D. Thesis, University of Adelaide.
Thong, Y. H. (1983). "Inaugural Lecture Series. Germ Wars: Immunological Strategy *versus* Microbial Tactics." University of Queensland Press, St Lucia.
Thong, Y. H. and Ferrante, A. (1978). *Am. J. Trop. Med. Hyg.* **27**, 354-356.
Thong, Y. H. and Ferrante, A. (1979*a*). *Clin. Exp. Immunol.* **35**, 443-446.
Thong, Y. H. and Ferrante, A. (1979*b*). *Clin. Exp. Immunol.* **35**, 10-12.
Thong, Y. H. and Ferrante, A. (1980*a*). *Clin. Exp. Immunol.* **39**, 728-732.
Thong, Y. H. and Ferrante, A. (1980*b*). *Clin. Exp. Immunol.* **39**, 190-194.
Thong, Y. H. and Ness, D. (1977). *Lancet* **ii**, 568.
Thong, Y. H. and Rowan-Kelly, B. (1978*a*). *IRCS Med. Sci.* **6**, 21.
Thong, Y. H. and Rowan-Kelly, B. (1978*b*). *Br. Med. J.* **1**, 149.
Thong, Y. H., Ferrante, A. and Rowan-Kelly, B. (1978). *Trans. R. Soc. Trop. Med. Hyg.* **72**, 537-539.
Thong, Y. H., Ferrante, A., Rowan-Kelly, B. and O'Keefe, D. E. (1979). *Trans. R. Soc. Trop. Med. Hyg.* **73**, 388-390.
Thong, Y. H., Ferrante, A. and Secker, L. K. (1980). *Immunol. Letters* **2**, 119-121.
Thong, Y. H., Ferrante, A. and Secker, L. K. (1981). *Trans. R. Soc. Trop. Med. Hyg.* **75**, 108-109.
Tizard, I. R. and Holmes, W. L. (1974). *Arch. Appl. Allergy Clin. Immunol.* **46**, 867-879.
Tosato, G., Magrath, I., Koski, I., Dooley, N. and Blese, M. (1979). *N. Engl. J. Med.* **301**, 1133-1137.

Tracy, J. W. and Mahmoud, A. A. (1982). *Am. J. Trop. Med. Hyg.* **31**, 1201-1212.
Traub, W. H. and Sherris, J. C. (1970). *Chemotherapy* **15**, 70-83.
Tripodi, D., Parks, L. C. and Brugmans, J. (1973). *N. Engl. J. Med.* **289**, 354-357.
Tsang, V. C. W., Hubbard, W. J. and Damian, R. T. (1977). *Am. J. Trop. Med. Hyg.* **26**, 243-247.
Ugazio, A. G., Burgio, G. R. and Astaldi, A. (1974). *Postgrad. Med. J.* **50** (Suppl. 5), 94-96.
Umezawa, H. (1983). *Proc. R. Soc. Lond. (Biol.)* **217**, 357-376.
Van den Bossche, H., Willensens, G., Cools, W., Lauwers, W. F. and Lejeune, L. (1978). *Chem. Biol. Interact.* **21**, 59-78.
Van den Bossche, H., Willensens, G., Cools, W. and Cornelissen, F. (1979). *Arch. Int. Physiol. Biochem.* **87**, 849-851.
Van Eygen, M., Znamensy, P. Y., Heck, E. and Raymaekers, I. (1976). *Lancet* **i** 382-385.
Van Ginckel, R. F. and Holbecke, J. (1976). *Eur. J. Immunol.* **6**, 305-307.
Van Ginckel, R. and De Brabander, M. (1979). *J. Reticuloendothel. Soc.* **25**, 125-131.
van Wauwe, J. and van Nijen, G. (1977). *Clin. Exp. Immunol.* **30**, 465-468.
Vindel, J. A. and Khoury, B. (1974). *Postgrad. Med. J.* **50** (*Suppl.*), 108-110.
Waisbren, B. A. and Brown, I. (1964). *Am. J. Med. Sci.* **248**, 56-60.
Walker, R. I. and Willemze, R. (1980). *Rev. Infect. Dis.* **2**, 282-292.
Wall, R. and Kuehl, M. (1983). *Ann. Rev. Immunol.* **1**, 393-422.
Walls, E. V. and Kay, J. E. (1982). *Immunology* **47**, 115-121.
Warren, G. H., Mills, L. and Friedman, H. (1979). *Immunopharmacology* **1**, 269-276.
Waxman, D. J. and Strominger, J. L. (1983). *Ann. Rev. Biochem.* **52**, 825-869.
Webster, L. T., Jr., Butterworth, A. E., Mahmoud, A. A. F., Mngola, E. N. and Warren, K. S. (1975). *N. Engl. J. Med.* **292**, 1144-1147.
Weisberger, A. S., Daniel, T. M. and Hoffman, A. (1964). *J. Exp. Med.* **120**, 183-196.
Weissmann, G., Smolen, J. E. and Korchak, H. M (1980). *N. Engl. J. Med.* **302**, 27-34.
Welch, W. D., Davis, D. and Thrupp, L. D. (1981). *Antimicrob. Agents Chemother.* **20**, 15-20.
Whichard, L. P., Morris, C. R., Smith, J. M. and Holbrook, D. J., Jr. (1968). *Mol. Pharmacol.* **4**, 630-639.
Whitcomb, M. E., Merluzzi, V. J. and Cooperband, S. R. (1976). *Cell. Immunol.* **21**, 272-277.
White, D. J. and Calne, R. Y. (1982). *Immunol. Rev.* **65**, 115-131.
Williamson, J. and Macadam, R. F. (1965). *Trans. R. Soc. Trop. Med. Hyg.* **59**, 367-368.
Wilson, R. A. and Barnes, P. E. (1977). *Parasitology* **74**, 61-71.
Wilson, W. R. (1977). *Mayo Clin. Proc.* **52**, 635-640.
Wingard, J. R., Hess, A. D., Stuart, R. J., Saral, R. and Burns, W. H. (1983). *Antimicrob. Agents Chemother.* **23**, 573-597.
Wittek, A. E., Cohen, P. S., Arvin, A. M., Smith, S. D., Korochak, C. M. and DeClercq, E. (1983). *Antimicrob. Agents Chemother.* **24**, 803-806.

Woods, D. D. (1962). *J. Gen. Microbiol.* **29**, 687-702.
Wozencraft, A. O., Dockrell, H. M., Taverne, J., Targett, G. A. T. and Playfair, J. H. L. (1984). *Infect. Immun.* **43**, 664-669.
Yang, L. C., Soprey, P. R., Wittner, M. K. and Fox, E. N. (1977). *J. Exp. Med.* **146**, 344-360.
Youmans, A. S., Youmans, G. P. and Cahall, D. (1976). *Infect. Immun.* **13**, 127-132.
Yourtee, E. L., Metcalf, J. and Rost, R. K. (1980). *Clin. Res.* **28**, 383A.
Yunis, A. A. (1973). *Semin. Hematol.* **10**, 225-234.
Ziegler, H. K. and Unanue, E. R. (1982). *Proc. Natl. Acad. Sci. U.S.A.* **79**, 175-178.
Zinkernagel, R. M. (1979). *Parasite Immunol.* **1**, 91-109.
Zinkernagel, R. M. and Doherty, P. C. (1979). *Adv. Immunol.* **27**, 51-177.

Chapter 5

Interaction of Antibiotics with Granulocytes and Lymphocytes

Hakan Gnarpe and Judy Belsheim
Department of Clinical Bacteriology,
Gävle Central Hospital, S-801 17 Gävle, Sweden

I. INTRODUCTION

A multitude of various host factors are important for defence against infections. The mechanical barriers, including the intact skin and mucous membranes fed by the circulatory system, are important, as well as a balance between the normal microbial flora and invading microbes. When the host barriers are disrupted, the invading, replicating microbes stimulate both non-specific and specific cellular defences by polymorphonuclear leucocytes (PMN) and later by monocytes, macrophages and lymphocytes. The intricate interplay of defence mechanisms in normal healthy individuals usually leads to rapid healing of the infection.

It has been shown that granulocytes and lymphocytes are of great importance for the defence, both directly through phagocytosis and indirectly, as demonstrated by studies of specific defects in granulocytes (Hill and Quie, 1974; Odeberg and Olsson, 1976; Quie and Cates, 1977) and lymphocytes (Cooper and Lawton, 1972; Bardana, 1981; Donabedian and Gallin, 1982) in various clinical syndromes. The advances of modern chemotherapy, resulting in increased survival rates for seriously ill patients, has contributed to an increased number of immunocompromised patients with severe infections (Feigin and Shearer, 1975; Christou and Meakins, 1979) which their own defence mechanisms cannot resolve. Appropriate

Antimicrobial agents and immunity
ISBN 0-12-383830-4

antibiotic treatment has therefore become even more crucial than earlier in many situations. It is also important to be aware of any possible side effects of antibiotics on the host defence mechanisms, since many of these patients are already in a compromised state which should not be made worse unnecessarily.

This chapter presents a review of the current knowledge of the way in which antibiotics influence the activity of granulocytes and lymphocytes.

II. NORMAL GRANULOCYTE ACTIVITY

A. Adherence

Polymorphonuclear leucocytes are released from the bone marrow, as a result of a stimulus which is regulated partly by complement factors. They then enter the peripheral circulation where they generally have a short lifetime of a few days to a week. There is evidence for at least two functionally different sets of polymorphonuclear granulocytes: one adhering to the endothelial lining of the blood vessels and the second circulating passively (Gallin, 1980; Horvath and Leonard, 1982). Some findings indicate that the adhering subset of the granulocytes is functionally the more important (Gallin, 1980). This complicates the interpretation of all *in-vitro* experiments done with granulocytes prepared from peripheral blood and makes it difficult to assess whether experimental results have clinical relevance. In any case, it is clear that the ability of the PMNs to adhere not only to the endothelial linings of blood vessels, but also to a phagocytic particle, is of essential importance for all subsequent leucocyte functioning.

B. Migration

Movement of granulocytes may be controlled by three separate yet interrelated functions. Random migration, or undirected migration, is a characteristic of the resting cell and is not affected by chemotactic stimuli. Chemokinesis is a term given to the type of general, undirected, stimulated movement of granulocytes in resting states when exposed to some chemotactic factors. Chemotaxis is the energy-dependent migration of granulocytes in direct response to a gradient of chemotactic stimuli, which emanates *in vivo* from the infectious focus.

Chemoattractants may be either of endogenous or exogenous origin, including complement activation components (C3a, C5a, C567), immune complexes, products of tissue and collagen breakdown and also by-products of bacterial growth (e.g. lipopolysaccharide, LPS), to name just a few. Once the inflammatory process has begun, a multitude of positive as well as negative feedback mechanisms are triggered, leading to the attraction of monocytes (macrophages) and lymphocytes to the focus. In addition to providing a cellular and humoral response to the invading microorganisms, these other cells may produce substances (e.g. lymphokines) which are stimulatory or inhibitory for granulocyte function. There are many factors serving to modify the inflammatory response. Only some of these have been identified and may be derived from either host or bacteria. For example bacterial lipopolysaccharides, which may act in efficient chemotactic factor activation via the complement system, may be toxic for leucocytes in high concentrations and impair chemotaxis. Other bacterial factors, for example pneumolysin (Paton and Ferrante, 1983), have been shown to impede chemotaxis even at low concentrations.

Chemotaxis is triggered by several different receptors in the cell membrane. When the PMNs are stimulated, they decrease their negative surface charge (Gallin and Rosenthal, 1974; Gallin *et al.*, 1974; Gallin and Wolff, 1975; Gallin, 1980) with a resulting increase in the deformability of the membrane. Both Ca^{2+} and Mg^{2+} take part in this procedure. An increase in deformability is a prerequisite for the type of cell migration that is an energy-requiring process (Lichtman and Weed, 1972; Miller, 1978). Reductions of the deformability invariably lead to an impaired migration.

Chemotactic deactivation may be due to two different mechanisms, as suggested by Nelson *et al.* (1978). Depending on the prevailing circumstances, this deactivation may be beneficial to the host or to the invading bacteria. It may be specific, resulting in cells which are unresponsive to a specific bacterial stimulus, or it may be more general, leading to cells unresponsive to a variety of chemotactic factors.

The chemotactic migration of granulocytes towards a specific stimulus does not occur in a straight path. As demonstrated by Zigmond and Hirsh (1973) with time-lapse cinematography, there may be several turns in the cell direction before the goal is reached. This may be explained by the continuous activation/deactivation of the receptors in the cell membranes.

C. Phagocytosis

In order to phagocytose and kill bacteria, opsonization is necessary. This can be accomplished in different ways: either by activation of the classical complement pathway as for protein A-containing *Staphylococcus aureus* strains (Verhoef *et al.*, 1977*a*, *b*), or through the alternative pathway of complement activation in the presence of serum IgG (C3b).

According to Verbrugh *et al.* (1983), the opsonization capacity of serum is reflected by its IgG ad C3 concentrations.

1. Granulocyte-microbe attachment

There are two important phases in the phagocytic process—attachment of the granulocyte to the opsonized microbe and ingestion (engulfment). According to Hed (1977), these two phases are controlled by different mechanisms, in which the opsonizing molecule plays an important part. Opsonization by IgG has been found to stimulate a more active ingestive phase with a dependence on actin polymerization, while opsonization with C3 provides a more passive, inactive stimulus (Ehlenberger and Nussenzweig, 1977; Forslid and Hed, 1982). When the granulocytes have migrated towards the source of the chemoattracting factor, specific receptor sites on the granulocyte membrane attach to specific sites on the microbe. Through an energy-requiring process, the PMN starts reforming its membrane to engulf and invaginate the microbe into its interior.

2. Engulfment

The attached microbe is invaginated into the interior of the granulocyte where a vacuole is formed. This process also requires energy and can be disturbed at several levels, which will be shown later in this chapter.

D. Intracellular Killing

The microbe is invaginated into a phagolysosome, into which lysosomal enzymes are released, which are destructive to the microbe (Weissmann *et al.*, 1979; Eaton and Rest, 1983). Microbial killing may be effected by two types of mechanisms. The first, which is oxidative, involves the myeloperoxidase-halide-hydrogen peroxide mechanism (Klebanoff and Clarke, 1978) or it may result from toxic products derived from the PMN oxygen metabolism (e.g. free radicals). The second mechanism may involve cationic compounds, proteins that alter permeability or neutral proteases (Odeberg and Olsson, 1976; Weiss *et al.*, 1978; Rest *et al.*, 1982; Wetherall *et al.*, 1984). Intracellular microbial killing is difficult to assess because of its dependence on the preceding sequence of events. Leijh *et al.* (1981) found the rate of ingestion to be the major determinant for the rate of killing in normal cells.

E. Techniques for the Measurement of Granulocyte Activity

One of the most difficult problems involved with studies of granulocyte function is the lack of standardization between laboratories, necessitating a detailed description of all variables and techniques before any assessment of the results may be made.

Granulocyte adhesion to surfaces is usually measured either as adherence to glass (or other surfaces, including tissue cells) where a direct count of the adhering cells is made (Belsheim *et al.*, 1983), or as retention in nylon fibre columns (MacGregor *et al.*, 1978) where not only the innate ability of granulocytes to adhere is measured, but also where an impairment of membrane deformability will be reflected as increased retention (i.e. adherence). A technical variation of the adherence to glass technique has been used by Belsheim *et al.* (1983) using scanning electron microscopy. This enables the investigator to study the morphology of the adhering cells as well as the number.

An important criterion for the choice of a method to be used for measurements of chemotactic response is that the method must be adaptable to larger cell populations to ensure that a representative sample is taken. Another is that the responding cell type should be able to be identified, particularly where unpurified cell suspensions are used.

Granulocyte migration may be investigated by several methods. The most popular and widely used techniques are the Boyden chamber technique and the leucocyte migration under agarose technique (LMAT). The general principle for the Boyden technique is as follows: by adding PMNs to one side of a filter membrane and a chemoattractant on the other side, it is possible to get an accurate measurement of the granulocytes' ability to deform and migrate actively through the pores in the filter (Boyden, 1962). This method, and variations thereof, has been used widely. The major disadvantages of this technique are the difficulties involved with the standardization of the filters and the problem of assessing absolute quantitative changes. All measures are given as ratios, and the procedure is considerably tedious. The second technique for the measurement of granulocyte migration, also adaptable for other cell types, is the LMAT, which was originally described by Nelson *et al.* (1975). Various modifications of this method have been used extensively for clinical research. The LMAT is particularly advantageous for studies of antibiotic effects on granulocyte populations because of the relative ease of replicate determinations. In most of our studies, we have used a modified and strictly controlled LMAT (Belsheim, 1981).

Most investigators have measured phagocytosis either by counting the number of bacteral colony-forming units remaining after leucocytes and bacteria have been mixed, or by measuring the uptake of isotope-labelled bacteria. Although permitting replicate determinations, neither of these methods permits any differentiation between what it just adherent or attached to the PMNs and what is actually engulfed. Methods using radioisotopes are especially difficult, since it is impossible to distinguish between leakage of isotopes from labelled ingested microbes and attached microbes.

Hed (1977) devised a method based on the quenching of fluorescence of extracellular fluorescein isothiocyanate-labelled microbes by crystal violet. With this technique, it is possible to distinguish between extracellularly adherent and internalized particles. Unfortunately, this method also has its limitations: it is only practical when using large particles such as yeast cells and it is also tedious due to the microscopic examination required.

Intracellular killing can be measured in direct and indirect ways (Beckerdite *et al.*, 1974; Bridges *et al.*, 1980; Tomita *et al.*, 1981). In order to make comparisons, it is necessary to compensate for the quantitative phagocytosis regardless of the method used. An indirect method for evaluating the intracellular killing capacity is the measure of the oxidative burst following PMN phagocytosis by determination of the light emission through chemiluminescence (Starkebaum *et al.*, 1981; Bender and van Epps, 1983; Robinson *et al.*, 1984). This technique is easy to perform, but is influenced by a multitude of factors. When studying patient groups, it is reproducible only when luminol, a light intensity augmenter, is omitted. Luminol may be used to magnify the responses with advantage where direct comparisons are made between antibiotic-influenced cells and untreated cells.

III. NORMAL LYMPHOCYTE ACTIVITY

The PMN is probably the most important cell involved in the initial, immediate inflammatory reaction. Accumulation of granulocytes at an infectious focus sets in motion a sequence of events resulting in migration of monocytes and, later, lymphocytes to the area. On being activated, some of these monocytes undergo a morphological transformation to activated macrophages, cells which are not only phagocytes but are also essential for presenting antigen to lymphocytes. The mononuclear cell infiltration takes place at a slower rate than PMN accumulation; however, when mobilized, it is responsible for the long-lasting cell-mediated and humoral host defence mechanisms.

Presentation of antigen to lymphocytes by macrophages is part of a complicated process having as a final goal the activation of cytotoxic lymphocytes and B lymphocytes capable of synthesizing specific immunoglobulins, which in turn may aid in opsonizing microbes for PMN phagocytosis.

It is difficult to standardize lymphocyte function tests, just as it is for PMN function tests. Enumeration of B and T lymphocyte cell ratios is generally the first step in the investigative process, and is usually accomplished by use of sedimentation/centrifugation techniques based on rosette formation of sheep or ox red blood cells around T or B lymphocytes (Jondal *et al.*, 1972). Recently, a number of commercially available monoclonal reagents have become available and, although expensive, these simplify the procedure of identification. However, variations of the rosette test are still very widely used, and these allow easy purification of the red blood cell-laden lymphocytes from mononuclear cell suspensions. Most investigators do not separate null cells or killer cells from the suspensions, but this can also be done using advanced techniques.

DNA synthesis, or blast transformation of B or T lymphocytes, using specific cell mitogens is a common procedure giving some information about the general ease of lymphocyte activation. In most methods, radiolabelled thymidine is added to purified B or T cell cultures which have first been stimulated with mitogens, of which the two most commonly used may be Cowan 1 protein A for B lymphocytes (Banck and Forsgren, 1980) and phytohaemagglutinin for T lymphocytes (Nowell, 1960).

Antibody synthesis by stimulated B lymphocytes is a useful parameter to measure, and this is most often carried out using plaque tests (Fauci and Pratt, 1976; Ginsburg *et al.*, 1978). These are based on the haemolysis of red blood cells in agar matrices where B lymphocytes are present, adding complement where applicable dependent on the type of immunoglobulin production to be measured. Cytotoxicity of lymphocytes is another valuable function to measure, and this is usually done by mixing two cell populations, one of which is designated the target cell and has been treated with an inhibitor, thereby providing appropriate inactive prey for the aggressive effector cells (Parish *et al.*, 1976). Measurement is very simply carried out by scoring cells strained with trypan blue, as viable cells do not permit dye uptake.

The diversity of tests for measuring different aspects of lymphocyte functioning is too large to enable a detailed presentation; however, suffice to say that the individual laboratory may choose techniques sufficient for the assessment of specific functions, and which are suited, both practically and economically, to their own purposes.

IV. ANTIBIOTIC INFLUENCES ON GRANULOCYTES AND LYMPHOCYTES

A. Cell Wall Antibiotics

1. Penicillin derivatives

The cell wall of growing bacteria is subject to constant building and rebuilding as part of the continuous adjustment to a changing cell mass and to replication. Parts of molecular aggregates meant to be built into the cell wall are usually lost into the surroundings and act *in vivo* as chemotaxins with the resulting accumulation of different types of phagocytic cells. When bacteria are exposed to β-lactam antibiotics, the regular addition of pieces to the peptidoglycan of the cell wall is blocked, resulting in sphaeroplast formation and eventual cell lysis in Gram-positive organisms, and filament formation with eventual lysis in Gram-negative organisms. The mode of action of specific β-lactams is dependent on the penicillin-binding proteins (PBPs) present in the bacterial cell membrane, and so is different from species to species. When the antibiotic concentration is too low to induce a total block of cell wall synthesis, cell growth continues with an increased leakage of cell wall constituents into the surroundings. These cell-derived molecules may act as chemoattractants.

It has been shown (Friedman and Warren, 1974; Belsheim and Gnarpe, 1981) that subinhibitory concentrations of some but not all β-lactam antibiotics cause an increased migration of granulocytes (Table 1). The substances most stimulatory at subinhibitory concentrations were the second generation cephalosporins (Table 1) and mecillinam, while ampicillin, penicillin V and benzyl penicillin did not cause a significant increase in migration. As yet, no explanation has been presented for the different effects of the various β-lactams other than that, to some extent, the activity must depend on the PBP structure of the bacterium.

Gemmell *et al.* (1983) have shown that *Bacteroides fragilis* exposed to subinhibitory concentrations of clindamycin are more readily phagocytosed by granulocytes than when untreated. As suggested by the authors, this is most likely due to alterations in the capsule of the bacterium, rendering

Table 1
Influence of subinhibitory concentrations of β-lactam antibiotics (0·1 MIC) on the release of chemoattractants from *Escherichia coli*. The results are expressed in terms of the chemotaxis elicited as a percentage of the antibiotic-free control

Antibiotic	Chemotactic differential[a]
Benzyl penicillin	107
Ampicillin	106
Mecillinam	125[b]
CPW 86 363	124[b]
Ceftazidime	115[b]
Cefroxadin (CGP 9000)	128[b]
Imipenem	132[b]

[a] Chemotactic differential = directed − random migration.
[b] $P \leq 0·01$.

it more easy to ingest, and not to any influences of the antibiotic on the granulocyte *per se*. Similar studies done on other bacteria, for example *Streptococcus pyogenes*, using not only clindamycin, but also penicillin and erythromycin, have also revealed an enhanced phagocytic response when bacteria are exposed to subinhibitory concentrations. However, the mechanisms vary from antibiotic to antibiotic and within species. Other investigators have studied the effect of subinhibitory antibiotic concentrations on the adherence of bacterial species to tissue cells and found that many antibiotics cause a change in the cell membrane of bacteria, even at low concentrations, resulting in an augmented adherence to cells. This may be a factor adding to the pathogenicity of certain bacteria, but it may also fix the bacteria more efficiently for eventual destruction by PMNs.

Due to technical difficulties it has not been shown conclusively that bacteria damaged but not killed by β-lactam antibiotics are more efficiently killed by leucocytes, although this is probably true, and has been suggested in reports where great pains have been taken to correct for technical factors (Gemmell *et al.*, 1982; Pruul *et al.*, 1984; Andreana *et al.*, 1984). Horne and Tomasz (1981) have found that group B streptococci are more effectively killed when previously exposed to subinhibitory concentrations of β-lactam antibiotics. On the other hand, Lorain and Atkinson (1980) found an increased survival of staphylococci exposed to oxacillin. In these reports, the overall figures are presented but they are not corrected for the possible increase in granulocyte uptake of bacteria.

The results presented by Grant *et al.* (1983) are also interesting. They report that cefaclor but not ampicillin stimulates the intracellular killing of bacteria. It was suggested that this may be explained by the depression of peroxidase enzymes seen with ampicillin (Rentz *et al.*, 1972).

2. Cephalosporins and cephamycins

Only a few and inconclusive clinical observations have been made regarding the action of these antibiotics on host defence mechanisms, at least in subminimal inhibitory concentrations. The newer cephalosporins with short half-lives could have a dual action: while the antibiotic concentrations are above the actual bacterial minimal inhibitory concentration (MIC), prevention of bacterial growth is effective, and at sub-MIC levels, increased leakage of cell substances may be stimulated. When the antibiotic concentration falls below the MIC the bacterial growth is resumed almost immediately (Ryan, personal communication, 1980). Although no documentation is available, it may be that mechanisms like this one of increased leakage of cell constituents could contribute to the possibility of using antibiotics with short half-lives for dosage every 8 h, even though the concentrations attained are below the known MICs for the pathogens.

Recently, Ohnishi *et al.* (1984) reported another indirect mechanism for the stimulation of granulocyte activity by a new, semisynthetic cephalosporin (AC-1370). Peritoneal macrophages were activated by the drug and released trypsin-sensitive but heat-stable factors that were capable of stimulating PMNs. Our own findings with imipenem (Gnarpe *et al.*, 1984) are as yet the only report where a direct stimulatory effect on PMN activity is documented with a β-lactam antibiotic. The mechanism of this stimulation is unknown. On the other hand, inhibition of granulocyte activity has been reported by several authors with different derivatives (Chaperon and Sanders, 1978; Majeski *et al.*, 1978 Forsgren, 1981; Manzella and Clark, 1983).

3. Fosfomycin

Fosfomycin is a preparation active against the cell wall that does not belong to the group of β-lactam derivatives. The antibiotic is bactericidal and inhibits early stages of muramic acid synthesis (Hendlin *et al.*, 1969). It has been found to be active against a broad spectrum of various clinical isolates (Forsgren and Walder, 1983). We have not found any publications concerning granulocyte activity and fosfomycin. In our own investigations, we found that fosfomycin, at a very high concentration, 100 μg/ml, had a slight stimulatory effect on the granulocyte chemotactic migration.

B. Inhibitors of Protein Synthesis

1. Aminoglycoside antibiotics

This group of antibiotics has been used extensively for the treatment of serious infections. A great number of more or less specific side effects, some of which are serious and irreversible, have been recorded; this has limited the use of these drugs. None of these antibiotics (including streptomycin, gentamicin, amikacin, tobramycin, sisomycin and netilmycin) penetrate into mammalian cells. Their effect is greatly reduced at acid pH levels, as found in abscesses containing large amounts of acidic granulocyte mucopolysaccharides. When they are active, they are bactericidal and inhibit protein synthesis.

Not much is known regarding the effects of the aminoglycosidic antibiotics' activities on granulocytes and lymphocytes. Goodhart (1977) and Sacchi *et al.* (1981) reported a reduction of granulocyte migration at concentrations of 10–33 μg/ml of gentamicin. Later these findings were extended to other members of this group of antibiotics. In a report from 1977, Forsgren and Schmeling could not detect any significant reduction of granulocyte activity by gentamicin. A decreased penetration of gentamicin into bacterial cells has been found in the presence of divalent cations (Bryan and van den Eizen, 1977), but gentamicin has also been found not to chelate divalent cations (Kohlhepp *et al.*, 1982). The mechanism of action is probably different from that of the tetracyclines. In a report on the influence of aminoglycosidic antibiotics on granulocyte migration, Gnarpe and Belsheim (1979) were able to show only a limited depression, and then only at high clinical concentrations, especially with amikacin. This depression was found only for male blood donors. In later investigations, Gnarpe and Belsheim (unpublished observations), found that both netilmicin and amikacin increased the adherence of granulocytes to glass and that amikacin also significantly increased the retention of cells on nylon fibre columns in a dose-dependent manner. The mechanism(s) of action are yet to be resolved as are the apparent differences in effect on granulocytes from males and females.

To our knowledge, no reports have been published on the influence of these antibiotics on quantitative phagocytosis or on intracellular killing.

2. Tetracyclines

Since the tetracyclines came onto the market approximately 30 years ago, they have undergone a pronounced development, and the derivatives most in use today have little in common with the earlier substances, excepting the mode of action. The most important difference in the context of their influence on leucocytes is the change in solubility. Earlier preparations were water-soluble while the modern preparations (doxycycline, minocycline) are highly lipid-soluble (Colazzi and Klink, 1969; Barza *et al.*, 1975). Because of this, these are differences in pharmacokinetic behaviour, some of which are relevant for the effects of tetracyclines on granulocytes and lymphocytes.

The basic mechanism by which all tetracyclines act on microbes is the formation of chelate bonds to ribosomes which causes a misreading of messenger RNA and consequentially a decreased protein synthesis as well as the production of defective proteins leading to a halt in cell growth (Pato, 1977). All tetracyclines bind to the cell membranes of cells and are actively transported into the cell interior (McMurray and Levy, 1978).

The tetracyclines are also taken up by mammalian cells, e.g., granulocytes and lymphocytes (Shils, 1963; Park and Dow, 1970). It seems likely that chelate binding to metal-containing enzymes occurs in these cells as well as in microbial cells. As this binding between antibiotic and cell constituent is strong, it may be expected that there would be an accumulation of tetracycline molecules in the cell. This has been shown to be the case by Forsgren (personal communication, 1982), who measured an increase in antibiotic concentrations within human granulocytes of 3–5 times the environmental concentrations. Therefore it is to be expected that the tetracyclines should effect both granulocyte and lymphocyte activities over a broad range of functions, including adherence, migration, phagocytosis and intracellular killing.

In a study using scanning electron microscopy (SEM), Belsheim *et al.* (1983) found that granulocytes preincubated for 30 min in 10 μg/ml doxycycline adhered slower and to a lesser extent than did control cells (up to 40%). The same slow adhesion was also found with other techniques and was paralleled by the results of retention in nylon fibre columns. In the SEM study we also found that doxycycline-incubated granulocytes had

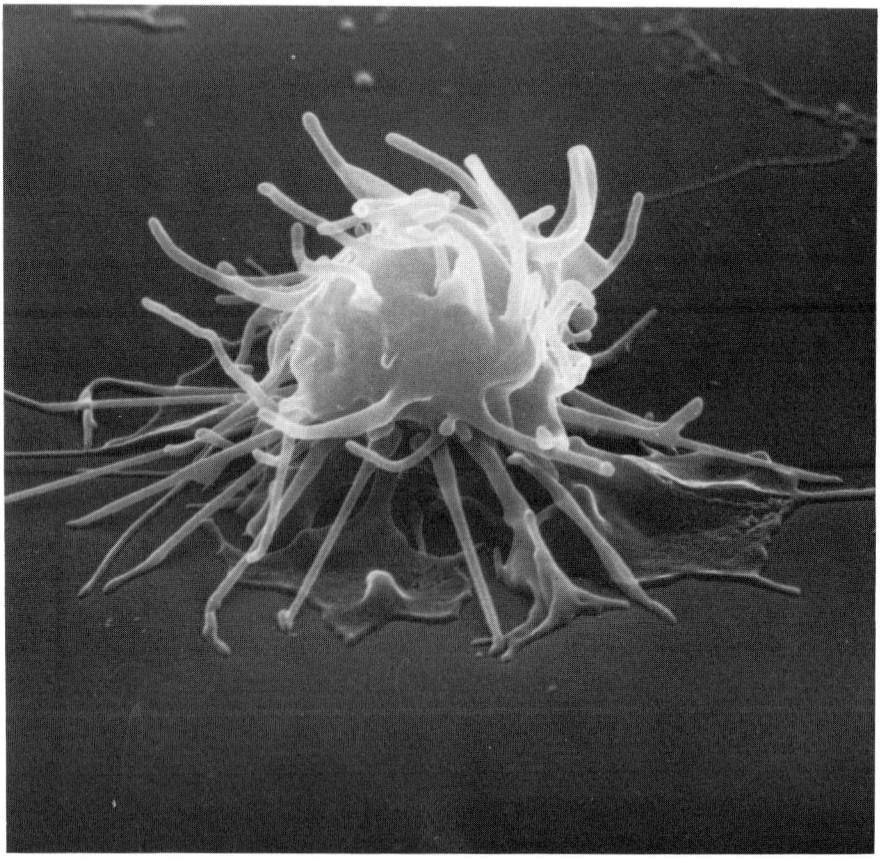

Fig. 1. Normal granulocyte after 10 min of adherence to glass. Note numerous filopods reached out from the membrane surface.

significantly fewer and shorter filopods (pseudopods) than did control cell preparations (see Figs 1, 2).

We have seen that the tetracyclines influenced both the undirected and the directed (stimulated) migration of granulocytes. This influence is dose-dependent with increasing depressions of both kinds of migration with increasing drug concentrations (Belsheim *et al.*, 1979*a*, *b*). This influence is also drug dependent: equimolar concentrations of the different tetracyclines cause increasing depression with increasing lipid solubility of the drugs (Belsheim *et al.*, 1979*a*, *b*). This effect can be observed both on *in-vitro* incubations and in experimental '*in-vivo*' tests with healthy volunteers (Belsheim *et al.*, 1979*a*) and with patients undergoing

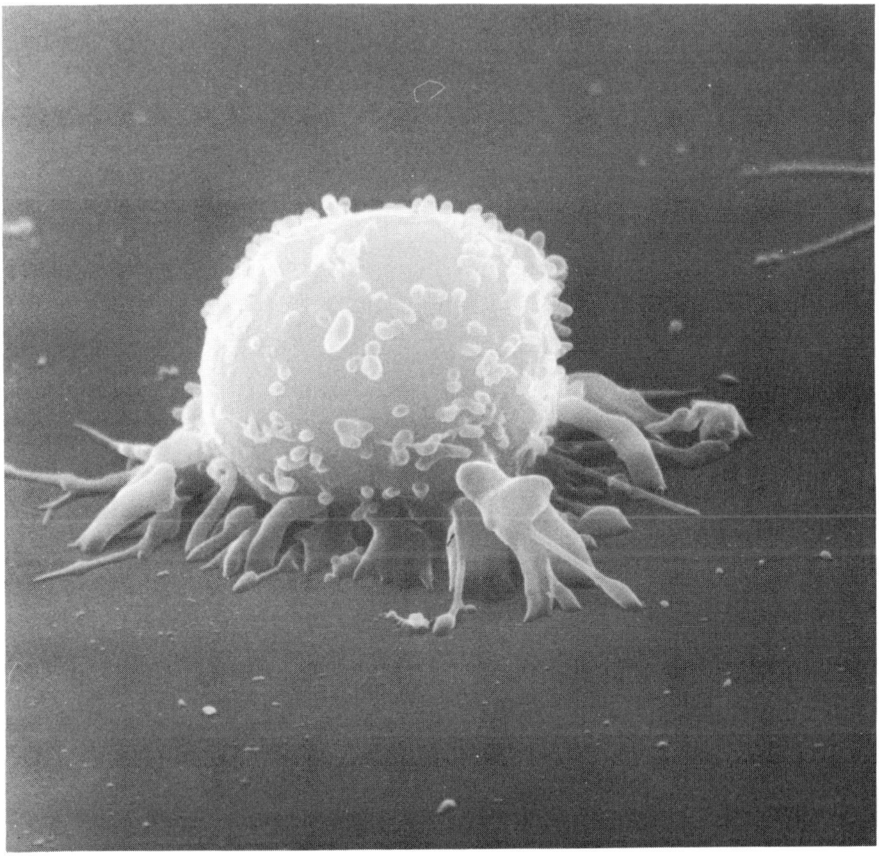

Fig. 2. A granulocyte, prepared from the same individual as that shown in Fig. 1, but incubated for 30 min with 10 μg/ml of doxycycline.

surgery (Belsheim *et al.*, 1979*b*). Using a skin blister technique, Hellum and Solberg (1977) and, later, Forsgren *et al.* (1980) showed a reduced migration of granulocytes into the blisters when the patients are given tetracyclines (Solberg *et al.*, 1983).

Several investigators have shown a reduced phagocytosis caused by tetracycline antibiotics (Munoz and Geister, 1950; Hoeprich and Martin, 1970; Forsgren *et al.*, 1974; Martin *et al.*, 1974; Forsgren and Schmeling, 1977; Siegel and Remington, 1982). Using a method described by Hed (1977), we have found a decrease in the quantitative phagocytosis, measured as the total number of ingested as compared to attached yeast cells. This depression increases with increasing concentrations of tetracyclines, more so with doxycycline than with lymecycline (Belsheim *et al.*, 1983). In SEM

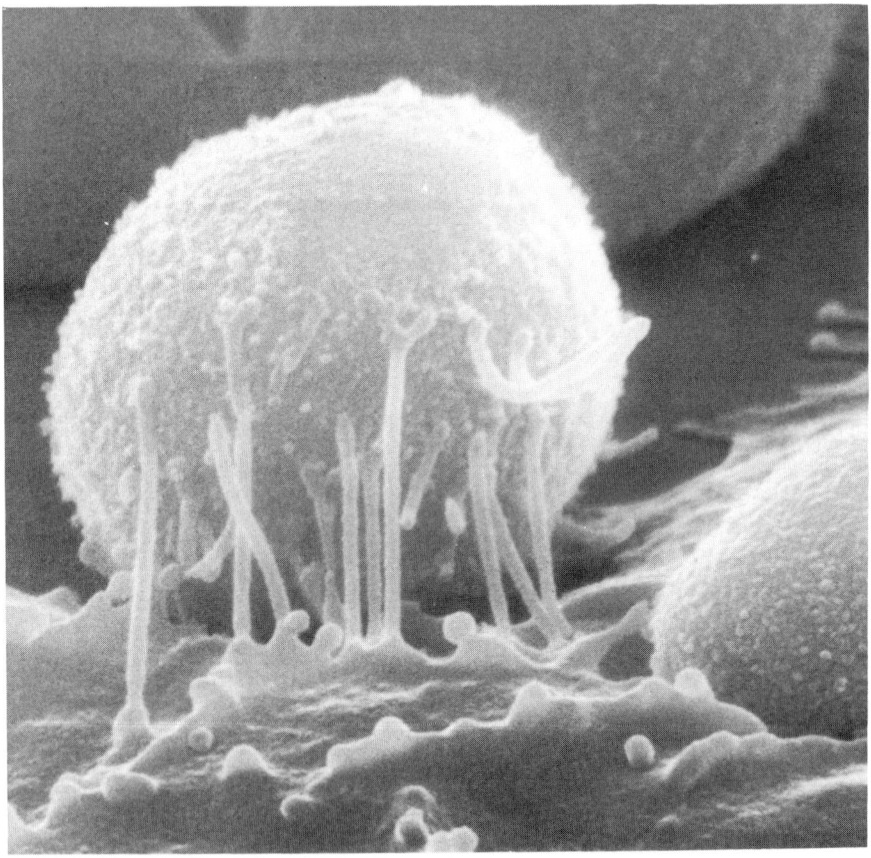

Fig. 3. Early stage of normal granulocyte phagocytosis of yeast cells (8 min). Note the number of filopods reaching up to the yeast cell.

studies we have shown that, while there is an ongoing phagocytosis in control and lymecycline-containing preparations, the doxycycline-incubated granulocytes appear to have come to a reduced, delayed and, in many cases, incomplete ingestion (see Figs 3, 4).

Other workers have reported a slight stimulation of phagocytosis by tetracyclines at some concentrations. The obviously divergent results are to a large extent explained by the different techniques used: most of these studies have been done with isotope-labelled bacteria (Melby and Midtvedt, 1977) and, as mentioned above, these do not discriminate between bacteria adhering to granulocytes and bacteria actually ingested. In many cases, the increase of 'phagocytosed' bacteria may still be localized on the granulocyte membrane. This is also supported by

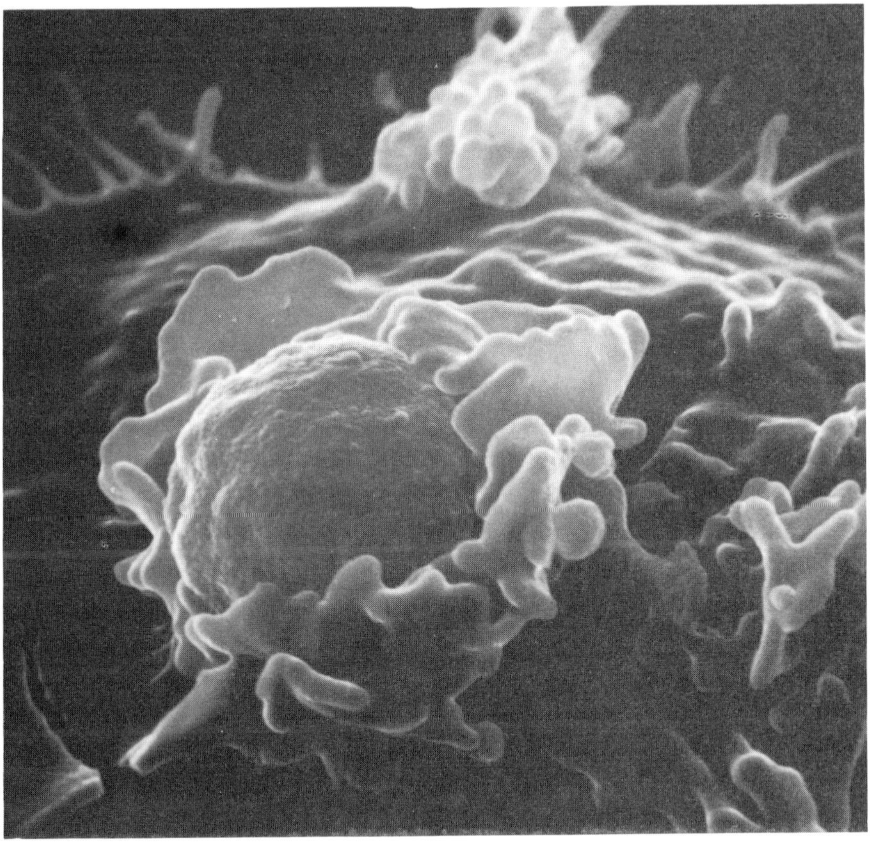

conditions may be different when bacteria are used instead of killed yeast cells.

Chemiluminescence does give an overall view of the intracellular granulocyte metabolic activity when stimulated (Bender and van Epps, 1983; Robinson *et al.*, 1984). Measuring the chemiluminescence for granulocytes preincubated in lymecycline and doxycycline gave results indicating a much more pronounced depressive effect from doxycycline (Belsheim *et al.*, 1982). Similar depressions, though not as pronounced, have been published by Siegel and Remington (1982). Yanai and Quie (1981) have shown that a prerequisite for chemiluminescence is membrane activation, and, in this manner, the active adherence may influence several other functions (Gallin, 1980).

Several authors have reported a suppression of the lymphocyte activity caused by tetracyclines (Banck and Forsgren, 1979; Thong and Ferrante, 1979). Gnarpe and Belsheim (1985) have found differences between different tetracyclines that are related to the lipid solubility of the preparation in the same manner as for granulocytes.

3. *Aminotriazolemutilin (TDM 85-530)*

TDM 85-530 is a derivative of the tricyclic diterpene pleuromutilin (Hildebrandt *et al.*, 1983) that acts as an inhibitor of bacterial protein synthesis at the ribosomal level (Högenauer and Brunowsky, 1983). TDM 85-530 has been found to be effective in the treatment of experimental infections (Wenzel *et al.*, 1983). Its antibacterial spectrum is similar to that of doxycycline (Hildebrandt *et al.*, 1983). In equimolar concentrations, TDM 85-530 has effects on granulocyte and lymphocyte activity that make it intermediate between lymecycline and doxycycline (Gnarpe and Belsheim, 1984).

4. *Erythromycin*

Erythromycin is a macrolide antibiotic which acts as an inhibitor of protein synthesis and has a reduced activity at acidic pH levels. Forsgren and Schmeling (1977) found that at high concentrations erythromycin had a depressive effect on the leucocyte migration. Banck and Forsgren (1979) later found that erythromycin also depressed the mitogenic response of human T and B cells. Melby and Midtvedt (1977) used an isotope method to show that high concentrations of erythromycin seemed to impair phagocytosis. In a conflicting report, van Rensburg *et al.* (1981) found that when erythromycin was taken by healthy volunteers, it could cause a slight stimulation of the directed migration and also a stimulation of lymphocyte transformation (Anderson *et al.*, 1982), which they ascribed to the antioxidant activity of the drug. Martin *et al.* (1980) reported that erythromycin did not influence chemiluminescence to a measurable extent. A reasonable conclusion on the basis of these different results is that, in normal clinical concentrations, erythromycin probably has no important effect on granulocyte and lymphocyte functioning.

5. Fusidic acid

Fusidic acid is a steroid antibiotic which suppresses bacterial growth by preventing translocation of messenger RNA on the ribosome. Fusidic acid is protein-bound to a high degree (Guttler and Tybring, 1971). Fusidic acid penetrates readily into blood cells (Brown and Percival, 1978). It has been used primarily in the treatment of staphylococcal infections.

However, very little and only incomplete information exists on how fusidic acid may interact with the host defence mechanisms. Forsgren and Schmeling (1977) observed that fusidic acid *in vitro* had a pronounced effect on leucocyte chemotaxis even at clinically attainable levels. The basic mechanism at work behind this depression is still unexplained; Forsgren and Schmeling (1977) suggest that the synthesis of a protein, necessary for the release of the chemotactic response, may be blocked at the level of transcription or at a later stage. Carruthers' early findings (1967) suggest that antibiotics with inhibitory effects on RNA and protein synthesis seem to have insignificant effects on random granulocyte migration, but very pronounced inhibitory effects on directed migration. Forsgren *et al.* (1980) later extended these observations to study the quantitative incorporation of ^{14}C-leucine into granulocytes in a trichloroacetic acid-insoluble form, and fusidic acid was also found to be inhibitory in this system. No reports have been published regarding the effects of fusidic acid on phagocytosis and intracellular killing.

The T-lymphocyte mitogenic response to fusidic acid has been investigated by Banck and Forsgren (1979) and later *in vitro* and *in vivo* by Forsgren *et al.* (1980). They found that there was a pronounced inhibitory effect on the mitogenic responses of B and T lymphocytes and on *in-vitro* antibody production as well as on the rejection of heart allograft transplants in an animal experimental model.

6. Chloramphenicol

Perhaps because of the well known side effects of chloramphenicol resulting in bone marrow aplasia, this antibiotic has not been investigated extensively as regards its effects on granulocyte and lymphocyte function. However, chloramphenicol has been found to exert slight depressive effects on granulocyte migration (Forsgren and Schmeling, 1977) and granulocyte phagocytosis (Lehrer, 1973). The studies of Pruul *et al.* (1981) demonstrated that there is an increased efficiency in granulocyte killing of *Escherichia coli* after bacterial preexposure to chloramphenicol. Banck and Forsgren (1979) found no depression of lymphocyte function *in vitro* after incubation with chloramphenicol.

7. Clindamycin

Clindamycin is a recent addition to the group of antibiotics that act by inhibition of protein synthesis, acting in the same manner as lincomycin. The microbial protein synthesis is blocked at the 50S ribosomal subunit. The drug has come into widespread use in the treatment of serious anaerobic infections and for treatment of staphylococcal infections.

Clindamycin is readily taken up by phagocytic cells and, according to Klempner and Styrt (1981), seems to be concentrated manyfold (up to 40 times the extracellular concentration). This intracellular accumulation seems to be against a pH gradient (Klempner and Styrt, 1983) and is localized primarily in the lysosomes.

In contrast with other inhibitors of protein synthesis, clindamycin has not been found to affect granulocyte chemotaxis adversely (Forsgren and Schmeling, 1977). According to Gemmell *et al.* (1981*a*, *b*), bacteria which have been preexposed to subinhibitory concentrations of clindamycin (¼ to ½ MIC) are more efficiently phagocytosed. Steinberg and Hand (1984) recently reported that the phagocytosis procedure itself stimulates an increased uptake of clindamycin by an increased activity of the nucleoside transport system, which is responsible for the uptake of clindamycin (Hand and King-Thompson, 1982). The very high intracellular concentrations of the drug may explain the finding that intracellular killing is more effective.

Banck and Forsgren (1979) as well as Bellasène and Forsgren (1980*a*, *b*) found that clindamycin in high concentrations (above therapeutic levels) does impair the incorporation of ^{3}H-thymidine into human T-lymphocytes stimulated by phytohaemagglutinin and into B lymphocytes stimulated by *Staphyloccoccus aureus* protein A. So far, these experiments have not been reproduced *in vivo*.

8. Rifampicin

Rifampicin acts by inhibition of the bacterial DNA-dependent RNA polymerase (Hartman, 1967). It is readily soluble in lipids and effectively penetrates into human cells (Mandell, 1973). In an early work from 1970, Paunescu reported that rifampicin had a depressive effect on delayed hypersensitivity in rabbits and guinea pigs, and also that the antibody production was depressed after injections of serum albumin. Later, Dajani *et al.* (1973) reported reduced cutaneous reactions to *Mycobacterium bovis* BCG and DNCB in guinea pigs treated with rifampicin in doses comparable to those used in humans. They also found this depression to be reversible on withdrawal of the antibiotic. Bassi *et al.* (1973) noticed a depression of the primary antibody response in mice only after large doses. Bellasêne and Forsgren (1980*a*, *b*) found that rifampicin markedly prolonged the survival of split-heart allografts, depressed the number of antibody-producing cells and gave a lower level of antibody as compared to control animals. This was confirmed by Scharre *et al.* (1981).

Banck and Forsgren (1979) also found that rifampicin impaired the incorporation of ^{3}H-thymidine into human T lymphocytes and B lymphocytes, stimulated by phytohaemagglutinin and protein A respectively. They also found that the incorporation of ^{14}C-leucine into a trichloroacetic acid-insoluble form in human granulocytes was depressed. The mechanism was not clearly defined at that time, but in a recent report Gray *et al.* (1983) have suggested that rifampicin competes with small peptide chemoattractants for granulocyte membrane receptors, but not with serum-derived chemoattractants like C5a. Their data seem convincing. The mechanism by which rifampicin depresses the lymphocyte activity is not yet fully delineated.

C. Nitroimidazole Derivatives

It has been observed that nitroimidazole derivatives have the potential to stimulate some granulocyte functions. In our own earlier investigations, we were unable to find any stimulation of the granulocyte migration response in normal control cells as a result of exposure to the drugs (Gnarpe and Belsheim, 1985).

Ursing and Kamme (1975) published findings on the treatment of patients with Crohn's disease with metronidazole, with resultant clinical improvement. They suggested that the favourable response to the treatment was due to the effects on the anaerobic bowel flora, which proved to be a controversial hypothesis. We suggest that the improvements seen may be due to a combination of factors: reduction of Gram-negative anaerobic bowel flora and a stimulation of host defence responses.

Using the modified LMAT, Belsheim *et al.* (1981) found that patients with Crohn's disease had a pronounced reduction of random as well as of directed granulocyte migration. This reduction was related to the stage of the disease; the more active the phase, the more pronounced the reduction in the chemotactic responses. When granulocytes from these patients were incubated *in vitro* with metronidazole, tinidazole, ornidazole or levamisole (Gnarpe *et al.*, 1978), the migration capacity was improved and in some cases normalized. The same phenomenon was not seen with cells from patients with ulcerative colitis. Our findings are partly contradictory to those of Binder and Riis (1977), who found that the undirected migration of granulocytes from ulcerative colitis patients was increased, while the chemotaxis decreased. This discrepancy is probably explained by the different techniques used, as the Boyden chamber, used by Binder and Riis, is not well suited to detect decreased undirected migration. Furthermore, we found that when patients with Crohn's disease in an acute stage were given test doses of metronidazole or tinidazole, they demonstrated a rapid trend toward normalization of directed and undirected PMN migration, following the serum concentration level curve. This effect could be found up to 5 h after a single oral dose (Gnarpe *et al.*, 1978). The same observations could not be made with cells from ulcerative colitis patients, from healthy volunteers or from Crohn's disease patients in inactive phases. Using nitroimidazole derivatives for an *in-vitro* preincubation of granulocytes, it was possible to use the normalization to differentiate between acute Crohn's disease and ulcerative colitis. We suggested that in the acute phases of Crohn's disease, the granulocytes were suffering from a defect in membrane function, which impeded mechanical movement (Gnarpe *et al.*, 1978; Belsheim *et al.*, 1984). We have indications that the nitroimidazole derivatives may act by removing complexes or aggregates from the membrane surface (Gnarpe *et al.*, 1978). Hogan and Hill (1978) suggested that levamisole could cause an elevation of the cellular nucleotide levels, which may affect the cell mobility. This may also be a credible hypothesis, though if it were the only mechanism, normal cells should also have been affected in our system.

Levamisole had earlier been reported to stimulate phagocytic responses of normal granulocytes (Molin and Stendahl, 1977). It has also been found to enhance the blast transformation of normal lymphocytes (Pabst and Crawford, 1975).

V. SUMMARY

This chapter has presented a review of the information available on the influence of antibiotics on granulocytes and lymphocytes. Most of the accumulated data have been collected from experimental *in-vitro* studies or from *in-vivo* animal studies. Only a few investigations have been done in human volunteers or in patients. The lack of relevant *in-vivo* studies may be attributed to the practical problems involved. At present, the only techniques at hand for *in-vivo* investigations of granulocyte chemotaxis, for example, are the skin window and skin (suction) blister techniques.

It is obvious from the above presentation that antibiotics do interact with and in some cases alter the behaviour of granulocytes and lymphocytes, at least under *in-vitro* conditions. The main problem remains the interpretation and correlation of findings to the clinical situation. Even assuming that the *in-vivo* effects of certain antibiotics are comparable to those found *in vitro*, it is still difficult to form an opinion as to whether a specific antibiotic should be regarded as having positive or negative effects on the immune system. In all likelihood, the clinical status of the patient is the determining factor. For example, antibiotics like the tetracyclines, which exert inhibitory effects on leucocyte functions, may play a dual role in some cases, and thereby not only have an effect on the microbial population, but also act as antiinflammatory agents. This may be the explanation for the good clinical effects obtained by treatment of pelvic inflammatory disease with tetracyclines. It is most probable that only the immunocompromised patient with multiple severe defects in the immune system may be unduly negatively influenced by the careless choice of an antimicrobial agent.

REFERENCES

Anderson, R., van Rensburg, C. E. J., Eftychis, H., Jooné, G. and van Rensburg, A. J. (1982). *J. Antimicrob. Chemother.* **10**, 409-417.

Andreana, A., Perna, P., Utili, R., Dilillo and M., Ruggerio, G. (1984). *Antimicrob. Agents Chemother.* **25**, 182-186.

Banck, G. and Forsgren, A. (1979). *Antimicrob. Agents Chemother.* **16**, 554-560.

Banck, G. and Forsgren, A. (1980). *Clin. Exp. Immunol.* **42**, 530-534.

Bardana, E. J., Jr. (1981). *Med. Clin. North Am.* **65**, 959-975.

Barza, M., Brown, R. B., Shanks, C., Gamble, C. and Weinstein, L. (1975). *Antimicrob. Agents Chemother.* **8**, 713-720.

Bassi, L., DiBernadino, L., Arioli, V., Silvestri, L. G. and Ligniere, E. L. C. (1973). *J. Infect. Dis.* **128**, 736-744.

Beckerdite, S., Mooney, C., Weiss, J., Franson, R. and Elsbach, P. (1974). *J. Exp. Med.* **140**, 396-409.

Bellasène, A. and Forsgren, A. (1980*a*). *Infect. Immun.* **27**, 15-20.

Bellasène, A. and Forsgren, A. (1980*b*). *Infect. Immun.* **29**, 873-878.

Belsheim, J. (1981). *Acta Path. Microbiol. Scand. Sect. C* **89**, 167-174.

Belsheim, J. and Gnarpe, H. (1981). *Acta Path. Microbiol. Scand. Sect. C* **89**, 217-221.

Belsheim, J., Gnarpe, H., Persson, S. (1979*a*). *Scand. J. Infect. Dis.* **11**, 141-145.

Belsheim, J., Gnarpe, H. and Löfberg, J. (1979*b*). *Scand. J. Infect. Dis.* **11**, 287-290.

Belsheim, J., Gnarpe, H. and Persson, S. (1981). *Acta Chir. Scand.* **147**, 197-200.

Belsheim, J., Blomqvist, C., Löfberg, J. and Gnarpe, H. (1982). *In* "Antibiotics in Tissues", pp. 37-47 (Holm, S., ed.). Carlo Erba S.p.A., Italy.

Belsheim, J., Blomqvist, C., Löfberg, J., Gnarpe, H. (1983). *Acta Oto-Rhino-Laryngol. Belg.* **37**, 635-648.

Belsheim, J., Gnarpe, H. and Swahn, Å. (1984). *Acta Path. Microbiol. Scand. Sect. C.* **92**, 75–79.
Bender, J. C. and van Epps, D. E. (1983). *Infect. Immun.* **41**, 1062–1070.
Binder, V. and Riis, P. (1977). *Scand. J. Gastroenterol.* **12**, 141–144.
Boyden, S. (1962). *J. Exp. Med.* **115**, 453–466.
Bridges, C. G., DaSilva, G. L., Yamamura, M. and Valdimarsson, H. (1980). *Clin. Exp. Immunol.* **42**, 226–233.
Brown, K. N. and Percival, A. (1978). *Scand. J. Infect. Dis.* **14** *(Suppl.)*, 251–260.
Bryan, L. E. and van den Eizen, H. M. (1977). *Antimicrob. Agents Chemother.* **12**, 163–177.
Carruthers, B. M. (1967). *Can. J. Physiol. Pharmacol.* **45**, 269–280.
Chaperon, E. A. and Sanders, W. E. (1978). *Infect. Immun.* **19**, 378–384.
Christou, N. V. and Meakins, J. L. (1979). *Ann. Surg.* **190**, 557–564.
Colazzi, J. L. and Klink, P. R. (1969). *J. Pharmacol. Sci.* **58**, 1184–1189.
Cooper, M. D. and Lawton, A. R. (1972). *Am. J. Pathol.* **69**, 513–528.
Dajani, B. M., Kasik, J. E. & Thomson, J. S. (1973). *Antimicrob. Agents Chemother.* **3**, 451–455.
Donabedian, H. and Gallin, J. I. (1982). *J. Clin. Invest.* **69**, 1155–1163.
Eaton, L. J. and Rest, R. F. (1983). *Infect. Immun.* **42**, 1034–1040.
Ehlenberger, A. G. and Nussenzweig, V. (1977). *J. Exp. Med.* **145**, 357–371.
Fauci, A. S. and Pratt, K. R. (1976). *Proc. Natl Acad. Sci. U.S.A.* **73**, 3676–3679.
Feigin, R. D. and Shearer, W. T. (1975). *J. Pediatr.* **87**, 507–514.
Forsgren, A. (1981). *J. Antimicrob. Chemother.* **8** *(Suppl. B)*, 183–186.
Forsgren, A. and Banck, G. (1978). *Infection* **6** *(Suppl. 1)*, 91–97.
Forsgren, A. and Schmeling, D. (1977). *Antimicrob. Agents Chemother.* **11**, 580–584.
Forsgren, A. and Walder, M. (1983). *J. Antimicrob. Chemother.* **11**, 467–471.
Forsgren, A., Schmeling, D. and Quie, P. G. (1974). *J. Infect. Dis.* **130**, 412–415.
Forsgren, A., Banck, G., Beckman, H., Bellasène, A. (1980). *Scand. J. Infect. Dis. Suppl.* **24**, 195–203.
Forslid, J. and Hed, J. (1982). *Infect. Immun.* **38**, 811–816.
Friedman, H. and Warren, G. H. (1974). *Proc. Soc. Exp. Biol. Med.* **146**, 707–711.
Gallin, J. I. (1980). *Ann. Intern. Med.* **92**, 520–538.
Gallin, J. I. and Rosenthal, A. S. (1974). *J. Cell Biol.* **62**, 594–609.
Gallin, J. I. and Wolff, S. M. (1975). *Clin. Hematol.* **4**, 567–607.
Gallin, J. I., Durocher, J. R., Kaplan, A. P. (1974). *J. Clin. Invest.* **55**, 967–974.
Gemmell, C. G., Peterson, P. K., Schmeling, D., Kim, Y., Matthews, J., Wannamaker, L. and Quie, P. G. (1981*a*). *J. Clin. Invest.* **67**, 1249–1256.
Gemmell, C. G., Peterson, P. K., Rigelman, W., Schmeling, D., Hoidal, J. R. and Quie, P. G. (1981*b*). *Infect. Immun.* **32**, 1298–1300.
Gemmell, C. G., Peterson, P. K., Schmeling, D. and Quie, P. G. (1982). *Drugs Exp. Clin. Res.* **8**, 235–240.
Gemmell, C. G., Peterson, P. K., Schmeling, D., Matthews, J. and Quie, P. G. (1983). *Eur. J. Clin. Microbiol.* **2**, 327–334.
Ginsburg, W. W., Finkelman, F. D., Lipsky, P. E. (1978). *J. Immunol.* **120**, 33–39.

Gnarpe, H. and Belsheim, J. (1979). *Drugs Exp. Clin. Res.* **5**, 1-4.
Gnarpe, H. and Belsheim, J. (1985). *Zbl. Bakt.* **13** (Suppl.), 123-140.
Gnarpe, H., Persson, S. and Belsheim, J. (1978). *Infection* **1** *(Suppl.)*, 107-110.
Gnarpe, H., Belsheim, J., Blomqvist, C. and Lundbäck, A. (1984). *Antimicrob. Agents Chemother.* **25**, 179-181.
Goodhart, G. L. (1977). *Antimicrob. Agents Chemother.* **12**, 540-542.
Grant, M., Raeburn, J. A., Sutherland, R., Harkness, R. A., Gormley, J. P. and Kowolik, M. J. (1983). *J. Antimicrob. Chemother.* **11**, 543-554.
Gray, G. D., Smith, C. W., Hollers, J. C., Chenoweth, D. E., Fiegel, V. D. and Nelson, R. D. (1983). *Antimicrob. Agents Chemother.* **24**, 777-783.
Guttler, F. and Tybring, L. (1971). *Br. J. Pharmacol.* **43**, 151-160.
Hand, W. L. and King-Thompson, N. L. (1982). *Antimicrob. Agents Chemother.* **21**, 241-247.
Hartman, G., Honikel, K. O. and Knüsel, J. (1967). *Biochim. Biophys. Acta* **145**, 843-844.
Hed, J. (1977). *FEMS Lett.* **1**, 357-361.
Hellum, K. and Solberg, C. O. (1977). *Acta Path. Microbiol. Scand. Sect. C* **85**, 413-423.
Hendlin, D., Frost, B. M., Thiele, E., Kropp, H., Valiant, M. E., Pelak, B., Weissberger, B., Corin, C. and Miller, A. K. (1969). *Antimicrob. Agents Chemother.* **9**, 297-302.
Hildebrandt, J., Berner, H., Laber, G., Schütze, E. and Turnowsky, F. (1983). Abstracts of the 13th International Congress on Chemotherapy, Vienna.
Hill, H. R. and Quie, P. G. (1974). *Lancet* **i**, 183-187.
Hoeprich, P. D. and Martin, C. H. (1970). *Clin. Pharmacol. Ther.* **11**, 418-422.
Hogan, N. A. and Hill, H. R. (1978). *J. Infect. Dis.* **138**, 437-444.
Högenauer, G. and Brunowsky, W. (1983). Abstracts of the 13th International Congress on Chemotherapy, Vienna.
Horne, D. and Tomasz. A. (1981). *Antimicrob. Agents Chemother.* **19**, 745-753.
Jondal, M., Holm, G. and Wigzell, H. (1972). *J. Exp. Med.* **136**, 207-215.
Horvath, L. and Leonard, E. J. (1982). *Infect. Immun.* **36**, 443-449.
Klebanoff, S. J. and Clark, R. A. (eds) (1978). *In* "The Neutrophil: Function and Clinical Disorders", pp. 409-488. North Holland, Amsterdam.
Klempner, M. S. and Styrt, B. (1981). *J. Infect. Dis.* **144**, 472-479.
Klempner, M. S. and Styrt, B. (1983). *J. Antimicrob. Chemother.* **12**, *(Suppl. C)*, 39-50.
Kohlhepp, S. J., Plant, S. B., McCarron, D. A. and Gilbert, D. N. (1982). *Antimicrob. Agents Chemother.* **21**, 668-669.
Lehrer, R. (1973). *J. Infect. Dis.* **127**, 40-48.
Leijh, P. C. J., van den Barselaar, M. T. and van Furth, R. (1981). *Scand. J. Immunol.* **13**, 159-174.
Lichtman, M. A. and Weed, R. J. (1972). *Blood* **39**, 301-315.
Lorian, V. and Atkinson, B. (1980). *Antimicrob. Agents Chemother.* **18**, 807-813.
MacGregor, R. R., Macarek, E. J. and Kefalides, W. A. (1978). *J. Clin. Invest.* **61**, 696-702.

Majeski, J. A. Morris, M. J. and Alexander, W. J. (1978). *J. Antibiotics* **31**, 1059-1062.
Mandell, G. L. (1973). *J. Clin. Invest.* **52**, 1673-1679.
Manzella, J. P. and Clark, J. K. (1983). *Antimicrob. Agents Chemother.* **23**, 360-363.
Martin, R. R., Warr, G. A., Couch, R. B., Yeager, H. and Knight, V. (1974). *J. Infect. Dis.* **129**, 110-116.
Martin, R. R., Putman, M., Greenberg, S. B., Wallace, R. J., Jr. and Wilson, S. Z. (1980). *J. Med.* **11**, 39-48.
McMurray, L. and Levy, S. B. (1978). *Antimicrob. Agents Chemother.* **14**, 201-209.
Melby, K. and Midtvedt, T. (1977). *Scand. J. Infect. Dis.* **9**, 9-12.
Miller, M. E. (1978). *In* "Leukocyte Chemotaxis: Methods, Physiology and Clinical Implications" (Gallin, J. I. and Quie, P. G., eds), pp. 379-388. Raven Press, New York.
Molin, L. and Stendahl, O. (1977). *Scand. J. Hematol.* **19**, 93-98.
Munoz, J. and Geister, R. (1950). *Proc. Soc. Exp. Biol. Med.* **75**, 367-370.
Nelson, R. D., Quie, P. G. and Simmons, R. L. (1975). *J. Immunol.* **115**, 1650-1656.
Nelson, R. D., McCormack, R. T., Fiegel, V. D., Simmons, R. L. (1978). *Infect. Immun.* **22**, 441-444.
Nowell, P. C. (1960). *Cancer Res.* **20**, 462-466.
Odeberg, H. and Olsson, I. (1976). *Infect. Immun.* **14**, 1269-1275.
Ohnishi, H., Inaba, H., Mochizuki, H., Kosuzune, H. (1984). *Antimicrob. Agents Chemother.* **25**, 88-92.
Pabst, H. and Crawford, J. (1975). *Clin. Exp. Immunol.* **21**, 468-473.
Parish, C. R., Chilcott, A. B., McKenzie, I. F. C. (1976). *Immunogenetics* **3**, 113.
Park, J. K. and Dow, R. C. (1970). *Br. J. Exp. Pathol.* **51**, 179-182.
Pato, M. L. (1977). *Antimicrob. Agents Chemother.* **11**, 318-323.
Paton, J. C. and Ferrante, A. (1983). *Infect. Immun.* **41**, 1212-1216.
Paunescu, E. (1970). *Nature* **228**, 1188-1190.
Pruul, H., Wetherall, B. L. and McDonald, P. J. (1981). *Antimicrob. Agents Chemother.* **19**, 945-951.
Pruul, H., Hill, N. and McDonald, P. J. (1984). *J. Antimicrob. Chemother.* **14**, 19-31.
Quie, P. G. and Cates, K. L. (1977). *Amer. J. Pathol.* **88**, 711-724.
Rebuck, J. W. and Crowley, J. H. (1974). *Ann. N.Y. Acad. Sci.* **59**, 757-805.
Rentz, M., Nicol, A. D. and Harkness, R. A. (1972). *In* "Host Resistance to Commensal Bacteria (MacPhee, T., ed.), pp. 246-253. Longman, Edinburgh.
Rest, R. F., Fischer, S. H., Ingham, Z. Z. and Jones, J. F. (1982). *Infect. Immun.* **36**, 737-744.
Robinson, P., Wakefield, D., Breit, N., Easter, J. F. and Penny, R. (1984). *Infect. Immun.* **43**, 744-752.
Sacchi, F., Marseglia, G., Fietta, A., Marchi, A. and Siccardi, A. G. (1981). *Antimicrob. Agents Chemother.* **20**, 258-259.
Scharre, K. A., Eckels, D. D. and Gershwin, M. E. (1981). *J. Infect. Dis.* **143**, 832-835.

Shils, M. E. (1963). *Ann. Intern. Med.* **58**, 389-408.

Siegel, J. P. and Remington, J. S. (1982). *J. Antimicrob. Chemother.* **10**, 505-515.

Solberg, C. O., Halstensen, A., Digranes, A. and Hellum, K. B. (1983). *Rev. Infect. Dis.* **5** *(Suppl. 3)*, 468-473.

Starkebaum, G., Stevens, D. L., Henry, C. and Gavin, S. E. (1981). *J. Lab. Clin. Med.* **98**, 280-291.

Steinberg, T. H. and Hand, W. L. (1984). *J. Infect. Dis.* **149**, 397-403.

Thong, Y. H. and Ferrante, A. (1979). Clin. Exp. Immunol. **35**, 443-446.

Tomita, T., Blumenstock, E. and Kanegasaki, S. (1981). *Infect. Immun.* **32**, 1242-1248.

Ursing, B. and Kamme, C. (1975). *Lancet* **i**, 775-776.

van Rensburg, C. E. J., Anderson, R., Jooné, G., vander Merwe, M. and van Rensburg, A. J. (1981). *J. Antimicrob. Chemother.* **8**, 467-474.

Verbrugh, H. A., Keane, W. F., Hoidal, J. R., Freiberg, M. R., Elliott, G. R. and Peterson, P. K. (1983). *J. Infect. Dis.* **147**, 1018-1029.

Verhoef, J., Peterson, P. K., Kim, Y., Sabath, L. D. and Quie, P. G. (1977*a*) *Immunology* **33**, 191-197.

Verhoef, J., Peterson, P. K. and Quie, P. G. (1977*b*). *Immunology* **33**, 231-239.

Weiss, J., Elsbach, P., Olsson, I. and Odeberg, H. (1978). *J. Biol. Chem.* **253**, 2664-2672.

Weissmann, G., Korchak, H. M., Perez, H. D., Smolen, J. E., Goldstein, J. M. and Hoffstein, S. T. (1979). *J. Reticuloendothel. Soc.* **26** *(Suppl.)*, 687-700.

Wenzel, A. F., Hildebrandt, J., Laber, G. and Schütze, E. (1983). Abstracts of the 13th International Congress on Chemotherapy, Vienna.

Wetherall, B. L., Pruul, H. and McDonald, P. J. (1984). *Infect. Immun.* **43**, 1080-1084.

Yanai, M. and Quie, P. G. (1981). *Infect. Immun.* **32**, 1181-1186.

Zigmond. S. H. and Hirsh, J. G. (1973). *J. Exp. Med.* **137**, 387-410.

Chapter 6

Effect of Sublethal Concentrations of Antibiotics on the Immune System

Rodger P. Silletti

Bronx-Lebanon Hospital Center, Microbiology Division,
1276 Fulton Avenue, Bronx, New York 10456, U.S.A.

I. INTRODUCTION

With the increasing incidence of serious opportunistic infections in immunocompromised patients, and the necessity for intensive and prolonged prophylactic and therapeutic antimicrobial regimens, it has become increasingly important to consider the effects of antimicrobial therapy on the immune system. Antimitotic agents are well known for their depressant effect on the immune system and are used to advantage in both organ transplantation and in the management of immune-mediated disease. The similarity of the chemical structures of certain antibiotics to the structures of antimetabolites and cytotoxic drugs (Ghilchik *et al.*, 1970; Hartmann *et al.*, 1967) and the bone-marrow suppressive effects and allergic reactions caused by commonly employed antimicrobial agents (Best, 1967; Spath *et al.*, 1971) has led to the investigation of the effects of antibiotics on certain parameters of the immune system. That certain antibiotics can diffuse into mammalian cells (Lobo and Mandell, 1973; Mandell, 1973; Johnson *et al.*, 1980; Klempner and Styrt, 1981) raises the possibility of both deleterious and beneficial effects on leucocytes and lymphocytes.

Antimicrobial agents and immunity
ISBN 0-12-383830-4

The investigation of the immunomodulating effects of antibiotics is fraught with difficulties. Data obtained *in vitro* are very dependent on the methods employed, and the attempt to limit variables renders any correlation with the *in-vivo* situation speculative. *In-vivo* results depend upon the animal model chosen, and the possibility that the response is due in part to individual host factors must always be considered. For example, *in vivo*, results will generally depend upon whether the drug is being tested in normal individuals or in those with a defect in their host defence mechanism. In the compromised patient, a positive effect of the drug may more readily be demonstrated. Since it is more difficult to show augmentation in normal individuals, studies on healthy subjects frequently demonstrate only a negative effect of drugs on host defence parameters.

The incompatibility of *in-vitro* and *in-vivo* results may be due to these modifying influences of individual host factors and the following differences in the test conditions:

(1) The bacterial inoculum of the *in-vitro* system is uniform and generally in the logarithmic phase. In contrast, the inoculum at the focus of an infection may vary from much less to much more than in an *in-vitro* system, and the maximal growth rate has slowed in many clinical settings.
(2) The temperature of the *in-vitro* system is generally kept at 37°C, whereas at the site of infection it may vary due to fever or peripheral location.
(3) The antibiotic concentration in the *in-vitro* system is fairly constant, but *in vivo* the concentration rises and falls as the antibiotic is delivered, and may be much higher or lower at the site of action due to secretory cells or barriers respectively.
(4) The differences in the chemical and physical composition between the *in-vitro* and *in-vivo* test systems are among the most important factors. *In vitro* the medium is either uniformly solid or liquid, and the pH and cation concentration may not approximate the *in-vivo* situation.

The significance of *in-vivo* results cannot be questioned, and they generally support present therapeutic regimens. However, they cannot easily be extrapolated to other infections, underlying disorders or even other individuals, since the effects of individual host factors cannot be determined. Host factors remain the major determinants of the outcome of antimicrobial therapy (Weinstein and Dalton, 1968; Sabath, 1982).

Therefore it is important to recognize the different contributions made by *in-vivo* and *in-vitro* experiments. Results of *in-vivo* experiments will add information necessary to treat empirically, and the universality of the empiric therapy will be proportional to the volume of data available from *in-vivo* experiments. In contrast, data from *in-vitro* experiments will elucidate the specific mechanism for inhibition or potentiation of various parameters of the immune system. Whether these effects will be seen *in vivo* can then be determined by considering the pharmacokinetics of the drug, the site of the infection, the infecting organism and any underlying disorder.

For this reason, the *in-vitro* system need not attempt to mimic the situation *in vivo*. Physical and chemical parameters should be varied to determine their effects, and this will aid in predicting the behaviour of the drug *in vivo*.

With this in mind, we need not lament the diversity of test conditions employed *in vitro* in examining the effects of antibiotics on leucocytes and lymphocytes, and though the results are often contradictory, they merely point to variables that remain to be elucidated and controlled to further refine the *in-vitro* test system. When the test system is fully refined, the specific mechanism of action of antibiotics that alter the immune response, as well as the various factors involved in the immune response that contribute to the present contradictory results, will become clear.

A. Sublethal Concentrations of Antibiotics

1. Effects on bacteria

As early as 1940, Gardner (1940) observed unsegmented filaments of *Clostridium perfringens* when the organism was grown in the presence of small amounts of penicillin. *Staphylococcus aureus* and *Streptococcus pyogenes* grew as large cells with incomplete fission in the presence of one-quarter of the minimum inhibitory concentration (MIC) of penicillin. Gram-negative bacilli were also shown to exhibit altered morphology when grown in the presence of sub-MIC of penicillin (Duguid, 1946; Dienes, 1949; Fleming *et al.*, 1950; Pulvertaft, 1952). Pulvertaft also studied the effects of low concentrations of tetracycline, chloramphenicol and streptomycin on *Escherichia coli* and Goss *et al.* (1964) noted the effects of nalidixic acid. Eagle and Musselman (1948) reported a reduction in the growth rate of spirochaetes and cocci after exposure to sub-MIC of penicillin, and Ciak and Hahn (1959) reported that the initial growth of *E. coli* was decreased by sub-MIC of penicillin.

Salmonella typhimurium exposed to low concentrations of gentamicin showed a decrease in ribosomes (Lorian and Atkinson, 1975), except at the ends of the bacillus. A decrease in ribosomal density was also reported when *Proteus mirabilis* was exposed to sub-MIC of ampicillin and cephalothin (Lorian, 1975; Lorian and Atkinson, 1975). Viano *et al.* (1981)

demonstrated a qualitative and quantitative alteration of cytoplasmic protein induced by sub-MICs of ampicillin and cefoperazone. Gemmell (1978) showed that the biosynthesis of staphylococcal toxins and enzymes were influenced by sub-MIC of clindamycin, and Gemmell and Dowd (1983) showed that one-half the MIC of clindamycin and one-quarter the MIC of fusidic acid reduced the amount of protein A on the staphylococcal cell surface.

Abraham (1949) recognized three effects of low concentrations of antibiotic which could occur for a given drug:

(1) a prolongation of the lag phase;
(2) a reduction in the rate of the logarithmic phase;
(3) a decrease in the size of the population at stationary phase.

Lorian and Popoola (1972) and Lorian *et al.* (1983*b*) reported in detail the morphologic effects of antibiotics on Gram-negative and Gram-positive bacteria.

Most of the investigations of the effects of sub-MICs of antibiotics on bacteria could be placed in one of two categories:

(1) those producing a morphological change as observed by Gram stain, interference phase microscopy or ultrastructural changes observed by electron microscopy;
(2) those that result in a decrease in the number of microorganisms.

Bacterial surface determinants, toxins or enzymes, and rapid growth rate or high bacterial density are all virulence factors that determine in part the outcome of a particular infection. Since in many cases these factors have been shown to be altered by sublethal concentrations of antibiotics, it was of interest to investigate the effects of low concentrations of antibiotics on infections *in vivo*.

2. In-Vivo *effects*

Until recently little was known about the *in-vivo* effects of sub-MICs of antibiotics with the exception of studies of antibiotic combinations. In mice, Comber *et al.* (1977) showed that half were protected from infection with *E. coli* when a concentration of one-quarter the MIC of amoxicillin was maintained in the blood. The same concentration of ampicillin in the blood and peritoneal fluid did not protect the mice (Zak *et al.*, 1977). This was shown to be the result of the greater bacteriolytic activity of amoxicillin over ampicillin in mice (Rolinson *et al.*, 1977).

Zak *et al.* (1977) and Zak and Krandolfer (1979) also demonstrated that maintaining one-third the MIC of ampicillin or cephaloridine, or one-sixth the MIC of gentamicin in the peritoneal exudate protected 50% of

P. mirabilis-infected rabbits from death. The survival time of those that did die was prolonged when compared with the control animals.

However, the effects of one-third the MIC of ampicillin in the peritoneal exudate of rabbits infected with *S. typhimurium* showed that the animals died sooner than the controls. Similarly, Smith and Kong (1979) reported that sub-MIC of nafcillin enhanced the virulence of *S. aureus* in mice. Chloramphenicol, lincomycin and penicillin produced no significant difference in the survival time of the animals. Low doses of rifampicin were sufficient to cure listeriosis in normal mice, but this efficiency was lost in athymic mice (Bakker-Woudenberg *et al.*, 1984). This is an indication that normal host defences are necessary and may be modifiers of *in-vivo* antibacterial activity.

Studies of treatment with sub-MICs of antibiotics in humans have demonstrated favourable results. In immunocompetent patients with Gram-negative sepsis being treated with gentamicin, the rate of mortality was the same whether the serum concentration was higher or lower than one-eighth the MIC of the infecting organism (Reymann *et al.*, 1979). Ben Redjeb *et al.* (1981) reported good therapeutic results when 10 mg/day of ampicillin and 2 of water, which resulted in a sub-MIC of ampicillin in the urine, was used to treat *E. coli* urinary tract infections.

3. Antibiotic levels in vivo

Many factors determine the amount of an antibiotic that actually reaches the site of an infection and is therefore available to kill or inhibit the growth of the infecting organism. Serum protein binding is a major influence, with some antibiotics 95% bound to serum proteins and many 50% bound (Benet and Sheiner, 1980). Tissue binding, lipid solubility and poor absorption will also contribute to the lowering of the level of antibiotic.

The effects of sublethal concentrations of antibiotics in patients have been shown by Lorian and Waluschka (1972). Abnormal forms of *Enterobacter cloacae*, *E. coli* and *Klebsiella pneumoniae* have been found in the blood cultures of patients treated with sublethal concentrations of antibiotics. These have also been found by Magnussen and Hruska (1980). Filaments (see Fig. 1, p. 188) and aberrant forms of bacteria have also been reported from urine specimens by Lorian (1980) and from cerebrospinal fluids by Louria and Kaminski (1969) in patients receiving antibiotics. Recently I have found multiseptate staphylococci in the sputum of a patient with staphylococcal pneumonia who was receiving penicillin, and rod-like pneumococci have been observed in sputa (Lorian *et al.*, 1980).

These aberrant forms are probably present in many more cases than are reported in the literature. Though these forms can be caused by changes in pH and serum factors, the influence of sublethal concentrations of antibiotics is, for the most part, the predominant mechanism. Indeed, the presence of these forms in a clinical specimen should alert the physician that the antibiotic concentration is suboptimal.

II. EFFECTS ON LYMPHOCYTES

Because of the interactions between lymphocytes and other host factors, including macrophages, *in-vivo* determinations of antibiotic action on lymphocyte function through measurements of delayed type hypersensitivity generally fail to differentiate among lymphocyte effects, effects on serum factors and macrophage effects.

The action of antibiotics *in vivo* is also modified by the pharmacokinetics of the drug. This was suggested as the mechanism for the similarity *in vivo* of the immune response to both rifamycin SV and rifampicin despite the greater suppression *in vitro* of lymphocyte transformation by rifamycin SV (Bassi and Bolzoni, 1982). In addition, since rifampicin immunosuppression appears to be due to the inhibition of macrophage phagocytic activity (Bassi *et al.*, 1973) and rifamycin SV seems to be cytotoxic, thus requiring high concentrations for activity, rifampicin reduces antibody production *in vivo* to a greater extent than does rifamycin SV (Bassi and Bolzoni, 1982).

As the concentration of antibiotic can be determined more accurately and the influence of modifying host factors can be reduced significantly in *in-vitro* systems, this chapter will focus on the results of these studies.

A. *In vitro* Effects

1. *β-Lactam antibiotics*

(a) Penicillins

Banck and Forsgren (1979) found no effect of penicillin or carbenicillin on transformation of normal human lymphocytes induced by phytohaemagglutinin (PHA). Similarly, no effect was found when transformation was induced by the Cowan I strain of *S. aureus*, a B-lymphocyte mitogen. As expected, neither penicillin nor carbenicillin affected protein synthesis in normal lymphocytes, and these antibiotics were used as controls in tests of antibody production because of their lack of effect. Larson *et al.* (1980) and Finch (1980) also found no effect of 5 μg/ml of penicillin on mitogen-stimulated lymphocyte transformation.

(b) Cephalosporins and related antibiotics

Although Chaperon and Sanders (1978) have shown suppression of lymphocyte transformation by PHA and concanavalin A (ConA) at high concentrations of cephalothin, cephalexin and cephradine, and by pokeweed mitogen (PWM) by high concentrations of cephalexin, cephradine and cefoxitin, Forsgren and Banck (1978) and Banck and Forsgren (1979) failed to show any effect of cephalothin or cefazolin on the PHA response. The response to B-lymphocyte mitogens was not determined.

Larson *et al.* (1980) showed no suppression of thymidine incorporation by unstimulated, nitogen-stimulated or antigen-stimulated lymphocytes with a cephalothin concentration of 5 μg/ml. In addition, no effect on protein synthesis was noted at this concentration. Similarly, Finch (1980) could not demonstrate any significant suppressive effect of cephalothin, cephalexin, cefamandole, cefazolin or cefoxitin on PHA-, PWM- or conA-stimulated lymphocyte transformation unless high concentrations were used.

In 1982, Chaperon (1982) reported that 12·5 μg/ml of cephalexin or cephradine significantly suppressed thymidine incorporation by peripheral blood lymphocytes following PHA stimulation.

The fact that Chaperon and Sanders used Eagle minimal essential medium supplemented with 10% fetal calf serum as a culture base and 8·5 μg/ml PHA and Banck and Forsgren used serum-free RPMI 1640 medium supplemented with L-glutamine and 1 μg/ml PHA could have contributed to the contradictory results. Larson *et al.* (1980) found that he could suppress PHA-induced lymphocyte transformation with 100 μg/ml of cephalothin only when the amount of PHA used was suboptimal for lymphocyte stimulation. Leyhausen *et al.* (1984) reported a stimulation of Molt-4 cells (a human T-cell-derived tumour cell line) as measured by thymidine incorporation with cefotaxime and cefodizime at concentrations as low as 0·3 μmol/l. The medium used was RPMI 1640 supplemented with 10% fetal calf serum, and the stimulation was greater when conA was not used. Ceftizoxime had no effect in this sytem. It was also noted that none of the drugs displayed any significant effect on the growth of mouse lymphoma cells (terminal deoxynucleotidyl transferase negative) at any concentration, but cefodizime did stimulate murine splenic lymphocytes.

It appears that the interaction of lymphocyte, mitogen and antibiotic is a complex phenomenon influenced at least by media composition, concentration or presence of mitogens or antigens and chemical structure of the antibiotic. Although no structure-function relationship can be derived from the study of three antibiotics, Leyhausen *et al.* (1984) do suggest that the replacement of the bulky derivatized thiazole group attached via the thiomethyl linker to the thiazolidine ring (cefodizime) by a hydrogen atom (ceftizoxime) resulted in a loss of the growth-stimulating activity. In addition, the two antibiotics that Chaperon (1982) reported to have the greatest suppressive effect on lymphocyte transformation, cephradine and cephalexin, share a similar structure (Finch, 1980).

Gillissen (1982), using mice immunized with sheep red blood cells and treated with antibiotics *in vitro*, determined the number of antibody-forming spleen cells in the plaque assay. Cephalothin, cephradine, cephaloridine, cephalexin, cefoperazone, ceftazidime, cefamandole, cefazolin, cefotaxime and cefoxitin had no effect on IgM-producing cells in this system at a concentration of 10 μg/ml.

2. Tetracyclines

Munster *et al.* (1977) reported the suppression of PHA-induced lymphocyte transformation by low concentrations of tetracycline and, to a greater extent, minocycline. Banck and Forsgren (1979) found no decrease in thymidine incorporation with tetracycline chloride or lymecycline up to 25 μg/ml. However, minocycline caused a suppression of transformation above 10 μg/ml and doxycycline did so at concentrations above 1 μg/ml. The suppression of thymidine incorporation in response to both B- and T-cell mitogens was identical. Furthermore, the suppression of transformation elicited by the Cowan I strain of *S. aureus* and PHA by doxycycline was irreversible, as shown by washing the cells and reincubating with the antigen and mitogen. Protein synthesis and antibody production were similarly depressed by concentrations of doxycycline between 1 and 10 μg/ml.

Thong and Ferrante (1979) also showed a suppression of lymphocyte transformation to both PHA and PWM by low concentrations of doxycycline. It appears that the extent to which the tetracyclines can suppress lymphocyte function correlates with their lipid solubility. In this way, doxycycline and minocycline exert the greatest effect, tetracycline and oxytetracycline suppress transformation to a lesser extent, and lymecycline has no effect.

Because tetracyclines inhibit protein synthesis in bacteria, this has been proposed as its mechanism of action on lymphocytes. Banck and Forsgren (1979) did show a depression of protein synthesis with doxycycline, and, due to its lipid solubility, doxycycline might be expected to accumulate within lymphocytes. However, Thong and Ferrante (1979) demonstrated that the effect of doxycycline could be completely abrogated by washing the cells prior to culture with the mitogens. This competitive effect could more easily be explained on the basis of a surface interaction rather than an inhibition of accumulation of doxycycline.

3. Aminoglycosides

In three separate studies (Forsgren and Banck, 1978; Banck and Forsgren, 1979; Forsgren *et al.*, 1980) no effect of gentamicin or kanamycin could be found on lymphocyte transformation by PHA or of gentamicin on *in-vitro* antibody synthesis by B lymphocytes stimulated with the Cowan I strain of *S. aureus*.

4. Rifamycins

Engle *et al.* (1970) found that oral administration of rifampicin to hamsters initiated 24 h prior to H-1 virus infection could suppress virus-specific antibody production. Though this effect could be correlated directly with an inhibition of virus replication, the effect was limited since only a partial suppression of virus proliferation could be demonstrated despite the use of very high doses of rifampicin. Since rifampicin is toxic to mammalian cells, this toxicity must be considered when the drug is found to have an inhibitory effect on an intracellular organism.

Paunescu (1970) found that DNA-dependent RNA polymerase was not inhibited in cell-free mammalian systems unless rifampicin concentrations of 200 μg/ml are used. However, as little as 1 μg/ml in culture delays antibody production by lymphocytes. Dajani *et al.* (1972) found that although very high concentrations of rifampicin inhibited *in-vitro* stimulation of peripheral blood lymphocytes by PHA, low concentrations (1–10 μg/ml) slightly stimulated lymphocyte transformation. Serrou (1974) reported that low concentrations of rifampicin significantly inhibited PHA stimulation of lymphocytes as well as secretion of migration inhibition factor. The suppression was also found, albeit to a lesser extent, by Banck and Forsgren (1979) with 10 μg/ml of rifampicin.

Bassi and Bolzoni (1982) found that rifamycin SV suppressed thymidine incorporation by mouse spleen cells to PHA, ConA and lipopolysaccharide (LPS) at a concentration of 5 μg/ml. Rifampicin also resulted in a dose-dependent suppression, but this was evident only at concentrations that are toxic to eucaryotic cells.

5. Trimethoprim and sulphamethoxazole

Although Gaylarde and Sarkany (1972) demonstrated a suppression of PHA-induced human lymphocyte transformation by *in-vitro* concentrations of trimethoprim (TMP) and sulphamethoxazole (SMZ) as low as 1 and 5 μg/ml respectively, as might be expected from the structural similarity of TMP to the immunosuppressive agent azathioprine, Forsgren *et al.* (1980) and Banck and Forsgren (1979) could not find any suppression of mitogen-induced lymphocyte transformation over a wide range of concentrations of either antibiotic alone. Anderson *et al.* (1980) found suppression only at very high concentrations of the antibiotic combination, and Arvilommi *et al.* (1976) reported that the lowering of the secondary antibody response to tetanus vaccination that occurred with the administration of a combination of TMP–SMZ could not be duplicated with either TMP or SMZ alone.

6. Antifungal antibiotics

Tarnvik and Ansehm (1974) could not demonstrate an effect of low concentrations of amphotericin B (amp B) or clotrimazole (CTZ) on human lymphocytes stimulated by PHA, PWM, ConA or purified protein derivative. Though higher concentrations of the drugs did affect thymidine incorporation, the effect was negated by serum concentrations of 45% or more.

Roselle and Kauffman (1978) observed that spontaneous transformation of human lymphocytes was significantly depressed by concentrations of amp B varying from 0·2 to 5·0 μg/ml. In fact, concentrations as low as 0·05 μg/ml suppressed spontaneous transformation to as much as 40% of the controls. In contrast, the same concentrations failed to inhibit PHA- and ConA-stimulated transformation but did suppress thymidine incorporation stimulated by streptokinase–streptodornase at concentrations of 1–10 μg/ml. They found that 5-fluorocytosine had no effect. Banck and Forsgren (1979) also found no effect of 5-fluorocytosine on lymphocytes stimulated by PHA and the Cowan I strain of *S. aureus* in a serum-free medium.

Although stimulation of lymphocyte transformation has not been found in studies with human lymphocytes, it has been found with murine lymphocytes. Klein *et al.* (1980) have reported an increase in thymidine incorporation with nystatin concentrations of 0·01–1·0 mg/kg in mice.

7. Other antibiotics

(a) Chloramphenicol

While no effect on PHA-stimulated human lymphocyte transformation has been shown with low concentrations of chloramphenicol (Forsgren and Banck, 1978; Banck and Forsgren, 1979; Forsgren *et al.*, 1980), DaMert and Sohnle (1979) demonstrated that low doses strongly suppress blastogenesis induced by Candida antigen and streptokinase–streptodornase. No effect on PHA-, PWM- or ConA-stimulated lymphocytes was seen in this study, and leucocyte migration inhibition factor production was also unaffected. Chaperon and Sanders (1978) also found no effect on mitogen-stimulated lymphocyte transformation with low concentrations of chloramphenicol.

(b) Erythromycin

Erythromycin at therapeutic levels did not suppress stimulation by PHA (Banck and Forsgren, 1979). In another study, however, lymphocyte transformation by PHA from healthy donors treated with low concentrations of erythromycin was stimulated *in vitro* (van Rensburg *et al.*, 1981).

(c) Fusidic acid

Banck and Forsgren (1979) have shown that fusidic acid significantly suppresses the mitogenic response of B and T lymphocytes at a concentration of 1 μg/ml.

Table 1
Effects on lymphocyte transformation[a]

Stimulus	Drug	Effect[b]	Reference
PHA	Cephalexin/cephradine	D	Chaperon, 1982
PHA	Cefotaxime/cefodizime	I	Leyhausen *et al.*, 1984
PHA	Tetracycline/ minocycline	D	Munster *et al.*, 1977
PHA, SA[c]	Doxycycline/ minocycline	D	Banck and Forsgren, 1979
PHA, PWM	Doxycycline	D	Thong and Ferrante, 1979
PHA	Rifampicin	I	Dajani *et al.*, 1972
		D	Serrou, 1974
PHA, ConA, LPS	Rifamycin SV	D	Bassi and Bolzoni, 1982
PHA	TMP/SMZ combination	D	Gaylarde and Sarkany, 1972
S-S[d]	Amphotericin B	D	Roselle and Kauffman, 1978
none	Nystatin	I	Klein *et al.*, 1980
Candida, S-S	Chloramphenicol	D	DaMert and Sohnle, 1979
PHA, ConA	Fusidic acid	D	Banck and Forsgren, 1979

[a]Representative positive or negative effects only. Null effects are described in the text.
[b]D, Decrease; I, Increase.
[c]Cowan I strain of *S. aureus*.
[d]Streptokinase-streptodornase.

(d) Nitrofurantoin and clindamycin

Both of these antibiotics did suppress lymphocyte transformation and antibody production, but only at very high concentrations (Banck and Forsgren, 1979).

Table 1 summarizes the effects of antibiotics on lymphocyte transformation by various mitogens.

B. Mechanism of Antibiotic Action

The question of whether the antibiotic enters the lymphocyte to exert its immunosuppressive effects or acts predominantly on the surface is still unanswered. The difficulty is in determining how much, if any, antibiotic penetrates the lymphocyte.

Using radiolabelled antibiotics in conjunction with scintillation counting or autoradiography alone does not distinguish between internalized antibiotic and membrane-bound drug. Intracellular death by viable counts of phagocytosed bacteria, the method of choice for phagocytic cells, cannot for obvious reasons be used with lymphocytes (Eltahawy, 1983).

Valinomycin and nonactin, a potassium ionophore, cause the disappearance of a specific and reproducible group of proteins from the map of labelled lymphocyte proteins (Anderson, 1981), and a calcium ionophore induced the production of immune interferon in the absence of DNA synthesis (Dianzani *et al.*, 1980).

The synthesis of cytochrome oxidase has been shown to be depressed in animal cells by tetracycline (Pious and Hawley, 1972), and human blood leucocytes have been shown to accumulate tetracycline to considerably higher levels than exist extracellulary (Park and Dow, 1970). However, the reversal of the inhibition of PWM- and PHA-induced lymphocyte transformation by tetracyclines by washing the cells with the mitogens before culture indicates that some surface effect may be responsible for the suppression of blast formation (Thong and Ferrante, 1979). If lymphocyte transformation is mediated through calcium flux, the chelating properties of the tetracyclines could easily account for their mode of action.

Cefodizime profoundly stimulated the growth of Molt-4 cells, but had no effect on L 5178y cells *in vitro* (Leyhausen *et al.*, 1984). It was shown by studies with radioactive drug that Molt-4 cells and not L 5178y cells bound cefodizime, and this binding was not inhibited by the presence of ceftizoxime. The presence of ConA, however, decreased the growth stimulation by cefodizine. Because trypsin treatment resulted in the loss of all cell-associated radioactivity, the authors suggest that cefodizime binds to the cell surface only and is not taken up.

Gemmell *et al.* (1982) have shown that staphylococcal alpha-toxin binds to the membranes of human and rabbit granulocytes. Petrini and Mollby (1981) demonstrated that purified staphylococcal alpha- and gamma-toxin caused an activation of lymphoid cells from adult human donors as measured by ^{3}H-thymidine incorporation. The lymphocyte-activating properties were shown to be independent of the haemolytic activity, and they suggested that the mechanism involves a non-specific triggering via surface acting properties of the toxins.

Rifamycins inhibit bacterial DNA-dependent RNA polymerase and appear to be more toxic to proliferating cells than resting cells (Benezra *et al.*, 1972). Due to their lipid solubility they may penetrate lymphocytes and affect DNA synthesis directly, but because the effect is reversible by washing the cells (Hauser and Remington, 1982), it is unlikely that this is the primary mode of action. In fact, Paunescu (1970) has shown that in cell-free mammalian systems rifampicin does not inhibit DNA-dependent RNA polymerase unless concentrations in excess of 200 μg/ml are used. Since this concentration is toxic to mammalian cells, any inhibition of DNA synthesis must be evaluated with care. Concentrations much less than this are necessary to demonstrate a suppression of lymphocyte transformation (Banck and Forsgren, 1979) and, in fact, a slight stimulation is seen with 10 μg/ml (Dajani *et al.*, 1972). Effects on antibody production are also seen at concentrations much less than those required for inhibition of DNA-dependent RNA polymerase in cell-free systems (Paunescu, 1970).

Although Wilhelm *et al.* (1978) demonstrated that aminoglycoside antibiotics containing the paronamine moiety can exert a miscoding effect on the translation of natural messengers in extracts of cultured human cells, Forsgren and Banck (1978) and Banck and Forsgren (1979) showed no effect on lymphocyte transformation *in vitro* at 50 μg/ml of gentamicin or kanamycin.

The hallmark of lymphocyte transformation is increased DNA synthesis; however, it appears that this effect can be mediated through the cell membrane. Antibiotics that interact with the lymphocyte membrane or its surface receptors can thus affect lymphocyte transformation and, possibly, other lymphocyte functions as well.

Experimental evidence is consistent with a model of antibiotic modulation of lymphocyte function by interaction with the cell membrane and its receptors. It appears that the antibiotic concentration within the lymphocyte is insignificant in terms of quantity or mechanism of action. The only possible exception to this interpretation involves the antifungal antibiotics which, because they are directed against eucaryotic cells, might be expected to enter lymphocytes in a metabolically active form.

III. EFFECTS ON PHAGOCYTES

Neutrophils and mononuclear phagocytes serve as the cornerstone of defence against invading bacteria because of their ability to phagocytose and kill microorganisms. The process of phagocytosis can be divided into a number of distinct phases: chemotaxis to the site of infection, attachment to opsonized bacteria, ingestion of the bacterium via pinocytosis and intracellular killing (see Fig. 2, p. 188).

Microbicidal activity involves both oxygen-dependent mechanisms, including the production of toxic oxygen radicals and hydrogen peroxide, and oxygen-independent mechanisms, which include the membrane-damaging enzymes lysozyme and lactoferrine.

Several antimicrobial agents have been shown to interfere with phagocytic activity directly by influencing the chemotactic, phagocytic or bactericidal activity of the phagocytic cell, or indirectly by introducing changes in the target organism itself. For a proper assessment of the direct effects of antibiotics on phagocytes, assays using inorganic phagocytosible particles, heat- or formalin-killed microorganisms or measuring various biochemical parameters are employed. When live bacteria are used, it is important to distinguish between direct effects and indirect effects. This can be accomplished by preincubating either the white cell or the bacteria with the antibiotic and assaying in the absence of drug. Care must be taken in proposing a mechanism of action if the drug is present during the assay.

A. *In-Vitro* Effects

1. β-Lactam antibiotics

(a) Penicillins and ampicillin

Gerald Mandell (1973) reported that penicillin did not enter polymorphonuclear leucocytes (PMNs), and that intraleucocytic bacteria were unaffected by its presence. In a later study, Lobo and Mandell (1973) showed that ampicillin killed only extraphagocytic *E. coli*. Low concentrations of nafcillin, oxacillin, methicillin and penicillin (0·1 μg/ml) increased phagocytosis of penicillin-resistant staphylococci if the bacteria were preincubated with the drug for more than 1 h (Friedman and Warren, 1974). If the time of preincubation was less, no effect was noted.

Root *et al.* (1981) demonstrated that *S. aureus* pretreated with low concentrations of penicillin were killed better than untreated controls. In fact, at one-quarter the MIC, the organisms were killed without phagosome formation. Easmon and Desmond (1982) showed that when *S. aureus* was pregrown in sublethal concentrations of penicillin, chemiluminescence was unaffected, but the survival rate of phagocytosed bacteria was half that of untreated controls.

Hand *et al.* (1984) reported that preincubation of *S. aureus* with inhibitors of protein synthesis led to increased phagocytosis and early intracellular killing by alveolar macrophages, but preincubation with penicillin had no effect. These contradictory results might be a consequence of the fundamental differences among phagocytes from different body site of a given species (Pesanti, 1980). Alveolar macrophages are able to phagocytose and kill M-protein positive *S. pyogenes* after opsonization in 10% serum for 15 min while monocytes and PMNs could not (Gemmell *et al.*, 1981*a*). Miller (1969) showed that leucocytes from cord blood phagocytose less efficiently than those from maternal blood.

Proctor *et al.* (1983*a*, *b*) showed that low concentrations of penicillin increased the number of fibronectin binding sites on *S. aureus*, while inhibitors of protein synthesis decreased them. Activation of macrophages results in the production of fibronectin, which is an attractant for connective tissue fibroblasts (Tsukamoto *et al.*, 1981). Verbrugh *et al.* (1981) and Proctor *et al.* (1982) have shown that fibronectin mediates the attachment of staphylococci to human neutrophils. Although chemiluminescence is increased in mixtures of staphylococci and neutrophils when fibronectin is present, the organisms are not killed.

Silva *et al.* (1983) have recently demonstrated that when chronic granulomatous disease granulocytes are preincubated *in vitro* with subinhibitory concentrations of methicillin, microbicidal activity against *S. aureus* is increased. Since clindamycin has no effect in this system, it is improbable that methicillin accumulated in the granulocyte and exerted its activity intracellularly. In addition, no increase in microbicidal activity was noted when only the bacteria were preincubated with the drug.

When *Streptococcus faecalis* was grown in the presence of sub-MIC of penicillin Lorian and Atkinson (1978) reported an increase in the bactericidal activity of serum and plasma. However, Kennedy *et al.* (1983) reported than when *S. faecalis* was preincubated with subinhibitory concentrations of penicillin and moxalactam, no increase in phagocytosis was seen in a serum-free assay.

Ginsburg *et al.* (1982) demonstrated an enhancement of phagocytosis of both opsonized and unopsonized *S. pyogenes* by mouse peritoneal macrophages in the presence of low levels of penicillin. Though inhibitors of protein synthesis did not affect the susceptibility of Group B streptococci to the bactericidal activity of a mixture of human leucocytes and normal human serum, one-third the MIC of penicillin increased killing and resulted in the release of substantial quantities of lipoteichoic acid, lipid and polysaccharide into the medium (Horne and Tomasz, 1981).

Sutton and Weiss (1966) have shown that *in-vitro* culture of blood monocytes results in morphological and functional activities similar to those occurring *in vivo* during transformation into tissue macrophages at extravascular sites. When cultured human macrophages were incubated with ^{3}H-listeria and low concentrations of ampicillin, phagocytic activity was enhanced significantly. No effect was seen when the macrophages were only exposed to the drug prior to the assay (Adam *et al.*, 1974; Adam, 1982).

Nishida *et al.* (1976) demonstrated that one-sixteenth the MIC of carbenicillin enhanced phagocytosis of two *Pseudomonas aeruginosa* strains by rabbit neutrophil granulocytes. The assay was performed in Hank's balanced salt solution (HBSS) to prevent bacterial growth and eliminate serum killing effects. Petit and Daquest (1981) showed that sub-MIC of carbenicillin and ticarcillin enhanced killing of *P. aeruginosa* by human PMNs, and Dalhoff (1984) found a similar increase when *P. aeruginosa* and *E. coli* were preincubated with low concentrations of mezlocillin.

The effect of mezlocillin was shown to be the result of drug interaction with the bacterial mannose-sensitive adhesions. The drug, through its action on the structure of the cell wall, exposed the adhesions tò the phagocytic cells.

Lorian and Atkinson (1979) reported that round cells of *Serratia marcescens* caused by sub-MIC of mecillinam were as susceptible as normal, untreated bacilli to fresh human serum but were more susceptible to the bactericidal effects of fresh defibrinated human blood. However, there was no demonstrable alteration in the antigenic determinants of mecillinam-induced ovoid cells of *S. typhimurium* (Viano *et al.*, 1980).

In 1983, Lorian *et al.* (1983*a*) found that mezlocillin-induced filaments of *E. coli* were phagocytosed as well as normal bacilli if compared on a basis of mass rather than colony-forming units (CFU). In a later study (Lorian and Atkinson, 1984), filaments of *E. coli* exposed to sub-MIC of mezlocillin and ampicillin and filaments of *P. aeruginosa* exposed to azlocillin were phagocytosed at a greater rate than normal, untreated bacilli if the mass of bacteria rather than the CFU is used for comparison. The authors suggested that, in phagocytic assays using β-lactam-induced filaments, counts of CFU to determine phagocytosis and intracellular killing may not be accurate. One bacillus has a mass of approximately 3×10^{-9} mg while a filament may have a mass of up to 50×10^{-9} mg. A single filament could contain up to 20 genomes and will readily separate into 20 bacilli when the drug is removed. However, this filament will give rise to only one colony when plated to agar despite its considerably greater mass. Comparison of phagocytosis and intracellular killing on the basis of CFU alone will greatly underestimate the phagocytic capacity of the PMN for filaments. Jabes *et al.* (1984) reported that the morphologic change induced in *E. coli* by a new Penem antibiotic, FCE22101, did not affect its rate of phagocytosis by human PMNs. However, the response to bacilli and filaments were compared on the basis of CFU.

Mandell (1982) reported an inhibitory effect of penicillin on chemotaxis of human PMNs to C5a and bacterial filtrate in the under agarose method. He also demonstrated a slight inhibitory effect on phagocytosis of diisodecyl phthalate Oil Red O particles, but there was no effect of low concentrations of penicillin on nitro blue tetrazolium reduction. Using the under agarose method and bacterial culture filtrate as a chemoattractant, Forsgren and Schmelling (1977) found no effect of penicillin on PMN chemotaxis.

Chemoattractant receptor-ligand binding promotes the assembly of both microtubules and microfilaments which are required for cellular orientation and migration (Hirata and Axelrod, 1980; Snyderman *et al.*, 1980; Snyderman and Goetzl, 1981). It would appear that any substance that can block the PMN receptor or remove or uncover the bacterial adhesion would affect chemotaxis. Chemotaxis *in vivo* may be influenced by the release of lipopolysaccharide-like substances from bacteria growing in the presence of subinhibitory levels of pencillin derivatives (Goodell and Tomasz, 1978).

Table 2 summarizes the effects of penicillins on phagocyte function.

Table 2
Effects of penicillins on phagocyte functions[a]

Drug	Organism	Effect[b,c]	Reference
Ampicillin	Listeria	I—P	Adam, 1982
Ampicillin	*E. coli*	I—P	Lorian and Atkinson, 1984
Azlocillin	*P. aeruginosa*	I—P	Lorian and Atkinson, 1984
Carbenicillin	*P. aeruginosa*	I—P	Nishida *et al.*, 1976
Carbenicillin	*P. aeruginosa*	I—K	Petit and Daquest, 1981
Methicillin	*S. aureus*	I—K	Silva *et al.*, 1983
Mezlocillin	*P. aeruginosa*	I—K	Dalhoff, 1984
Mezlocillin	*E. coli*	I—K	Dalhoff, 1984
Mezlocillin	*E. coli*	I—P	Lorian and Atkinson, 1984
Penicillin	*S. pyogenes*	I—P	Ginsburg *et al.*, 1982
Penicillin	*S. agalactiae*	I—K	Horne and Tomasz, 1981
Penicillin	*S. aureus*	I—K	Root *et al.*, 1981
Ticarcillin	*P. aeruginosa*	I—K	Petit and Daquest, 1981

[a,b]See footnotes to Table 1 for explanation and abbreviations.
[c]K, Intracellular killing; P, engulfment (phagocytosis).

(b) Cephalosporins and cephamycins

In 1980, Bar-Shavit *et al.* (1980) reported that filaments of *E. coli* grown in low concentrations of cephalexin had similar levels of attachment to macrophages as did normal bacilli in stationary phase. However, exponential phase normal bacilli had markedly reduced attachment. In addition, he found that internalization of filaments was less efficient than that of exponential phase bacilli, stationary phase bacilli or antibody-coated filaments. This was the first paper to show that β-lactam antibiotics can affect internalization and not attachment. It was suggested that, although antibiotic-induced filaments attach well to macrophages, because they are engulfed less efficiently, β-lactams may impair the elimination of certain bacteria by inducing filaments.

Cuffini *et al.* (1980), showed that one-half the MIC of cefazolin enhanced the phagocytosis of *E. coli* by mouse peritoneal macrophages. Intraphagolysosomal killing of *K. pneumoniae* by guinea pig alveolar macrophages was enhanced by the presence of subinhibitory concentrations of cephalothin provided opsonizing antibodies were present (Undeutsch and Brunner, 1981).

A new semisynthetic cephalosporin, AC-1370, killed *K. pneumoniae*, *P. aeruginosa* and *E. coli* at concentrations of one-sixth to one-eighth the MIC when human PMNs were present (Ohnishi *et al.*, 1983). By contrast, cefoperazone did so at one-half the MIC for *P. aeruginosa*, and not at all for *K. pneumoniae* or *E. coli*. In a later study, Ohnishi *et al.* (1984) showed that AC-1370 bound to macrophages and caused the release of a trypsin-sensitive, heat-stable factor that activated neutrophils.

Bassler *et al.* (1982) demonstrated an enhancement of phagocytosis of serum-resistant *P. aeruginosa* by one-quarter the MIC of ceftriaxone. However, the *in-vitro* activity is reduced by the presence of serum since the drug is 95% protein bound. Although Daschner *et al.* (1982) also showed an effect of serum on the enhanced phagocytosis of serum-resistant *E. coli* with ceftriaxone, the improved activity against serum-resistant *Acinetobacter anitratus* was not affected by the presence of serum. Preincubation of *E. coli*, *P. mirabilis*, *K. pneumoniae* and *P. aeruginosa* with subinhibitory concentrations of ceftriaxone reduced adherence to buccal epithelial cells and potentiated phagocytosis and killing (Lianou *et al.*, 1984). A similar effect was shown for *S. aureus* (Borowski *et al.*, 1984).

Low concentrations of cefotetan (Martinetto *et al.*, 1985), azthreonam (Mancini *et al.*, 1984) and ciprofloxacin (Bassaris *et al.*, 1984) were all shown to enhance the phagocytic and bactericidal activity of human PMNs. Although ceftazidime had no effect on PMN migration, the supernatant of *E. coli* grown in one-tenth the MIC of the drug was shown to be a potent

Table 3
Effects of cephalosporins on phagocyte functions[a]

Drug	Organism	Effect	Reference
AC-1370	*K. pneumoniae*	I—K	Ohnishi *et al.*, 1983
AC-1370	*P. aeruginosa*	I—K	Ohnishi *et al.*, 1983
AC-1370	*E. coli*	I—K	Ohnishi *et al.*, 1983
Cefazolin	*E. coli*	I—P	Cuffini *et al.*, 1980
Cefoperazone	*P. aeruginosa*	I—K	Ohnishi *et al.*, 1983
Ceftriaxone	*P. aeruginosa*	I—P	Bassler *et al.*, 1982
Ceftriaxone	*S. aureus*	I—K, P	Borowski *et al.*, 1984
Ceftriaxone	*E. coli*	I—K, P	Lianou *et al.*, 1984
Ceftriaxone	*P. mirabilis*	I—K, P	Lianou *et al.*, 1984
Ceftriaxone	*K. pneumoniae*	I—K, P	Lianou *et al.*, 1984
Ceftriaxone	*P. aeruginosa*	I—K, P	Lianou *et al.*, 1984
Cephalexin	*E. coli*	D—P	Bar-Shavit *et al.*, 1980
Cephalothin	*K. pneumoniae*	I—K	Undeutsch and Brunner, 1981

[a]See Tables 1 and 2 for explanation and abbreviations.

chemoattractant (Gnarpe and Belsheim, 1981). Neither doxycycline nor ampicillin improved the ability of the supernatant to attract PMNs. Fietta *et al.* (1983) could find no deleterious effects of low concentrations of cefotetan or ceftazidime on bactericidal activity or migration. However, cefoperazone markedly inhibited chemotaxis. Jabes *et al.* (1984) also reported a reduction of chemotaxis, but at 5 μg/ml cefoperazone.

Limbert *et al.* (1982) demonstrated no effect of low concentrations of cefotaxime or cefoxitin on opsonized *E. coli*-associated chemiluminescence.

These effects of the cephalosporins on phagocyte function are summarized in Table 3.

2. *Tetracyclines*

In 1950, Munoz and Geister (1950) reported the inhibition of phagocytosis of *Staphylococcus epidermidis* by chlortetracycline in a dose-dependent fashion. Twenty years later Hoeprich and Martin (1970) could not find any adverse effect on phagocytosis with any concentration of tetracycline. Forsgren and Gnarpe (1973) reported no effect of tetracycline hydrochloride, oxytetracycline, lymecycline or doxycycline on phagocytosis or killing, but did find a slight reduction of the bactericidal activity of human serum on *E. coli* with low concentrations of all the tetracyclines tested. When they used a different method a year later, Forsgren *et al.* (1974) now reported that tetracycline hydrochloride and doxycycline definitely inhibited the phagocytosis of bacteria and yeast in a dose-dependent fashion. Although the effect at sublethal concentrations was negligible, this does illustrate that the method has a significant effect on the results.

Martin *et al.* (1974) showed that low concentrations of tetracycline could inhibit both chemotaxis to mycoplasma and influenza antigen and random migration. Belsheim *et al.* (1979) found similar results in the agarose plate method using *E. coli* or *Bacteroides fragilis* LPS as chemoattractants. The antibiotics were not used to pretreat the leucocytes, but were incorporated in the agar. Forsgren and Schmeling (1977) had reported that when tetracyclines were used to pretreat the leucocytes for 30 min, an inhibitory effect on chemotaxis to *E. coli* culture filtrate could be seen at a concentration of 0·5 μg/ml, particularly with doxycycline. They also reported that preincubation was necessary to achieve this effect. Because tetracyclines accumulate considerably within PMNs (Park and Dow, 1970), the length of preincubation might influence the minimum concentration needed to inhibit chemotaxis.

When Limbert *et al.* (1982) pretreated guinea pig PMNs for 30 min at 30°C with low concentrations of tetracycline or doxycycline, they could not demonstrate any effect on *E. coli* phagocytosis-associated chemiluminescence. A similar lack of effect of low concentrations of doxycycline on chemiluminescence, tube migration and glucose oxidation, as well as on migration of PMNs into skin chambers *in vivo*, was shown by Glette *et al.* (1982). However, when the PMNs were irradiated with PUVA light (340–380 nm) a significant decrease in tube migration, chemiluminescence and glucose oxidation was seen. The authors suggested that calcium concentration and photodamage may affect the results of studies of the effects of tetracyclines on PMN function.

3. Aminoglycosides

Johnson *et al.* (1980) reported that gentamicin penetrated poorly into rabbit alveolar macrophages. Barber and Waterworth (1966) used a cell-free system to show that the low pH prevailing in the phagosome reduced the bactericidal activity of gentamicin. Vandaux and Waldvogel (1979) reported that phagocytosed staphylococci were unaffected by the presence of gentamicin, but since the intracellular concentration was approximately 21·5 μg/ml, they suggested that the resistance was due to an inactivation of gentamicin by the low intraphagosomal pH rather than poor penetration. Two years earlier, Bryan and Van den Elgen (1977) had shown that intraleucocytic *S. aureus* could become insensitive to gentamicin by a leucocyte-induced defect in its aerobic transport mechanism which inhibits the accumulation of bactericidal amounts of the drug.

Nishida *et al.* (1976) reported that no concentration of gentamicin affected the bactericidal activity of rabbit PMNs even though the bacteria were pretreated with the antibiotics. Similarly, Root *et al.* (1981) demonstrated that pretreatment of *S. aureus* with subinhibitory concentrations of gentamicin had no effect on subsequent killing by human neutrophils. However, Undeutsch and Brunner (1981) found that subinhibitory concentrations of gentamicin facilitated the intraphagolysosomal bactericidal activity of guinea pig alveolar macrophages when opsonizing antibody was present; in addition, Traub (1982*b*) demonstrated that low concentrations of amikacin, gentamicin and netilmicin enhanced the bactericidal activity of a mixture of human PMNs and defibrinated blood against *S. marcescens*.

Adam (1972) showed that low concentrations of streptomycin increased the phagocytosis of *E. coli* by mouse peritoneal macrophages. Ten years later, Brunner and Undeutsch (1982) reported that one-third the MIC of gentamicin did not affect phagocytosis, but it did reduce the number of viable intracellular bacteria.

When human neutrophils were pretreated with tobramycin and gentamicin, they were shown to have decreased candidacidal activity (Ferrari *et al.*, 1980). However, in contrast to Adam, Undeutsch, Traub and Ferrari, Mandell (1982) reported that low concentrations of gentamicin had no effect on nitro blue tetrazolium reduction, but did decrease phagocytosis of diisodecyl phthalate Oil Red O particles.

Unlike Forsgren and Schmeling (1977) and Mandell (1982), who found no inhibition of granulocyte migration by kanamycin or gentamicin, Seklecki *et al.* (1978) demonstrated that random migration and chemotaxis were inhibited by 1 μg/ml of aminoglycosides. They showed that there was no direct effect on the chemotactic factor. Concentrations of netilmicin, tobramycin and gentamicin as low as 0·25 μg/ml were shown to increase phagocyte adherence to nylon fibres. The contradictory results might be due to the two different methods used to measure migration, since the under agarose method used by Forsgren and Schmeling and Mandell is not as sensitive as the micropore filter technique used by Seklecki *et al.* Dierich and Weikel (1982), using the modified Boyden chamber, found that one-quarter the MIC of gentamicin reduced the chemotaxis of *P. aeruginosa* to 60% of that of the control.

In 1977, Goodhart (1977) reported that injectible gentamicin contains a preservative that could inhibit chemotaxis of human PMNs independently of the antibiotic. Using the under agarose method, a significant difference was found between the migration of granulocytes in the presence of injectible and powdered gentamicin.

4. Clindamycin and erythromycin

Johnson *et al.* (1980) have shown that clindamycin is concentrated 50-fold and erythromycin is concentrated 20-fold by human alveolar macrophages. Both antibiotics are actively transported but, since clindamycin utilizes the nucleoside transport system (Hand and King-Thompson, 1982), its accumulation is stimulated by phagocytosis (Hand *et al.*, 1983; Steinberg and Hand, 1984).

Howard and Soucy (1983) reported that, although preincubation of human neutrophils with one-half the MIC of clindamycin did not affect phagocytosis, preincubation of *B. fragilis* with one-fifth MIC significantly increased phagocytosis. Similarly, Gemmell *et al.* (1983) and Klempner (1984) found an increase in phagocytosis when *B. fragilis* was preincubated with subinhibitory concentrations of clindamycin. However, Wade *et al.* (1983) reported no effect on phagocytosis or intracellular killing of *B. fragilis* following preincubation with low concentrations of the drug. Chemotaxis toward the supernatant of preincubated bacteria was also unaffected.

Klempner and Styrt (1983) demonstrated that clindamycin transport by human PMNs was abolished at pH 5·0, which would be expected under anaerobic conditions or in abscesses. In addition, although they found neutrophil locomotion unaffected by the drug, they demonstrated that the alkalinization of the intraphagolysosomal pH by clindamycin, which is a weak base, inhibits the respiratory burst and enzyme secretion.

Milatovic (1982) reported that staphylococci pretreated with clindamycin were phagocytosed at a higher rate than were untreated organisms, but that killing was not enhanced. In contrast, Elliot *et al.* (1982) showed that when *S. aureus* is grown in subinhibitory concentrations of clindamycin, both phagocytosis and intracellular killing are enhanced, but that chemiluminescence is decreased. Killing in the absence of oxidative metabolism could be due to the accumulation of biologically active clindamycin within the phagocytes (Klempner and Styrt, 1981). However, Vosbeck *et al.* (1984) reported that clindamycin had no effect on phagocytosed *S. aureus* except when present in high concentrations.

Easmon and Desmond (1982) reported an increase in chemiluminescence when Group B streptococci, but not *S. aureus*, were preincubated in one-half the MIC of clindamycin. Gemmell and Dowd (1983) demonstrated an increase in chemiluminescence with *S. aureus* pretreated with one-half the MIC of clindamycin and showed that the degree of chemiluminescence depended on the amount of serum used for opsonization. The authors proposed that clindamycin reduced the amount of protein A on the surface of the staphylococci, resulting in the exposure of a greater number of receptor sites for C3b binding. This mechanism was shown for the enhancement of opsonization, phagocytosis and killing of *S. pyogenes* pretreated with clindamycin by human PMNs and macrophages (Gemmell *et al.*, 1981*b*). Doran and Rissing (1983) showed a decrease in both fibronectin binding to and phagocytosis of *S. aureus* pretreated with clindamycin. However, serum-mediated phagocytosis was unaffected by pretreatment with clindamycin.

Hand *et al.* (1984) found an increase in phagocytosis and intracellular killing by alveolar macrophages of *S. aureus* preincubated with clindamycin and erythromycin. When clindamycin was only present in the assay medium, no increase in phagocytosis of untreated bacteria was seen. It was suggested that the decrease in bacterial protein synthesis induced by clindamycin reduced antiphagocytic surface components.

Van Rensburg *et al.* (1981) and Privitera *et al.* (1984) found no effect of low concentrations of erythromycin on either phagocytosis, chemotaxis or postphagocytic hexose-monophosphate shunt activity. However, a reduction in myeloperoxidase-mediated iodination of *Candida albicans* was seen.

5. Other antibiotics

(a) Chloramphenicol

In 1973, Lehrer (1973) demonstrated a reduction in hexose-monophosphate shunt activity after the ingestion of heat-killed staphylococci or *C. albicans*, but not polystyrene, in the presence of 3·5 mmol/l chloramphenicol. Chloramphenicol also inhibited oxygen consumption regardless of the stimulus. Unlike the situation in granulocytes from patients with chronic granulomatous disease, uncoupling of phagocytosis and the respiratory burst by chloramphenicol depends upon the ingested particle.

Pruul *et al.* (1981) found that a 10-min exposure of *E. coli* to four times the MIC of chloramphenicol, which is sublethal, increased intracellular killing but not phagocytosis. McDonald *et al.* (1981) reported similar findings and noted that chloramphenicol does not enter PMNs to a significant degree. Its activity may be related to its ability to cause incomplete proteins of low molecular weight to be incorporated into the bacterial outer membrane, thereby disrupting its integrity and function and making it more susceptible to the oxidative attack of PMNs (Hirashima *et al.*, 1973).

(b) Rifampicin

Forsgren and Schmeling (1977) showed a significant reduction in chemotaxis of human PMNs preincubated in rifampicin. Bassi *et al.* (1973) reported that the main target of rifampicin in the immune system is the

Table 4
Effects of antibiotics on phagocyte function[a]

Drug	Organism	Effect	Reference
Aminoglycosides	*S. aureus*	I—P, K	Hand *et al.*, 1984
Aminoglycosides	*S. marcescens*	I—K	Traub, 1982*b*
Chloramphenicol	*E. coli*	I—K	McDonald *et al.*, 1981
Chlortetracycline	*S. epidermidis*	D—P	Munoz and Geister, 1950
Clindamycin	*B. fragilis*	I—P	Gemmell *et al.*, 1983
Clindamycin	staphylococci	I—P, K	Elliot *et al.*, 1982
Clindamycin	*S. pyogenes*	I—P, K	Gemmell *et al.*, 1981*b*
Cotrimoxazole	*S. marcescens*	I—K	Traub, 1982*a*
Doxycycline/ tetracycline	*E. coli*, yeast	D—P	Forsgren and Gnarpe, 1982
Gentamicin/ tobramycin	Candida	D—K	Ferrari *et al.*, 1980
Rifampicin	*S. aureus*	I—P, K	Hand *et al.*, 1984 Vosbeck *et al.*, 1984
Streptomycin	*E. coli*	I—P	Adam, 1972

[a]See Table 2 for explanation and abbreviations.

PMN, in which the drug affects pinocytosis and, consequently, chemotaxis and phagocytosis.

Hand *et al.* (1984) demonstrated that when *S. aureus* is preincubated with rifampicin, phagocytosis and intracellular killing is enhanced. Vosbeck *et al.* (1984) also demonstrated an enhanced intracellular killing with low concentrations of rifampicin.

Mandell (1983) has shown that the killing of *S. aureus* inside PMNs and macrophages in an anaerobic environment depends upon the accumulation of rifampicin and subsequent bactericidal activity. Ten years earlier, Mandell (1973) reported that the killing of bacteria inside PMNs by rifampicin requires that the bacteria be actively metabolizing. Rifampicin does not stimulate PMNs to kill bacteria, but exerts its own bactericidal effect intracellularly (Jacobs and Wilson, 1983).

(c) Sulphamethoxazole and trimethoprim

Anderson *et al.* (1980) reported no effects of SMZ or TMP on random migration, glycolysis, hexose monophosphate shunt activity, myeloperoxidase or hydrogen peroxide production of human PMNs. Traub (1982*a*) did find an enhancement of bactericidal activity of PMNs and defibrinated human blood with sublethal levels of cotrimoxazole against *S. marcescens*, but not against *E. coli*.

Table 4 summarizes the actions of various antibiotics on phagocyte function.

B. Mechanism of Antibiotic Action

Bryant (1969) supplied evidence for the necessity of calcium ions for normal functioning of neutrophil phagocytic and chemotactic responses. Alobaidi *et al.* (1981) and Lohr *et al.* (1984) have shown that chemotaxis, lysosomal enzyme release, aggregation and oxygen consumption depend upon calcium as a second messenger and neutrophil adherence, margination and bactericidal activity are regulated by calmodulin, a calcium-binding protein.

That extracellular calcium was not a requirement for stimulus-response coupling in human neutrophils was shown by Smolen *et al.* (1981, 1982) and DeChatelet and Shirley (1982). The level of intracellular calcium, regulated by calmodulin, controls the enzymic processes involved in the phagocytic response. Jones *et al.* (1982) have demonstrated that inhibition of calmodulin-stimulated NADPH oxidase resulted in the inhibition of production of oxygen radicals. Degranulation was shown to be dependent upon calcium (Densen and Mandell, 1980).

It is doubtful that antibacterial agents exert deleterious effects on leucocytes by the same mode of action useful against bacteria. Mammalian cells lack the structural wall components that are the target of β-lactam drugs, and the inhibitors of protein synthesis generally cannot penetrate mitochondria to attack the ribosomes.

It seems likely that the tetracyclines interfere with the regulation of intracellular calcium, and could, depending upon the degree of lipid solubility, affect leucocytes even at low concentrations *in vivo*. Other lipid-soluble antibiotics (e.g. rifampicin) could disrupt the cell membrane and disturb membrane-bound enzymes, and drugs such as clindamycin may accumulate intracellularly to high concentrations, raising the pH to the point where lysosomal release is inhibited.

The potentiating effects of antibiotics seem to fall into three major categories:

(1) altering the structure or integrity of the bacterial cell wall so that opsonization is improved or the cell is more susceptible to the toxic oxygen radicals and lytic enzymes of the PMN;
(2) slowing the growth rate or causing filamentous growth which improves the efficiency of phagocytosis;
(3) substantial intraphagolysosomal accumulation in a bioactive form and exerting antibacterial effects intracellularly.

Subinhibitory concentrations minimize the deleterious effects of antibiotics on the white cell and promote sufficient bacterial effects to potentiate elimination of the pathogen by the host's immune system. However, use of these levels therapeutically must depend upon clinical experience, as the pharmacokinetics of the drug and the immunologic status of the patient, among other factors, affect the outcome.

REFERENCES

Abraham, E. P. (1949). *In* "Antibiotics" (Abraham, E. P., ed.), pp. 1438–1447. Oxford University Press, London.

Adam, D. (1972). *Infect. Immun.* **5**, 537–541.

Adam, D. (1982). *In* "The Influence of Antibiotics on the Host-Parasite Relationship" (Eickenberg, H. U., Hahn, H. and Opferkuch, W., eds), pp. 67–74. Springer-Verlag, Berlin.

Adam, D., Schaffert, W. and Marget, W. (1974). *Infect. Immun.* **9**, 811–814.

Alobaidi, T., Naccahe, P. H. and Sha'afi, R. I. (1981). *Biochim. Biophys. Acta* **675**, 316–321.

Anderson, L. (1981). *Proc. Natl Acad. Sci. U.S.A.* **78**, 2407–2411.

Anderson, R., Grabow, G., Oosthulzen, R., Theron, A. and van Rensburg, A. J. (1980). *Antimicrob. Agents Chemother.* **17**, 322–326.

Arvilommi, H., Vuori, M. and Salmi, A. (1976). *Chemotherapy* **22**, 37–42.

Bakker-Woudenberg, I. A., deBos, M. P. and Michel, M. F. (1984). *Chemotherapy* **30**, 194–204.

Banck, G. and Forsgren, A. (1979). *Antimicrob. Agents Chemother.* **16**, 554–560.

Barber, M. and Waterworth, P. M. (1966). *Br. Med. J.* **1**, 203–205.

Bar-Shavit, A., Goldman, R., Ofek, I., Sharon, N. and Mirelman, D. (1980). *Infect. Immun.* **29**, 417–424.

Bassaris, H. P., Lianou, P. E., Votta, E. G. and Papavassiliou, J. T. (1984). 4th Mediterranean Congress of Chemotherapy, Rhodes, Greece. Abstract No. 239.

Bassi, L. and Bolzoni, G. (1982). *In* "The Influence of Antibiotics on the Host-Parasite Relationship" (Eickenberg, H. U., Hahn, H. and Opferkuch, W., eds), pp. 12–21. Springer-Verlag, Berlin.

Bassi, L., DiBernardino, L., Arioli, V., Silvestri, L. G. and Cherie-Ligniere, E. L. (1973). *J. Infect. Dis.* **128**, 734–744.

Bassler, M., Blaschke, H., Just, M. and Daschner, F. D. (1982). *Chemotherapy* **28**, 390–396.

Belsheim, J., Gnarpe, H. and Persson, S. (1979). *Scand. J. Infect. Dis.* **11**, 141–145.

Benet, L. Z. and Sheiner, L. B. (1980). *In* "The Pharmacological Basis of Therapeutics" (Gilman, A. G., Goodman, L. S., and Gilman, A., eds) 6th edn, pp. 1675–1737. Macmillan, New York.

Benezra, D., Heller, E., Pitaro, R. and Hochman, A. (1972). *Israel J. Med. Sci.* **8**, 897–900.

Ben Redjeb, S., Slim, A., Horchini, A., Zmerli, S., Boujnah, A. and Lorian, V. (1981). 12th International Congress of Chemotherapy, pp. 9–15. Florence, Italy.

Best, W. R. (1967). *J. Am. Med. Assoc.* **201**, 181-188.
Borowski, J., Chyrek-Borowska, S. and Jakoniuk, P. (1984). 4th Mediterranean Congress of Chemotherapy, Rhodes, Greece. Abstract No. 240.
Brunner, H. and Undeutsch, C. (1982). *In* "The Influence of Antibiotics on the Host-Parasite Relationship" (Eickenberg, H. U., Hahn, H. and Opferkuch, W., eds), pp. 129-138. Springer-Verlag, Berlin.
Bryan, L. E. and Van den Elgen, H. M. (1977). *Antimicrob. Agents Chemother.* **12**, 163-167.
Bryant, R. E. (1969). *Yale J. Biol. Med.* **41**, 303-310.
Chaperon, E. A. (1982). *In* "The Influence of Antibiotics on the Host-Parasite Relationship" (Eickenberg, H. U., Hahn, H. and Opferkuch, W., eds), pp. 22-32. Springer-Verlag, Berlin.
Chaperon, E. A. and Sanders, W. E., Jr. (1978). *Infect. Immun.* **19**, 378-384.
Ciak, J. and Hahn, F. E. (1959). *J. Bacteriol.* **75**, 125-129.
Comber, K. R., Boon, R. J. and Sutherland, R. (1977). *Antimicrob. Agents Chemother.* **12**, 736-743.
Cuffini, A. M., Corlone, N. A. and Cimino, F. (1980). *Microbiologica* **3**, 393-405.
Dajani, B. M., Canady, M. S., Thompson, J. S. and Kasik, J. E. (1972). *Lancet* **ii**, 1094-1099.
Dalhoff, A. (1984). *Am. J. Med.* **76**, 91-100.
DaMert, G. J. and Sohnle, P. G. (1979). *J. Infect. Dis.* **139**, 220-229.
Daschner, F. D., Langmaack, H., Bassler, M. and Wais, V. (1982). *J. Antimicrob. Chemother.* **9** (*Suppl. C*), 213-219.
DeChatelet, L. R. and Shirley, P. S. (1982). *Infect. Immun.* **35**, 206-212.
Densen, P. and Mandell, G. L. (1980). *Rev. Infect. Dis.* **2**, 817-838.
Dianzani, F., Monshan, T. M., Georgiades, J. and Alperin, J. B. (1980). *Infect. Immun.* **29**, 561-563.
Dienes, L. (1949). *J. Bacteriol.* **57**, 529-531.
Dierich, M. P. and Weikel, W. (1982). *In* "The Influence of Antibiotics on the Host-Parasite Relationship" (Eickenberg, H. U., Hahn, H. and Opferkuch, W., eds), pp. 139-140. Springer-Verlag, Berlin.
Doran, J. E. and Rissing, J. P. (1983). *J. Antimicrob. Chemother.* **12** (*Suppl. C*), 75-83.
Duguid, J. P. (1946). *Edinburgh Med. J.* **53**, 401-407.
Eagle, H. and Musselman, A. D. (1948). *J. Exp. Med.* **28**, 99-106.
Easmon, C. S. F. and Desmond, A. M. (1982). *In* "The Influence of Antibiotics on the Host-Parasite Relationship" (Eickenberg, H. U., Hahn, H. and Opferkuch, W., eds), pp. 202-207. Springer-Verlag, Berlin.
Elliot, G. R., Peterson, P. K., Verbrugh, H. A., Freiberg, M. R., Hoidal, J. B. and Quie, P. G. (1982). *Antimicrob. Agents Chemother.* **22**, 781-784.
Eltahawy, A. T. (1983). *J. Antimicrob. Chemother.* **11**, 293-298.
Engle, C. G., Lasinski, E. and Gelzer, J. (1970). *Nature* **228**, 1190-1191.
Ferrari, F. A., Pagoni, A., Marconi, M., Stefanoni, R. and Siccardi, A. G. (1980). *Antimicrob. Agents Chemother.* **17**, 87-88.
Fietta, A., Sacchi, F., Bersani, C., Grassi, F., Mangiarotti, P. and Grassi, G. C. (1983). *Antimicrob. Agents Chemother.* **23**, 930-931.
Finch, R. (1980). *J. Antimicrob. Chemother.* **6**, 691-699.
Fleming, A., Voureka, A. and Kramer, I. R. H. (1950). *J. Gen. Microbiol.* **4**, 257-261.

Forsgren, A. and Banck, G. (1978). *Infection* **6**, S91-S97.
Forsgren, A. and Gnarpe, G. (1982). *Scand. J. Inf. Dis.* **33**, 115-120.
Forsgren, A. and Schmeling, D. (1977). *Antimicrob. Agents Chemother.* **11**, 580-589.
Forsgren, A., Schmeling, D. and Quie, P. G. (1974). *J. Infect. Dis.* **130**, 412-415.
Forsgren, A., Banck, G., Beckman, H. and Bellahsene, A. (1980) *Scand. J. Infect. Dis.* **24**, 195-203.
Friedman, H. and Warren, G. H. (1974). *Proc. Soc. Exp. Biol. Med.* **146**, 707-711.
Gardner, A. D. (1940). *Nature* **146**, 837-840.
Gaylarde, P. M. and Sarkany, I. (1972). *Br. Med. J.* **3**, 144-146.
Gemmell, C. G. (1978). *In* "Current Chemotherapy" (Siegenthaler, W., and Luthy, R., eds), pp. 512-514. American Society of Microbiology, Washington, D. C.
Gemmell, C. G. and Dowd, A. O. (1983). *J. Antimicrob. Chemother.* **12**, 587-597.
Gemmell, C. G., Peterson, P. K., Regelman, W., Schmeling, D., Hoidal, J. R. and Quie, P. G. (1981*a*). *Infect. Immun.* **32**, 1298-3000.
Gemmell, C. G., Peterson, P. K., Kim, Y., Mathews, J., Wannamaker, L. and Quie, P. G. (1981*b*). *J. Clin. Invest.* **67**, 1249-1256.
Gemmell, C. G., Peterson, P. K., Schmeling, D. J. and Quie, P. G. (1982). *Infect. Immun.* **38**, 975-980.
Gemmell, C. G., Peterson, P. K., Schmeling, D., Mathews, J. and Quie, P. G. (1983). *Eur. J. Clin. Microbiol.* **2**, 327-334.
Ghilchik, M. W., Morris, A. S. and Reeves, D. S. (1970). *Nature* **227**, 393-394.
Gillissen, G. J. (1982). *In* "The Influence of Antibiotics on the Host-Parasite Relationship" (Eickenberg, H. U., Hahn, H. and Opferkuch, W., eds), pp. 5-11. Springer-Verlag, Berlin.
Ginsburg, I., Lahan, M., Bergner-Rabinowitz, S. and Ferne, M. (1982). *In* "The Influence of Antibiotics on the Host-Parasite Relationship" (Eickenberg, H. U., Hahn, H. and Opferkuch, W., eds) pp. 218-227. Springer-Verlag, Berlin.
Glette, J., Halstensen, A., Sandberg, S., Hopen, G., Hellum, K. B. and Solberg, C. O. (1982). *In* "The Influence of Antibiotics on the Host-Parasite Relationship" (Eickenberg, H. U., Hahn, H. and Opferkuch, W., eds) pp. 33-39.
Gnarpe, H. and Belsheim, J. (1981). *J. Antimicrob. Chemother.* **8** (*Suppl. C*), 71-78.
Goodell, E. W. and Tomasz, A. (1978). *Antimicrob. Agents Chemother.* **13**, 514-526.
Goodhart, G. L. (1977). *Antimicrob. Agents Chemother.* **12**, 540-542.
Goss, W. A., Dietz, W. H. and Cook, T. M. (1964). *J. Bacteriol.* **88**, 112-117.
Hand, W. L. and King-Thompson, N. L. (1982). *Antimicrob. Agents Chemother.* **21**, 241-247.
Hand, W. L., King-Thompson, N. L. and Steinberg, T. H. (1983). *J. Antimicrob. Chemother.* **12** (*Suppl. C*), 1-11.
Hand, W. L., King-Thompson, N. L. and Johnson, D. (1984). *J. Infect. Dis.* **149**, 271-276.

Hartmann, G., Honikel, K. O., Knusel, F. and Nuesch, J. (1967). *Biochim. Biophys. Acta* **145**, 843-844.
Hauser, W. E. and Remington, J. S. (1982). *In* "The Action of Antibiotics in Patients" (Sabath, L. D., ed.), pp. 127-147. Hans Huber, Bern.
Hirashima, A., Childs, G. and Inouye, M. (1973). *J. Mol. Biol.* **79**, 373-389.
Hirata, F. and Axelrod, J. (1980). *Science* **209**, 1082-1090.
Hoeprich, P. D. and Martin, C. H. (1970). *Clin. Pharmacol. Ther.* **11**, 418-422.
Horne, D. and Thomasz, A. (1981). *Antimicrob. Agents Chemother.* **19**, 745-753.
Howard, R. J. and Soucy, D. M. (1983). *J. Antimicrob. Chemother.* **12** (*Suppl. C*), 63-68.
Jabes, D., Debla-Brunner, C., Sanfilippo, A. and Carlo Erba, F. (1984). 4th Mediterranean Congress of Chemotherapy, Rhodes, Greece. Abstract No. 234.
Jacobs, R. F. and Wilson, C. B. (1983). *J. Antimicrob. Chemother.* **12** (*Suppl C*), 13-20.
Johnson, J. D., Hand, W. L., Francis, J. B., King-Thompson, N. and Corwin, R. W. (1980). *J. Lab. Clin. Med.* **95**, 429-439.
Jones, H. P ., Ghai, G., Petrone, W. F. and McCord, J. M. (1982). *Biochim. Biophys. Acta* **714**, 152-156.
Kennedy, E. M., Snowden, N., Westenfelder, G., and Phair, J. P. (1983). *J. Antimicrob. Chemother.* **12** (*Suppl. C*), 69-74.
Klein, D. L., Aszalos, A. and Pearson, J. W. (1980). *J. Immunopharmacol.* **2**, 367-380.
Klempner, M. S. (1984). *Rev. Infect. Dis.* **6**, S40-S44.
Klempner, M. S. and Styrt, B. (1981). *J. Infect. Dis.* **144**, 472-479.
Klempner, M. S. and Styrt, B. (1983). *J. Antimicrob. Chemother.* **12** (*Suppl. C*), 39-50.
Larson, S. E., DaMert, G. J., Collins-Lech, C. and Sohnle, P. G. (1980). *J. Infect. Dis.* **142**, 265-272.
Lehrer, R. I. (1973). *J. Infect. Dis.* **127**, 40-48.
Leyhausen, G., Seibert, G., Maidhof, A. and Muller, W. E. G. (1984). *Antimicrob. Agents Chemother.* **26**, 752-756.
Lianou, P. E., Bassaris, H. P., Votta, E. G. and Papavassiliou, J. T. (1984). 4th Mediterranean Congress of Chemotherapy, Rhodes, Greece. Abstract No. 801.
Limbert, M., Seibert, G. and Schrinner, E. (1982). *In* "The Influence of Antibiotics on the Host-Parasite Relationship" (Eickenberg, H. U., Hahn, H. and Opferkuch, W., eds) pp. 74-86. Springer-Verlag, Berlin.
Lobo, M. C. and Mandell, G. L. (1973). *Proc. Soc. Exp. Biol. Med.* **142**, 1048-1050.
Lohr, K. M., Feix, J. B. and Kurth, C. (1984). *J. Infect. Dis.* **150**, 643-652.
Lorian, V. (1975). *Bull N.Y. Acad. Sci.* **51**, 1046-1055.
Lorian, V. (1980). *In* "Antibiotics in Laboratory Medicine" (Lorian, V., ed.), chap. 12. Williams & Wilkins, Baltimore.
Lorian, V. and Atkinson, B. (1975). *Am. J. Clin. Pathol.* **64**, 678-686.
Lorian, V. and Atkinson, B. (1978). *J. Infect. Dis.* **138**, 865-871.
Lorian, V. and Atkinson, B. (1979). *Rev. Infect. Dis.* **1**, 797-806.

Lorian, V. and Atkinson, B. (1984). *J. Infect. Dis.* **149**, 719–727.
Lorian, V. and Popoola, B. (1972). *J. Infect. Dis.* **125**, 87–94.
Lorian, V. and Waluschka, A. (1972). *Am. J. Clin. Pathol.* **57**, 406–409.
Lorian, V., Atkinson, B., Kim, Y. and Waluschka, A. (1980). 20th Interscience Conference on Antimicrobial Agents and Chemotherapy Prog. Abstract No. 689.
Lorian, V., Atkinson, B. and Kim, Y. (1983*a*). *J. Antimicrob. Chemother.* **11** (*Suppl. C*), 71–75.
Lorian, V., Atkinson, B. and Kim, Y. (1983*b*). *Rev. Infect. Dis.* **5**, S418–S427.
Louria, D. B. and Kaminski, T. (1969). *Arch. Intern. Med.* **124**, 39–41.
Magnussen, C. R. and Hruska, J. F. (1980). *J. Clin. Microbiol.* **12**, 690–691.
Mancini, C., Cipriani, P., Lun, M. T., Giordano, A., Raponi, G. and Filadoro, F. (1984). 4th Mediterranean Congress of Chemotherapy, Rhodes, Greece. Abstract No. 241.
Mandell, G. L. (1973). *J. Clin. Invest.* **52**, 1673–1679.
Mandell, G. L. (1983). *Rev. Infect. Dis.* **5** (*Suppl. 3*), S463–S469.
Mandell, L. A. (1982). *In* "The Influence of Antibiotics on the Host-Parasite Relationship" (Eickenberg, H. U., Hahn, H. and Opferkuch, W., eds), pp. 40–55. Springer-Verlag, Berlin.
Martin, R. R., Wair, G. A., Couch, R. B., Yeager, H. and Knight, V. (1974). *J. Infect. Dis.* **129**, 110–116.
Martinetto, P., Gariglio, M., Scarsi, G., Vietti, G., Stradella, E. and Grosso, C. (1985). *In* "Cefotetan. A Long Acting Antibiotic for Polymicrobial Infections" (Lode, M., Periti, P. and Strachan, C. J. L., eds), pp. 74–79. Churchill Livingston, London.
McDonald, P. J., Wetherall, B. L. and Pruul, H. (1981). *Rev. Infect. Dis.* **3**, 38–44.
Milatovic, D. (1982). *Eur. J. Clin. Microbiol.* **1**, 97–101.
Miller, M. E. (1969). *J. Pediatr.* **74**, 255–259.
Munoz, J. and Geister, R. (1950). *Proc. Soc. Exp. Biol. Med.* **75**, 367–370.
Munster, A. M., Loadholdt, C. B., Leary, A. G. and Barnes, M. A. (1977). *Surgery* **81**, 692–695.
Nishida, M., Mine, Y., Nonoyama, S. and Yokota, Y. (1976). Chemother. **22**, 203–210.
Ohnishi, H., Kosuzume, H., Inaba, H., Okura, M., Mochizuki, H., Suzuki, Y. and Fujii, R. (1983). *Antimicrob. Agents Chemother.* **23**, 874–880.
Ohnishi, H., Inaba, H., Mochizuki, H. and Kosuzume, H. (1984). *Antimicrob. Agents Chemother.* **25**, 88–92.
Park, J. K. and Dow, R. C. (1970). *Br. J. Exp. Pathol.* **51**, 179–182.
Paunescu, E. (1970). *Nature* **228**, 1188–1190.
Pesanti, E. L. (1980). *Antimicrob. Agents Chemother.* **18**, 208–209.
Petit, J. C. and Daquest, C. L. (1981). *Biomedicine* **34**, 29–33.
Petrini, B. and Mollby, R. (1981). *Infect. Immun.* **31**, 952–956.
Pious, D. A. and Hawley, P. (1972). *Pediatr. Res.* **6**, 687–692.
Privitera, G., Lazzarin, A., Ortisi, G., Vigo, B., Capsoni, F. and DePascale, A. (1984). 4th Mediterranean Congress of Chemotherapy, Rhodes, Greece. Abstract No.238.
Proctor, R. A., Prendergast, E. and Mosher, D. F. (1982). *Blood* **59**, 681–687.

Proctor, R. A., Hamill, R. J., Mosher, D. F., Textor, J. A. and Olbrantz, P. J. (1983*a*). *J. Antimicrob. Chemother.* **12** (*Suppl. C*), 85-95.
Proctor, R. A., Olbrantz, P. J. and Mosher, D. F. (1983*b*). *Antimicrob. Agents Chemother.* **24**, 823-826.
Pruul, H., Wetherall, B. L. and McDonald, P. J. (1981). *Antimicrob. Agents Chemother.* **19**, 945-951.
Pulvertaft, R. J. V. (1952). *J. Pathol. Bacteriol.* **64**, 75-77.
Reymann, T. M., Bradac, J. A., Cobbx, C. G. and Dismukes, W. E. (1979). *Antimicrob. Agents Chemother.* **16**, 353-359.
Rolinson, G. N., MacDonald, A. C. and Nelson, D. A. (1977). *J. Antimicrob. Chemother.* **3**, 541-549.
Root, R. K., Istunz, R., Molavi, A., Metcalf, J. A. and Malech, H. L. (1981). *J. Clin. Invest.* **67**, 247-259.
Roselle, G. A. and Kauffman, C. A. (1978). *Antimicrob. Agents Chemother.* **14**, 398-402.
Sabath, L. D. (1982). *In* "The Action of Antibiotics in Patients" (Sabath, L. D., ed.), pp. 74-84. Hans Huber, Bern.
Seklecki, M. M., Quintiliani, R. and Maderazo, E. G. (1978). *Antimicrob. Agents Chemother.* **13**, 552-554.
Serrou, B. (1974). *Lancet* **ii**, 172.
Silva, J., Dembinski, S. and Schaberg, D. (1983). *J. Antimicrob. Chemother.* **12** (*Suppl. C*), 21-27.
Smith, I. M. and Kong, Y. L. (1979). 4th International Symposium on Streptococcal and Staphylococcal Infections, October, Warsaw, Poland.
Smolen, J. E., Korchak, H. M. and Weissmann, G. (1981). *Biochim Biophys. Acta* **677**, 512-520.
Smolen, J. E., Eisenstadt, B. A. and Weissmann, G. (1982). *Biochim Biophys. Acta* **717**, 422-431.
Snyderman, R. and Goetzl, E. J. (1981). *Science* **213**, 830-837.
Snyderman, R., Pike, M. C. and Kredich, N. M. (1980). *Mol. Immunol.* **17**, 209-218.
Spath, P., Garratty, G. and Petz, L. (1971). *J. Immunol.* **107**, 860-869.
Steinberg, T. H. and Hand, W. L. (1984). *J. Infect. Dis.* **149**, 397-403.
Sutton, J. S. and Weiss, J. (1966). *J. Cell Biol.* **28**, 303-332.
Tarnvik, A. and Ansehm, S. (1974). *Antimicrob. Agents Chemother.* **6**, 529-533.
Thong, Y. H. and Ferrante, A. (1979). *Clin. Exp. Immunol.* **35**, 443-446.
Traub, W. (1982*a*). *Chemotherapy* **28**, 369-380.
Traub, W. (1982*b*). *Chemotherapy* **28**, 434-443.
Tsukamoto, Y., Helsel, W. E. and Wahl, S. M. (1981). *J. Immunol.* **127**, 673-678.
Undeutsch, C. and Brunner, H. (1981). *Zbl. Bakt. Hyg. I. Abt. Orig. A.* **249**, 53-62.
Vandaux, P. and Waldvogel, F. A. (1979). *Antimicrob. Agents Chemother.* **16**, 743-749.
van Rensburg, C. E. J., Anderson, R., Joone, G., van den Merine, M. and van Rensberg, A. J. (1981). *Antimicrob. Agents Chemother.* **8**, 467-474.
Verbrugh, H. A., Peterson, P. K., Smith, D. E., Nguyen, B. T., Hoidal, J. R., Wilkinson, B. J., Verhoef, J. and Furcht, L. T. (1981). *Infect. Immun.* **33**, 811-819.
Viano, I., Amaral, L., Atkinson, B. and Lorian, V. (1980). *Curr. Microbiol.* **4**, 309-312.

Viano, I., Marchisio, M., Santiano, M. and Eandi, M. (1981). Proceedings of the 12th International Congress of Chemotherapy, Florence, Italy. p. 12.
Vosbeck, K., James, P. R. and Zimmermann, W. (1984). *Antimicrob. Agents Chemother.* **25**, 735-741.
Wade, B. H., Kasper, D. L. and Mandell, G. L. (1983). *J. Antimicrob. Chemother.* **17** (*Suppl. C*), 51-62.
Weinstein, L. and Dalton, A. C. (1968). *N. Engl. J. Med.* **279**, 467-473, 580-588.
Wilhelm, J. M., Jessop, J. J. and Pettitt, S. (1978). *Biochemistry* **17**, 1149-1153.
Zak, O. and Krandolfer, F. (1979). *Rev. Infect. Dis.* **1**, 862-866.
Zak, O., Vischer, W., Tosch, W. and Krandolfer, F. (1977). *Drugs Exp. Clin. Res.* **3**, 11-19.

NOTE ADDED IN PROOF

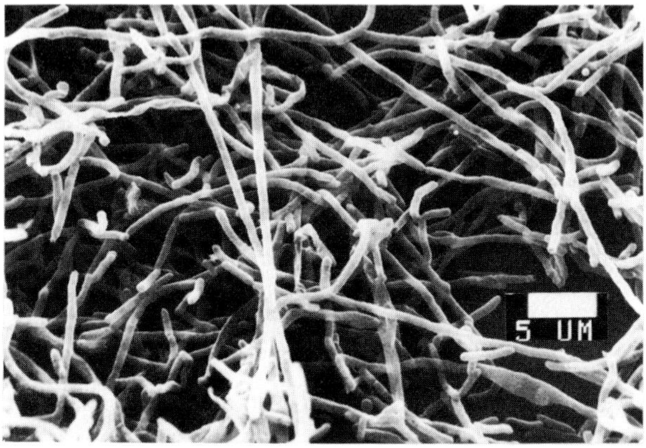

Fig. 1. Filaments of Gram-negative rods produced by low concentrations of ampicillin.

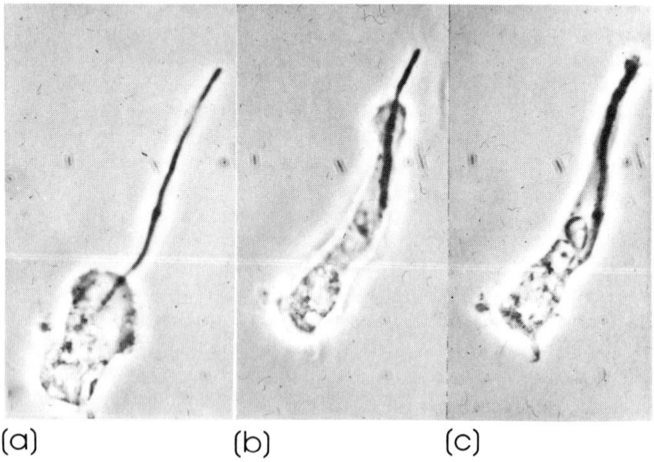

Fig. 2. Phagocytosis. (a) Attachment to opsonized bacteria. (b) Ingestion via pinocytosis. (c) Intracellular killing using oxygen-dependent mechanisms and membrane damaging enzymes.

Chapter 7

Development of Immunological Tolerance to the Mucosa-associated Flora: A Possible Prerequisite for Mitigation of Graft-*vs*-Host Disease in Bone-marrow Transplant Recipients

D. van der Waaij[1] and P. J. Heidt[2]

[1]*Laboratory for Medical Microbiology, University Hospital, Groningen, The Netherlands and* [2]*Radiobiological Institute TNO, Rijswijk, The Netherlands*

I. INTRODUCTION

Following lethal whole-body irradiation and subsequent infusion of allogeneic bone-marrow cells (including mature lymphocytes), the recipient may be immunologically attacked by this graft. The syndrome that follows is called graft-*vs*-host disease (GvHD) and is characterized by emaciation, dermatitis, pneumonitis and liver necrosis. This syndrome can develop acutely soon after transplantation when many mature T lymphocytes contaminate the graft or it may be delayed when a small number of lymphocytes are transplanted along with bone-marrow stem cells. Regardless of the risk of GvHD, transplantation of allogeneic or syngeneic bone marrow has become established as a therapeutic option of definite benefit to patients with acute leukaemia. For patients with an identical twin donor, (syngeneic) marrow transplantation appears to be the treatment of choice in view of the high rate of complete remission even in adult patients, but good results have also been obtained by transplanting allogeneic

Antimicrobial agents and immunity
ISBN 0-12-383830-4

bone-marrow cells from HLA-identical family donors (Bortin, 1984). Progress has been made towards resolution of the problems of transplantation biology that are associated with transplantation of bone marrow from an unrelated (allogeneic) donor (Wagemaker *et al.*, 1982). Efforts to reduce the incidence of recurrent leukaemia by transplantation in remission are still under study. Both the occurrence of GvHD and the eradication of leukaemia appear to be proportional to the number of bone-marrow cells that are transplanted per kilogram of body weight (Bortin *et al.*, 1983). Also the use of immunosuppressive drugs postgrafting has helped to reduce the severity and frequency of GvHD (Storb *et al.*, 1970; Powles *et al.*, 1980). However, both the delayed form of GvHD and the immunosuppressive treatment given to mitigate it involve suppression of the humoral and cell-mediated immunity to microorganisms. This may explain the relatively high incidence and severity of late posttransplantation infections, where this defence is mostly T-cell-dependent, i.e. against viruses, parasites or fungi. Indeed, patients with GvHD and those receiving corticosteroids do have a higher incidence of such infections occurring after day 30 posttransplantation (Atkinson *et al.*, 1979; Winston *et al.*, 1979). Many of these infections are viral and cannot be treated properly so that in about 10% of such patients they are the direct cause of death. Another late complication in these patients is the occurrence of interstitial pneumonia, the pathogenesis of which is not yet fully understood. However, there is evidence that cytomegalovirus (CMV) infection could play a role. Interstitial pneumonia is seen in a little more than half of the recipients who survive for more than 30 days and is associated with a mortality of 60%. Infections—viral, parasitic or fungal—therefore represent a major barrier to long-term survival. After day 30 posttransplantation, a successfully engrafted patient generally does well if GvHD and/or corticosteroid therapy are avoided (Atkinson *et al.*, 1979; Winston *et al.*, 1979). Corticosteroids suppress the cellular immune response to T-cell-dependent infections.

These observations in man show that the success of marrow transplantation is frequently hampered by one of its complications (GvHD) and/or the prophylactic immunosuppressive treatment administered to mitigate this complication. If GvHD could be mitigated without immunosuppressive treatment, late infections might occur less frequently, or not at all. This supposition is based on observations in experimental animals (Jones *et al.*, 1971; Heit *et al.*, 1973; Van Bekkum *et al.*, 1974; Van der Waaij and Heidt, 1977). Mortality among germ-free mice and mice decontaminated with oral non-absorbable antibiotics prior to transplantation of allogeneic H-2-incompatible bone-marrow grafts was significantly reduced as compared with mortality among conventionally maintained mice (Heit *et al.*, 1973; Van Bekkum *et al.*, 1974). The pathological lesions of

GvHD were rare in germ-free mice, although the acute form of GvHD was generally influenced much less by the germ-free conditions than was the delayed form (Van Bekkum *et al.*, 1974). These studies indicate that, at least in rodents, the absence of a microflora at the time of transplantation plays a decisive role in mitigating delayed GvHD without any immunosuppressive treatment. A comprehensive review of the literature on these and related observations may provide more insight into the pathogenesis of GvHD following engraftment of (mismatched) donor marrow, at least in mice. This in turn may provide indications on how to proceed in man in order to avoid delayed GvHD following allogeneic transplantation.

II. INTERACTIONS BETWEEN HOST (IMMUNE SYSTEM) AND MICROFLORA

As the microflora of the digestive tract appears to play an important role in the development of delayed GvHD, studies on interactions between the host and its microflora are reviewed in this section. This concerns investigations performed in normal mice as well as in those suffering from delayed GvHD or a wasting syndrome (WS). The pathological changes in the latter are similar to those of delayed GvHD and occur in animals that are thymectomized at birth (De Vries *et al.*, 1964; Miller and Howard, 1964) or in which the thymus is congenitally absent (Artzt, 1972). The interactions are reviewed systematically starting with the development of the normal flora, with special emphasis on colonization by potentially pathogenic microorganisms and the mechanism(s) which control their colonization pattern. One of the factors involved in this control is the gut-associated lymphoid tissue (GALT); the thymus plays an indirect role. The importance of the nutritional status on thymus function and the immune response is then briefly reviewed. Finally, the possible significance of these observations in the mouse for the understanding of the pathological changes typical for delayed GvHD and WS is discussed.

A. Development of the Microflora after Birth with Special Emphasis on Potentially Pathogenic Microorganisms

The course of the bacterial colonization of the digestive tract in newborns has been investigated in man by a number of investigators (Ehrenkranz, 1970; Bullen *et al.*, 1977; Long and Swenson, 1977; Rotimi and Duerden, 1981). This has also been done under more controlled circumstances in experimental animals (Ashburner and Mushin, 1962; Dubos *et al.*, 1965;

Savage *et al.*, 1968; Savage, 1979). In these studies, the investigators were interested in qualitative and quantitative analyses of the gastrointestinal tract microflora. Only a few studies have been performed in which the number of potentially pathogenic bacteria required for the intestinal colonization of 50% of orally challenged mice (ID_{50}) was investigated. Most of these studies involved adult animals. For example, Mushin and Dubos (1965) reported on the relative ease with which mice of less than 2 weeks of age were colonized with *Escherichia coli*. However, when the fate of 10^5 bacteria given orally to adult animals was followed for 24 h, it appeared that many organisms failed to survive in the entire (intestinal) environment as judged by their decrease in numbers at 3–12 hours after oral contamination. A similar disappearance of bacteria has been described by McGuirre and Floyd (1958) when *Shigella* bacteria were fed orally to mice. Kenny *et al.* (1970) compared the population pattern of resistant *E. coli* 0127 in infant mice, weanlings and adult mice. The weanlings and the adult animals were pretreated with broad-spectrum antibiotics so as to make them more susceptible to oral infection. It appeared that the ID_{50} for antibiotic-treated weanlings and adults was a little higher than 10^3 bacteria, whereas that for sucklings was lower—slightly more than 10^2 bacteria. Adult germ-free mice appear to have an ID_{50} for *E. coli* that is even lower than 10^2 bacteria (Van der Waaij *et al.*, 1971). Later studies by Abrams *et al.* (1963) as well as investigations by Freter (1972) indicated the great importance of the presence of a normal flora for the control of colonization with potentially pathogenic microorganisms following oral contaminations. These observations reported by different investigators indicate that baby mice already have a control mechanism for intestinal colonization. The power of this mechanism increases with age. Furthermore, this resistance to colonization appears to depend greatly on the indigenous intestinal flora, as it is susceptible to broad-spectrum antibiotics. The increase in resistance to colonization after birth has been confirmed and investigated in greater detail by Heidt and Van der Waaij (1979). These investigators performed experimental oral contamination studies in infant mice of 1–28 days of age. Before weaning, the ID_{50} for *E. coli* was found to be approximately 10^3 bacteria. This ID_{50} increased tenfold at weaning to reach its final value of 10^8 bacteria in mice of 4 weeks of age. In animals older than 4 weeks, no further changes were observed. Similar results have been reported by McGuirre and Floyd (1958) and by Bohnhoff *et al.* (1964) as well as from similar contamination studies in antibiotic-treated and normal mice with pathogenic microorganisms such as *Salmonella* and *Shigella* (Abrams and Bishop, 1966; Hentgens, 1967; Maier *et al.*, 1972). The significant differences in ID_{50} between adult mice with a normal flora and the antibiotic-treated animals with a disturbed gastrointestinal microecology have been the subject of investigation by our group since the 1960s. We have investigated which bacteria in the normal flora are involved in the process determining the ID_{50} (Ashburner and Mushin, 1962; Van der Waaij *et al.*, 1971; Van der Waaij and Berghuis, 1973) and also the role of the gut-associated immune system in this mechanism (Heidt and Van der Waaij, 1979) which we have called 'Colonization resistance'. In addition, the effect of several oral doses of different, potentially pathogenic bacteria above the ID_{50} on the occurrence of translocation into the cervical and mesenteric lymphnodes as well as into the spleen has been studied in both irradiated and unirradiated mice (Van der Waaij *et al.*, 1972, 1978; Berg and Garlington, 1979; Van der Waaij, 1981).

B. Colonization Resistance

Colonization resistance (CR) can be defined as the resistance encountered by pathogenic and potentially pathogenic bacteria or yeasts (fungi) when they attempt to colonize either one of the three tracts: the digestive tract, the respiratory tract or the urinary tract. The CR of these three tracts is the resultant of a myriad of cooperating mechanisms. In the urinary and respiratory tracts, these mechanisms are most likely to be excusively of host origin. In the digestive tract, however, host-mediated factors and the indigenous (mostly anaerobic) microflora appear to cooperate very efficiently in determining the chance of potentially pathogenic and pathogenic bacteria to colonize the digestive tract or part of it. Because the digestive tract may be regarded as the most important source of infection for both the respiratory tract (Eickhoff, 1979) and the urinary tract (Stamey *et al.*, 1971), it is of great practical importance to understand the mechanisms involved in the development of a superinfection or overgrowth by pathogenic microbes in the digestive tract. For example, large numbers of potentially pathogenic microorganisms in the oropharynx apparently increase the risk of infection in the respiratory tract (Johanson *et al.*, 1972). This is particularly the case if the mucosal lining is affected by a viral infection or allergies or if the normal flow of mucus is obstructed such as in tracheal intubation (Schwartz *et al.*, 1978).

A decrease in the CR of the alimentary canal will permit colonization of new—not yet colonizing—potentially pathogenic or pathogenic microbes following contamination with low numbers of bacteria. This means that an individual with a decreased CR has a decreased ID_{50} for pathogens and potential pathogens or, in other words, is easily colonized by many different organisms. In that case, these microorganisms (bacteria and/or fungi) will grow into relatively high densities not only in their natural habitat but even in parts of the digestive tract where they are absent under normal circumstances. High numbers of potentially pathogenic organisms may then exist in close association with the mucosa. This condition increases the chance of penetration of the mucosal lining (translocation), which may or may not be associated with an inflammatory response. Whether or not penetration of the mucosa occurs depends on the invasiveness of the organisms and on the condition of the mucosa. Whether or not the presence of potentially pathogenic or pathogenic microorganisms in the mesenteric lymph nodes is detectable is related to their number on the mucosa and on the number of circulating phagocytic cells (granulocytes). Whether or not penetration of the mucosa is associated with an inflammatory response may depend on how the defence apparatus of the host organisms regards the invaders (i.e. as 'foreign' or as 'related'). Not only antibody formation but also complement fixation, the availability of granulocytes and chemotaxis by the organisms may be important. This matter is much more complex than it seems at first. On the basis of animal experiments, it is to be expected that it may also have significance in the pathogenesis of a number of diseases (among which may be GvHD).

C. The Importance of Colonization Resistance

From the information provided so far, it is obvious that the development of a normal indigenous microflora in the digestive tract after birth is of great practical value. With such a microflora, the host organism is well protected against oral contaminations with modest numbers of pathogenic enteric organisms. Secondly, if potentially pathogenic bacteria such as *E. coli*, *Klebsiella*, *Proteus* and *Enterobacter* spp. colonize the intestines, they can do so only in a controlled manner (i.e. in moderate numbers). Like the potentially pathogenic *Enterobacteriaceae* sp. mentioned above, oral contaminations with other microorganisms such as *Pseudomonas*, *Actinobacter* and *Staphylococci* at below 10^4 bacteria may go clinically unnoticed, because the bacteria cannot multiply and adhere in sufficient numbers to the mucosa to enable them to colonize. In this respect, it is important to analyse why many different indigenous bacterial species—composing the normal flora—can adhere freely to the mucosa and live in close association with the host organism while others appear to be 'rejected' after some time. What selective processes are active from birth that give preference to those bacteria forming the autochthonous flora? This chapter will attempt to formulate a working hypothesis concerning the selection criteria determined by the host. For that purpose, the various mechanisms possibly involved from birth will be briefly reviewed.

III. THE IMMUNE SYSTEM AND THE MICROFLORA IN THE CONTROL OF MICROBIAL COLONIZATION OF THE DIGESTIVE TRACT

A. The Gut-associated Lymphoid Tissue

The gut-associated lymphoid tissue (GALT) consists of the tonsils in the oropharynx, the Peyer's patches in the intestinal wall, intraepithelial lymphocytes and the associated lymphoid organs such as the lymph nodes and perhaps the spleen. The effector system is formed by IgA-producing plasma cells, most of which are located directly underneath the epithelial lining of the intestines or the acini of the salivary glands (Craig and Cebra, 1971). A considerable number of investigations have indicated that the primary site of antigen induction of IgA precursor cells to orally administered antigen is in the GALT (André *et al.*, 1975; Kagnoff, 1978). Antigen stimulation of Peyer's patch cells followed by their selective migration to distant secretory tissues may provide an efficient mechanism for immune responses at mucosal surfaces. Joel *et al.* (1970) found that the amount of intragastrically administered carbon particles in the mucosal lining of the intestines was a fraction of that seen in the Peyer's patches. An antigen-sampling role has also been ascribed to the Peyer's patches by other investigators (Brockman and Cooper, 1973; Carter and Collins, 1974). In this context it is tempting to suggest that under normal circumstances IgA (IgM) precursors have—in the presence of T cells (Joel *et al.*, 1971)—their first encounter with antigen inside the Peyer's patches. There is evidence that IgA may have two major functions:

(1) interference with absorption of large immunogenic molecules by complexing with these molecules in the intestinal mucus;
(2) agglutination of bacteria and blocking of adherence pili.

Deleterious inflammatory responses by IgA antibodies have not been reported. On the contrary, these antibodies contribute to the resistance of the host by limiting colonization by microbial pathogens associated with mucosal epithelia. Comprehensive studies have emphasized the importance of selective bacterial adherence in the oropharynx area (Gibbons *et al.*, 1971; Van Houte *et al.*, 1971; Gibbons, 1974). Fubara and Freter (1972) found a marked limiting effect of IgA on the colonization of mice by *Vibro cholerae*. It is intriguing in this respect how the indigenous flora escapes from this control mechanism of colonization.

B. Tolerance by the Gut-associated Lymphoid Tissue

In the 1970s, it became likely that tolerance development to non-self antigens may also occur in the Peyer's patches. Although Chase (1946) had revealed long before that oral feeding of haptens such as picrylchloride diminished contact hypersensitivity to these molecules, it was not until 1975 that André *et al.* (1975) reported that prolonged oral administration of sheep erythrocytes to mice decreased the level of plaque-forming cells in the spleen after systemic challenge with this antigen. Extensive studies by Kagnoff (1978) demonstrated that prolonged feeding of sheep erythrocytes resulted in diminished delayed hypersensitivity due to the induction of suppressor cells. Mattingly and Waksman (1978) reported that oral administration of sheep red blood cells to rats induced T suppressor (T_S) cells in Peyer's patches. Subsequent migration of these cells into systemic lymphoid tissue led to decreased IgM and IgG splenic plaque-forming units to sheep erythrocytes *in vitro*. Finally, bacterial lipopolysaccharides (LPS) may have regulatory effects on the GALT. This has been made likely by Babb and McGhee (1980) in comparing the effect of LPS in LPS-non-responsive (C3H/HeJ) with that in LPS-responsive mice (C3H/HeN) mice. Only in LPS-non-responsive animals was an enhanced splenic immune response to sheep erythrocytes found after previous oral administration; in LPS-responsive animals, oral tolerance was found (Michalek *et al.*, 1982). This tolerance could be ascribed to T_s-cell formation, most probably in the GALT. These authors conclude that LPS from the indigenous gut microflora enhanced the formation of T_s cells during prolonged exposure to antigen. GALT-induced T_s cells would migrate to peripheral lymphoid tissue such as the spleen to account for oral tolerance.

C. Intestinal Flora and Thymocytes

The thymic cortex is a well known site of intensive lymphoregulation and there is evidence to suggest that the majority of the newly formed or instructed thymocytes migrate to other organs (Joel *et al.*, 1971, 1972, 1974). The magnitude of migration of thymocytes into the GALT has been studied by Laissue *et al.* (1976). They found that radioactively labelled thymus cells were rapidly catabolized in the small intestines. Furthermore, in the early periods of postnatal life of mice, the vast majority of the lymphocytes entering the GALT appeared to be of thymic origin (Joel *et al.*, 1972). Work of Cottier *et al.* (1975) has shown that it is likely that the growth of the GALT—and thereby the thymic activity—is largely antigen-driven in mammals. In germ-free mice, Peyer's patches and mesenteric lymph nodes are poorly developed but increase in size when stimulated via the intestinal route. No such reaction has been seen in germ-free animals when the antigens were administered parenterally (Pollard and Sharon, 1970).

The influence of the microflora on the immune system, including the thymus and the spleen, is well illustrated by the following observations made in antibiotic-decontaminated mice: if a mixture of non-absorbable broad-spectrum antibiotics is administered to mice via their drinking water, the digestive tract of the animals becomes free of bacteria in the course of about 4 days (Van der Waaij and Sturm, 1968). In conventional mice, the influence which the intestinal microflora apparently exerts on their immune system has appeared to be considerable. Gut decontamination causes a significant increase in the mean weight of the intestinal walls of the ileum and the colon and a concomitant decrease in the weights of the spleen and the thymus in the first 2 weeks of antibiotic decontamination of the digestive tract (Van der Waaij, 1969). The increase in the weight of the intestinal wall was found to be due to large accumulations of mononuclear cells (presumably lymphocytes) in the submucosa. The decrease in the weight of both the spleen and the thymus started rapidly after the initiation of antibiotic decontamination of the digestive tract. The thymus decreased from an average weight of 51 mg (s.d. = 2·7) before treatment to 40 mg (s.d. = 6·8) after 2 weeks of oral antibiotic treatment. The spleen lost 20 mg on the average in these 2 weeks. This suggests that the intestinal microflora has a regulatory influence on the lymphoid system (thymus). This conclusion is supported by the fact that in adult germ-free mice the mean weight of the thymus is significantly lighter than in their conventional counterparts (Wilson *et al.*, 1964; Bealmear and Wilson, 1966).

D. Concanavalin A and the Formation of T-suppressor Cells

Early studies by Dutton (1973) and Rich and Pierce (1974) indicated that splenic T cells can be activated by the T-cell mitogen concanavalin A (ConA) to become cells which suppress the immunological function of other cells. Furthermore, Rich and Pierce have shown that ConA-activated splenic cells produce a soluble immune response suppressor substance that is suppressive to humoral immune responses *in vitro*.

In the spleen of a mouse strain with genetically determined early thymus involution (NZB/W mice; Barthold *et al.*, 1974), Krakauer *et al.* (1976) found losses of precursors of T_s cells as these animals age. These authors showed that if spleen cells of adult and young (< 3 weeks old) normal mice such as BALB/c, C57BL and of adult or 18-week-old NZB/W mice were cultured *in vitro* in the presence of pokeweed mitogen—a B-cell mitogen—they produced significant quantities of IgM in the 7-day culture period. However, when 2 μg/ml of ConA was added to the cultures along with the pokeweed mitogen, there was an 80–94% suppression of IgM biosynthesis by the spleen cells from adult normal or young NZB/W mice. In contrast, addition of ConA to the cultures caused significantly less (only 27%) suppression of IgM synthesis by spleen cells of the adult NZB/W mice. Gershwin (1978) has reviewed data showing that formation of T_s cells occurred in mice if they had been previously injected with ConA. Suppression of immune responses against sheep red blood cells was evident both *in vivo* and *in vitro*.

E. The Effect of Dietary Protein Deficiency on Suppressor Cells

Deficiency in dietary protein during growth and development interferes not only with maturation of all organs and tissues but also with the development of T cells and particularly of T suppressor cells. Cooper *et al.* (1975) and later Kohrshidi and Mohagheghpour (1979) have shown this convincingly in mice, while experiments of Raffi *et al.* (1977) made it likely in malnourished children. This may imply that in protein-deprived newborns the development of tolerance in the GALT to antigenically related mucosa-associated bacteria (see later) can be reduced. Therefore, anaerobic bacteria in protein-deprived individuals may not form the normal protective blanket in the mucous layer on the mucosa. Absence of parts of this heterogenic mucosa-associated flora (e.g. due to immunological rejection by IgA instead of induction of tolerance) may interfere with the complex physiological regulatory function of this part of the intestinal flora.

F. Bacterial Adherence to Mucosal and Other Cells

Bacterial adherence involves both host and microbial factors. In the case of epithelial and blood cells, receptors are required for attachment, while microbes must have structures which fit into these receptors. Such structures on bacteria are called pili or fimbriae (Gibbons *et al.*, 1976). Pili are filamentous appendages on the cell wall of bacteria and are demonstrable by electron microscopy. They are smaller and more numerous than flagellae and unrelated to bacterial motility (Brinton, 1967). The mechanism of binding of potentially pathogenic Gram-negative bacteria to oral epithelial cells is not yet well understood. It appears to involve sugar-containing binding sites (Ofek *et al.*, 1977). The finding that ConA inhibits adherence in a dose-related manner (Johanson *et al.*, 1979) suggests a finite number of such binding sites on the cell surface. A similar conclusion can be drawn from the studies reported by Woods *et al.* (1980). These investigtors found that preincubation of buccal epithelial cells with purified bacterial pili before an adherence assay was performed caused a dose-related decrease in adherence of *Pseudomonas aeruginosa*.

G. The Intestinal Flora and Specific IgA Production

In man but also in animals, the anaerobic bacteria outnumber the so-called facultatively anaerobic or 'aerobic' bacteria in the ileum and in the large intestine. As mentioned earlier, there the anaerobes may have a crucial function in the control of the aerobic, potentially pathogenic intestinal population. They may do this largely by the blocking of receptor sites on the mucosa and/or by steric hindrance of adherence by potentially pathogenic bacteria. These CR-associated anaerobes appear to compose a bacterial 'wallpaper' or 'blanket' on the mucosa in the mucus layer, which may be a major source of nutrients for this flora. Irradiation (Van der Waaij and Berghuis, 1973; Van der Waaij *et al.*, 1978) and chemotherapy studies (Berg, 1983) have shown that it is likely that in mice the CR decreases possibly as a result of a decrease in the number of goblet cells in the mucosa. This reduced mucin secretion may result in a reduction of the 'feeder layer' of the anaerobic wallpaper of the gut. However, loss of T cells due to irradiation or chemotherapy may also have resulted indirectly in a reduction in mucus secretion (Lake *et al.*, 1979).

The GALT activity was studied in a more direct way in sublethally irradiated (6 Gy) mice (Van der Waaij and Heidt, 1977). In these animals, it was investigated whether and if so which bacteria in the intestinal flora (freshly voided faeces) were coated with IgA antibodies. This investigation of IgA coating of faecal bacteria started before irradiation and was repeated on alternate days for 6 weeks. Briefly, fresh faeces were suspended in water 1:3 (w/v), centrifuged and an aliquot of the supernatant was then mixed with fluorescent rabbit antimouse IgA. After incubation at 4°C for 3 h, drops of these suspensions were put onto McConkey agar covering microscopic slides. Subsequent observation of such a slide with an ultraviolet microscope revealed the presence and the location of IgA-coated bacteria on the agar layer. Overnight incubation of the slide at 37°C permitted the Gram-negative bacteria to form microcolonies, so that the location of the various IgA-coated bacteria directly after preparation of the slide could be compared with the location of colonies of *Enterobacteriaceae* on the slide. During the 6 weeks of this experiment in mice, the CR of the animals was monitored by investigating the concentration of *Streptococcus faecalis* and Gram-negative bacteria in the faeces of each mouse (Van der Waaij and Berghuis, 1973). The study revealed that, after irradiation, concomitantly with a decrease in the CR (increase in the concentration of the potentially pathogenic bacteria), the number of IgA-coated bacteria decreased to an undetectable low level in the first week. When in the third week the CR (i.e. the concentration of potentially pathogenic bacteria) returned to preirradiation values, IgA coating of Gram-negative bacteria returned to preirradiation levels in the fourth week.

A second point of importance in this study was that, before as well as long after irradiation, most (99%) of the faecal bacteria were not IgA-coated. In fact, only *Enterobacteriaceae* spp. and *S. faecalis* were found to be IgA-coated. More recent studies by Van Saene and Van der Waaij (1979), using essentially the same technique as described above, have shown that healthy human individuals also have only a fraction of their intestinal bacteria coated with IgA. As in mice, the anaerobic majority of the flora was found not to be IgA-coated. These observations in man and mice suggest that either anaerobic bacteria and/or their antigens do not enter the Peyer's patches or else that they are not immunogenic to their host species. No antigenic contact between anaerobes and the GALT seems very unlikely, since all kinds of antigens—even sheep erythrocytes and carbon particles (see previous paragraph)—appear to be picked up readily by the Peyer's patches in experimental animals. Consequently, the autochthonous anaerobic microflora may not be or be very slightly immunogenic to the GALT. This is in accord with observations reported by Foo and Lee (1972) in mice and rats. When their animals were parenterally injected with autochthonous *Bacteroides* vaccines, they did not respond immunologically, whereas high titres were found when an *E. coli* or a *Proteus mirabilis* strain was injected. Guinea pigs, rabbits and sheep responded well to the *Bacteroides* vaccine, so that the failure of mice to respond cannot be attributed to a lack of antigen. A possible explanation for the observations of Foo and Lee is that, because of the continued association of the organism with the rodent host, a state of immunological tolerance was achieved. This may not be induced directly after birth but a little later, since *Bacteroides* species normally do not establish in the mouse intestine until 2 weeks after birth (Savage *et al.*, 1968; Savage, 1977). Also other evidence supports the hypothesis that an animal's immunological response affects the composition of the indigenous flora. As predicted by Dubos *et al.* (1965), indigenous microorganisms not uncommonly prove to have a poor or a totally absent capacity to induce antibodies, especially when only present in the gastrointestinal canal. When investigated, such microorganisms often share antigens with the mucus or the mucosa of the gut in which they normally have their habitat (Van der Waaij, 1983). These and similar findings concerning antigenic similarities between intestinal microorganisms and their animal hosts suggest that such microbes have evolved to a close immunological relationship with the host animal. At least, the cell-wall components of the bacteria that contact the animal's mucosal cells must perhaps be sufficiently related to the host's antigens so as to render them recognizable as 'self' by the animal's immune system. Otherwise, bacteria that tend to colonize the mucosal membrane may elicit a GALT immune response and thereby their rejection. Being recognized as 'self' may provide microorganisms an enormous advantage over others and may permit them to become indigenous and colonize their natural habitats in the digestive tract.

IV. AETIOLOGY OF WASTING DISEASE IN THYMUSLESS MICE

As mentioned earlier, there is much in common between GvHD and wasting disease (WD). This justifies a brief discussion of the aetiology of WD. Removal of the thymus within a strictly determined short period after birth impairs the immune response of mice to skin allografts (Miller, 1962) and to grafts of foreign cells (Parrot, 1962; Parrot and East, 1962). Neonatally thymectomized and congenitally thymusless (nude) mice develop a wasting syndrome (WD) after a period of normal growth and development. The WD is characterized by a gradual deterioration in the physical condition of the animals. They suffer diarrhoea, progressive loss of weight and a severe depletion of lymphocytes in the lymph nodes, spleen and peripheral blood (Jutila, 1973). Although the onset of the WD in thymusless animals is not accompanied by any obvious bacterial invasion of tissues, the intestinal colonization pattern changes at the time that the physical deterioration begins. At that time, both the number of different *Enterobacteriaceae* biotypes that colonize the animals when maintained conventionally (not isolated) as well as the concentration of Gram-negative bacilli increases in their faeces. According to investigations of Nomura *et al.* (1974) and Owens and Berg (1980), translocation of these bacteria to the mesenteric lymph nodes may then occur. Implantation of a thymus reverses the situation.

Mice that suffer from WD not only compare well with those that suffer from delayed GvHD but also histologically and serologically have many characteristics of autoimmune phenomena (Monier *et al.*, 1974; Okudaira *et al.*, 1977; Holland *et al.*, 1978). Just as GvHD is strongly mitigated in bacteria-free mice, congenitally thymusless mice which are maintained germ-free do not develop WD (Wilson *et al.*, 1964), nor do they do so when the potentially pathogens or pathogens from their flora are eliminated by means of antimicrobial drugs (selective decontamination). WD also does not develop when nude mice harbour a microflora which is free of potentially pathogenic microorganisms and the animals are maintained isloated under specific pathogen-free conditions (Van der Waaij, 1981).

V. THE COLONIZATION PATTERN OF BIOTYPES OF *ENTEROBACTERIACEAE* SPECIES IN MAN AND MICE

To obtain a better insight into the needs of prophylactic treatment for Gram-negative infections in individual granulocytopenic patients, the faeces and oral washings of patients with acute leukaemia have been analysed (Van der Waaij, 1982). For a minimum of 5 weeks, biweekly oral washings and faecal samples were obtained for culturing and subsequent typing of the Gram-negative bacilli. Only the results of patients who either had received no antibiotic therapy during the period that they were on the study or had received it for less than 5 days were included. The results in 41 patients and in 14 healthy subjects indicated that in each individual the mean number of different biotypes per faecal sample did not change markedly during the 5-week period that they were on the study. Among patients as well as among healthy volunteers, however, significant differences were noticed. No obvious differences were observed between the two groups if they were regarded as a group. A similar result was obtained in a subsequent study in conventional inbred mice, although with lower average numbers of biotypes per faecal sample. The mice were maintained in a germ-free isolator during the observation period so as to guarantee that the only sources of Gram-negative contaminations were items inside the isolator (i.e. cage mates and the food pellets). These had a known total number of 12 biotypes of *Enterobacteriaceae* spp.

The results of this study showed that, although the animals were inbred (genetically identical), their Gram-negative (aerobic) flora was different. Some animals entered the study (first week) with an average of two different biotypes per gram of faeces, whereas others had only one. These differences between animals remained present during the 5-week study period. As in man, sublethal irradiation did not significantly change these results. In animals which had an average low number of different biotypes in their faeces before irradiation, this average did not change. Mice with an average of two different biotypes before irradiation increased very modestly in this respect to around three biotypes per week.

The intriguing points in these observations are: (1) different individuals with similar chances of becoming contaminated with biotypes of *Enterobacteriaceae* spp. yet appear to make their own selection out of a 'common contamination source'. Some individuals appear to permit more different biotypes to pass through their alimentary canal to appear in the faeces in detectable numbers than do others who are much more 'selective'; (2) this occurs not only in man in a hospital community but also among inbred mice inside an isolator, i.e. with a known contamination source (food and cage mates). This property of permitting fewer or more biotypes through the digestive tract is apparently phenotypically determined, as it was found not only in genetically unrelated individuals (man) but also in genetically related (inbred) mice. Since the mice entered the study with different numbers of biotypes in their faeces and remained so during the study period, they must have acquired this property before the experiment, most likely from their mothers in the breeding unit. However, we did not trace from which dams the animals originated, so that we can only speculate that some mice were exposed after birth to a flora that differed in some respect from that of others. Differences in the flora acquired between birth and weaning appear to be quite permanent, since the differences in the excretion of biotypes did not change when animals with different numbers of biotypes shared the cage during the experimental period. Cross-contamination with anaerobic (possibly CR-associated) flora will have occurred under these circumstances, as happened with *Enterobacteriaceae* spp. However, cross-contamination with anaerobes apparently did not result in colonization to equalize the CR of all mice in the cage.

Comparison of the results obtained in this study with those subsequently obtained in congenitally thymusless mice (Van der Waaij, 1981) makes it likely that the thymus plays a decisive role in the determination of the composition of the flora of mice. In a conventional room, they behaved differently to the likewise occurring oral contaminations with Gram-negative bacilli than did other animals of the same strain. The thymusless animals did all have a significantly increased turnover of different biotypes in their faeces from the age of 6 weeks onwards. However, no obvious individual differences in the mean number of biotypes were seen when thymusless mice were maintained isolated in a specific pathogen-free room. This implies that, during ageing, the animals can apparently not maintain a normal Gram-negative intestinal colonization pattern unless they are isolated so that there is no other serious contamination source in their environment. The increase in the turnover of biotypes in the faeces after the age of 6 weeks could be the consequence of a gradual rejection of components of the anaerobic CR-associated flora.

Recently, Van de Merwe *et al.* (1983) reported that in man not only the aerobic but also the anaerobic intestinal flora differs between individuals. In human twins, these investigators found differences only when they were not identical. This suggests that in man genetic identity may play a stronger role in the composition of the flora than in mice. On the other hand, each of the human twins studied by Van de Merwe *et al.* (1983) were obviously delivered by one mother, whereas the inbred mice employed in our study came from a minimum of eight different dams. As a consequence, these mice had been born and housed in eight different cages until weaning at 3 weeks of age. This suggests that in mice the colonization pattern of the Gram-negative intestinal flora observed later in life is perhaps largely determined by the composition of the indigenous anaerobic flora acquired in the first weeks after birth. This may concern not only the anaerobic but also some *Enterobacteriaceae* spp. of the maternal flora. Lack of IgA antibody production towards most bacteria acquired before weaning could be a determinant factor in their prolonged (possibly life-long) colonization of the gut.

VI. IMMUNOGENICITY OF BACTERIA

A. Cellular (Cytotoxic) Immunity to Cross-reactive Antigens

Delayed-type hypersensitivity to tissue antigen seems not to be induced by the presence of soluble cross-reactivity between microbial and tissue antigens. For eliciting a cellular lymphocytotoxic hypersensitivity, there must be large-sized common sites in both microbial and tissue antigens. The common sites must be larger than is required for a humoral cross-reactive response.

Ruddle and Waksman (1968) demonstrated *in vitro* that injury to tissues can still occur in the presence of cell-mediated reactions to microbial antigens. In contrast to foreign animal proteins, some bacterial antigens are capable of inducing prolonged delayed-type hypersensitivity (Salvin, 1958). No circulating antibodies are present in those cases. This reaction may be caused by the presence of lipid components in most bacteria which may serve as adjuvants enhancing cellular responses (Munoz, 1964; Chiller *et al.*, 1973; Peavy *et al.*, 1978). Thus, in contrast to soluble components, intact microbial cells may induce cellular immunity not only following inoculation via special routes (foot pad) but with any mode of penetration into the organism. Some cross-reactive antigens could thus evoke a pronounced and prolonged cytotoxic reaction which would promote the development of an autoimmune process.

B. Humoral Immunity to Antigens Common to Host and Microorganisms

Envelopes of *E. coli* have been found to cross-react with some animal mitochondrial membrane structures (Okuda and Weinbaum, 1969).

Common enterobacterial antigen (CEA) has been shown to possess an antigenic relationship with colon cell membranes and patients with inflammatory bowel disease have been found to have elevated titres of humoral antibody to this common antigen (Bull and Ignaczak, 1973). Others have found immunogenic cross-reactivity between human liver, kidney, muscle and heart tissues and CEA (Morgenstern and Gorzynski, 1977). Van de Rijn *et al.* (1977) reported the occurrence of (human) heart-reactive antibodies which also bind to skeletal muscle and smooth muscle of blood vessel walls following group A Streptococcal infection or inoculation into rabbits. The presence of cross-reacting antigens between *Lactobacillus casei* and neurological brain cells and between *Propionibacterium acnes* and kidney glomeruli has been reported by Stinson *et al.* (1977). Welsh *et al.* (1980) demonstrated cross-reactivity with human tissue typing sera in patients with ankylosing spondylitis. Cross-reactivity of *Streptococcus mutans* antigens and human heart tissue was also reported recently by two different groups (Ferretti *et al.*, 1980; Hughes *et al.*, 1980).

VII. BONE-MARROW TRANSPLANTATION STUDIES IN MICE

It is possible to recognize arbitrarily two types of graft-*vs*-host disease (GvHD) that may develop after lethal whole-body irradiation and transplantation of mismatched bone-marrow cells. These are the *acute type* and the *delayed type* of GvHD (Vos *et al.*, 1959; Grushka and Lapp, 1974; Korngold and Sprent, 1978). The acute type is seen when marrow grafts which contain a large number of T lymphocytes are transplanted. This results in mortality within 30 days after transplantation. Elimination of most of the T lymphocytes from the graft *in vitro* prior to infusing the marrow into the recipient results in a delay of GvHD if the recipient has a conventional microflora. There is an abolition of the syndrome if the flora is absent at the time of transplantation and for several weeks afterwards (see also the Introduction).

There is little doubt that GvHD is caused by donor T lymphocytes. The acute type of GvHD is caused by committed T lymphocytes in the graft, whereas the delayed type is ascribed to T cells which have been developed from the stem-cell level and which have matured in the recipient. However, the question of how these cells become sensitized is still open as long as the origin of the antigens involved is still uncertain. These antigens could be of host tissue origin but, on the basis of the information given above, they can very well be of bacterial origin; for example, they may originate from the mucosa-associated flora of the recipient animal. To investigate this assumption, we have performed a series of experiments attempting to elucidate the question of the involvement of the microflora. In the experimental protocol, we aimed to compare the incidence of GvHD following allogeneic marrow transplantation in a standardized donor/recipient combination. In all the experiments, the donor mouse strain was C57BL/Rij and the recipient mice (15–20 mice per group) were 12-week-old

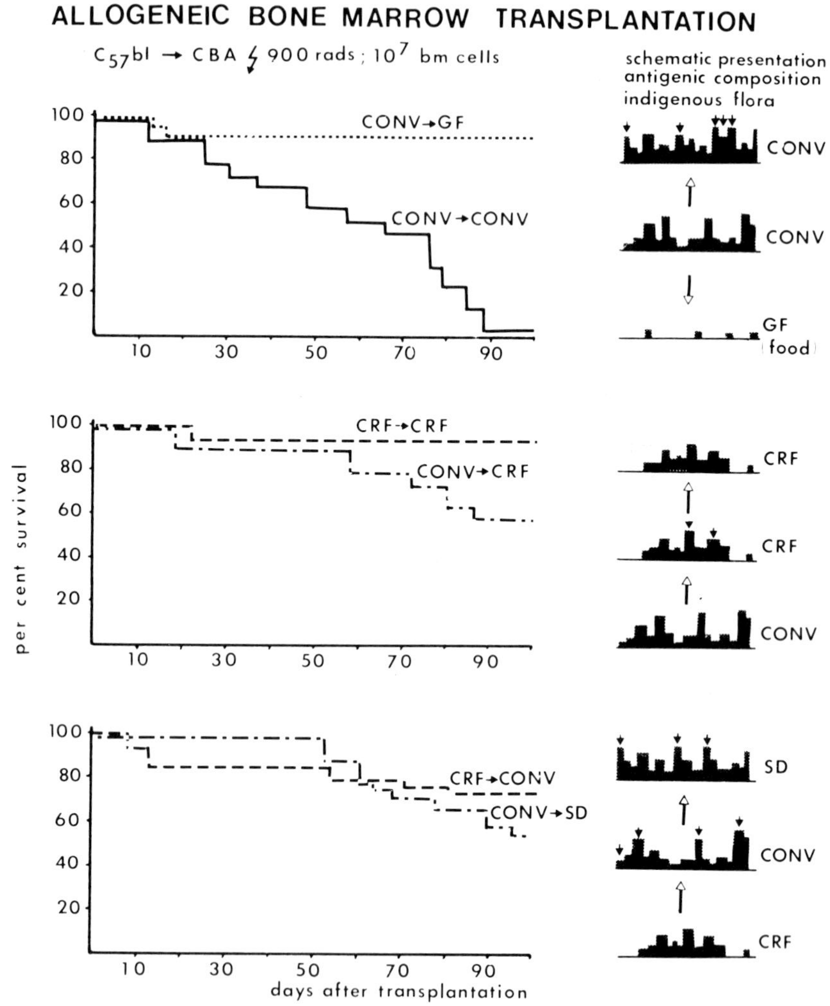

Fig. 1. Results of a pilot study in which allogeneic (C57BL) bone marrow was transplanted into (CBA) recipient mice. In the six experiments presented, the floras of donor and recipient differed, were identical (CRF CRF) or there were none in the recipient (GF). The skyline of the antigen composition of the flora is hypothetical and is presented only to illustrate the hypothesis forming the basis of the proposed investigation. The arrows mark differences in antigenic composition of the indigenous flora between donor and recipient mice.

CBA/Rij females. On the day before transplantation, the animals received 9 Gy whole-body irradiation. For transplantation, they were infused with 10^7 bone-marrow cells. From experiment to experiment, the donor and recipient animals had either no microflora, an identical indigenous flora or a different indigenous microflora. In using the term microflora, all microbial strains and species (mainly anaerobic bacteria) which colonized the digestive tract and skin are meant. Including the mice with a conventional flora, all animals originated from the same germ-free stock. Animals designated as CRF had been associated (at birth) with a mouse-derived anaerobic intestinal flora (Van der Waaij *et al.*, 1977) and were maintained isolated from birth. Mice indicated as conventional had for several generations been maintained in an open animal room and were originally conventionalized ex-CRF mice. Finally, animals with a flora indicated as SD were conventional mice that were treated with polymyxin E (colistin) in their drinking water so as 'selectively' to eliminate their aerobic Gram-negative potentially pathogenic flora (Emmelot and Van der Waaij, 1980). Polymyxin treatment was applied during the entire period of the experiment, i.e. from 2 weeks prior to irradiation up to day +100. The various floras in the donor/recipient combinations as well as their survival after transplantation are depicted in Fig. 1. Figure 1 also gives a schematic skyline of a hypothetical antigenic profile of the various mucosa-associated floras. The germ-free mice in this scheme were assumed to have some dead bacterial antigens originating from the diet in their digestive tract represented by the few small blocks that may form their skyline. Furthermore, on the basis of the data reviewed above, it was assumed but not proven by comprehensive culturing that mice of different mouse strains would have a different microflora.

The floras of the animals in our experiments may have differed in many respects, not only regarding the aerobic bacteria but also regarding the anaerobes. This assumption is realistic because the conventional donors and recipients were maintained under conventional conditions at different places. The mice of the two strains were found to have different *Enterobacteriaceae* biotypes in their faecal cultures.

The survival curves after transplantation depicted in Fig. 1 confirm previous experiments in germ-free (GF) and colonization resistance flora (CRF) mice (Van Bekkum *et al.*, 1974). Identity in microflora (CRF flora) between donor and recipient mice appeared to have the same preventative effect on the occurrence of GvHD and thus enhanced long-term survival as did the absence of a flora (GF) in the recipient. However, if the donor had a more complex (conventional) flora than the (CRF) recipient mice, almost 50% of the recipients died of delayed GvHD. Also in the reverse situation in an experiment in which the donor animals had a CRF flora and the recipients had been maintained conventionally since birth, a certain percentage of the mice developed signs of GvHD (i.e. diarrhoea, loss of weight and death after day +50). In the experiment in which SD mice were recipients, the results were comparable to those seen in the CRF recipients: about 40% mortality occurred, most likely due to GvHD.

Although these observations must be regarded with caution because no systemic autopsy study was done, with the result that no histological data confirming GvHD are available, these preliminary results are presented, as they may illustrate the complexity of the possible role of the microflora in the pathogenesis of chronic GvHD. The data were considered to be of value for us to formulate a working hypothesis for further investigations.

VIII. DISCUSSION

This chapter permits a number of tentative conclusions which are necessary for the formulation of a working hypothesis for future investigations. These conclusions are:

(1) Adult mice are markedly more resistant to oral contamination with *Enterobacteriaceae* spp. and other potentially pathogenic Gram-negative bacilli when they have an indigenous anaerobic microflora than when they lack this microflora.

(2) After weaning, conventionally maintained mice respond individually different to oral contamination with Gram-negative bacilli. However, the way each individual animal deals with such oral infections appears to be rather constant, at least for a (study) period of 5 weeks. This long-lasting constant handling of Gram-negative enterobacilli by the host and his indigenous flora appears to be phenotypically determined (e.g. after birth).

(3) For the establishment and maintenance of a constant indigenous flora (aerobes and anaerobes) a functioning thymus is apparently required, especially at the time of first association with bacteria (birth).

(4) It seems plausible to assume that bacteria entering the tonsils or the Peyer's patches either induce tolerance (indigenous mucosa-associated flora) or elicit an immune response (IgA antibodies) and may thereby become 'rejected'.

(5) In normal mice as well as in man, IgA coating of bacteria in the intestines appears to be almost confined to *Enterobacteriaceae* spp. Even within this group of facultative anaerobic Gram-negative bacilli, not all bacteria in the faeces are IgA-coated. It is unlikely that anaerobes which live in close association with the mucosa do not

come into contact with the GALT. The effect of penetration of Peyer's patches by antigenically host-related anaerobes after birth may be induction of tolerance rather than induction of humoral immunity (IgA).

(6) Concanavalin A can enhance formation of T suppressor (T_s) cells and also substitute for adherence pili to block receptor sites on buccal cells. Consequently, adherence pili may enhance the formation of T_s cells *in vivo*. T_s cell formation in mice has appeared to be more pronounced in the presence of lipopolysaccharides (endotoxins), which form the greater part of the cell wall of Gram-negative bacteria.

(7) Oral administration of high concentrations of foreign antigens such as sheep red blood cells to normal conventional mice mitigates the immune response following a subsequent parenteral administration of the same antigen.

(8) In the absence of a thymus since birth, mice maintained under conventional circumstances with all kinds of bacteria in the environment develop wasting disease and soon after weaning have an inconstant microflora. This flora then no longer has the individually determined characteristics of the flora of mice of the same age with a thymus.

(9) Delayed GvHD may be caused by T cells which mature in the recipient and are sensitized by a complex of antigens which are of bacterial origin and cross-reactive with host tissue and/or organ-specific antigens. Induction of reactivity in T cells of donor origin may be confined to antigens of bacteria which are absent in the indigenous flora of donor mice. This contact between matured T cells and foreign (to the donor) bacterial antigens should occur in the tissues (i.e. after invasion). A first contact in the Peyer's patches may lead to T_s cell formation. This is in agreement with the finding that to mitigate GvHD the bacteria-free status of the digestive tract should be maintained for a minimum of 3 weeks, the time required for repopulation of the Peyer's patches by donor cells and for the clearance of bacteria and bacterial fragments that invaded the recipient from the gut after irradiation. Soluble cross-reactive antigens appear to be associated generally with a humoral immune response. In the presence of a normally functioning GALT in addition to formation of T_s cells, T helper cells could develop and play a role in the control of intestinal colonization (mucosa associated) by antigenically unrelated microorganisms.

(10) Wasting disease may be caused by a T-cell-independent immune

(B-cell) response to bacterial antigens in host tissues and/or to organ- and/or tissue-specific antigens which are cross-reactive with bacterial antigens.

A. Working Hypothesis

On the basis of these ten points, the following sequence of events could occur in normally developing healthy individuals.

From birth, an individual is exposed to many different bacteria, the first ones coming primarily from the mother. If the thymus is functioning normally, bacteria which are antigenically related with the host may selectively colonize the mucosa lining the digestive tract, thereby rendering the host immunologically tolerant. This process of induction of tolerance may occur in the Peyer's patches and perhaps also in the tonsils. Induction of tolerance could be enhanced by adherence structures on the bacterial cell wall, the pili of (anaerobic) bacteria. Induction of tolerance may be promoted further by bacterial lipopolysaccharides (endotoxins). These lipopolysaccharides can be provided by either the tolerance-inducing mucosa-associated bacteria or come from the intestinal contents. Individuals born in an environment with a large number of different Gram-negative bacteria could become tolerant to more types of these bacteria (presumably, mostly *E. coli*, as this is the most common *Enterobacteriaceae* spp.) than those born and initially raised under very hygienic conditions in an environment with a very limited or no exposure to new enterobacteria. The first category of host individuals could later in life be the ones with a relatively high number of different biotypes of *Enterobacteriaceae* spp. in comparison with the second group.

A difference in immunological response between host individuals to antigenically related Gram-negative bacilli on the basis of early association may also be expressed in the incidence or absence of IgA coating of these bacteria. This has not yet been studied. It is conceivable that the situation becomes static by the time of weaning, since, as long as the thymus functions sufficiently, induction of tolerance to host-related bacterial antigens may continue: bacteria with antigens that cross-react with organ or tissue antigens of the host organism may also enter Peyer's patches later after birth and render the host more readily tolerant than if the microorganisms do not share antigens with host tissues.

These considerations make it likely that individual differences in immunological response to Gram-negative bacilli are due to the net result of a difference in numbers and species that comprise the much more complex anaerobic colonization resistance (CR), i.e. the indigenous mucosa-associated flora. The composition of this flora—'the anaerobic wallpaper of the intestines'—may be acquired and selected immunologically primarily in the first weeks after birth in the presence of a functioning thymus. Obviously, the intestinal feeder layer (intestinal mucus) may also play a role in the determination of which bacteria colonize the mucosa. Those bacteria which have the proper enzymes for digestion of mucus components will be at an advantage. Both the mucus and the type of immune response elicited in the GALT may play a role in the determination of the composition of the mucosa-associated flora. To summarize, the saliva and the mucus may to some extent represent decisive factors in determining the (animal) species specificity of the flora. The GALT response, which is determined to an important extent early in life, may define the interindividual differences in the 'intestinal wallpaper' within one species. During ageing, when the thymus involutes, the capacity to respond with tolerance to certain antigenically related bacteria in the 'intestinal wallpaper' may gradually decrease.

B. Possible Significance for Bone-marrow Transplantation

After bone-marrow transplantation in an irradiated recipient, repopulation of the Peyer's patches (and tonsils) by a complete set of lymphocytes and macrophages to ensure 'normal function' is perhaps a prerequisite for the development of tolerance to the mucosa-associated flora of the recipient. The more mature and sensitized lymphocytes of the donor contaminate the transplant, the higher the risk of an aggressive response to components or fragments of bacteria of the recipients indigenous flora which, after irradiation, have penetrated the mucosa and gained access to host tissues. If this assumption is correct, it may concern only fragments or components of bacteria which were not indigenous to the flora of the donor of the marrow. Differences in mucosa-associated flora between bone marrow donor and recipient obviously may only concern differences in serotypes (i.e. in the antigenic composition of microorganisms of the same species). Once the implanted bone marrow stem cells have produced sufficient T-lymphocyte precursor cells that can mature under control of the thymus populate GALT organs, the development of tolerance to a mucosa-associated flora of the recipient may again become possible.

Until that state of maturation of donor cells has been reached, bacterial antigens unrelated to the donor flora should not be present. This means in practice that, at the time of irradiation, microorganisms should be completely absent or else be of donor type in case allogeneic (mismatched) bone marrow is transplanted.

The mucosa-associated flora should also not alter when syngeneic marrow is used for transplantation, at least not during the interval required for functional repopulation of the Peyer's patches (tonsils). Our hypothesis concerning the role of bacteria in the pathogenesis of chronic GvHD may apply also to skin flora. However, in mice, the skin flora appears to be largely if not completely secondary to digestive tract microflora (Van der Waaij and Sturm, 1971). Therefore, if our hypothesis is correct, tolerance to skin flora may be induced in the intestines in mice. How this works in man is a matter of even greater speculation. Although we do not lick our skin to clean it like mice, in man there may be sufficient oral contamination of indigenous skin flora (perhaps of maternal origin) to bring skin flora into contact with the GALT. More experimental studies in mice with various controlled digestive tract microfloras must be performed to elucidate further the role of bacteria in GvHD. These experiments should be done in the absence of viruses—at least initially—since viruses may play their own (separate) role in the pathogenesis of GvHD. However, viruses should not be overlooked. But studies in mice infected with different viruses at the time of bone-marrow transplantation represent a separate category and do not fall within the slope of this chapter.

ACKNOWLEDGEMENT

The authors wish to thank Dr A. C. Ford for editing the English text.

REFERENCES

Abrams, G. D., Bauer, H. and Sprinz, H. (1963). *Lab. Invest.* **12**, 335-364.
Abrams, G. D. and Bishop, J. E. (1966). *J. Bacteriol.* **92**, 1604-1608.
André, C., Heremans, J. F., Vaerman, J. P. and Cambiaso, C. L. (1975). *J. Exp. Med.* **142**, 1509-1519.
Artzt, K. (1972). *Transplantation* **13**, 547-549.
Ashburner, F. M. and Mushin, R. (1962). *J. Hyg.* **60**, 175-181.
Atkinson, K., Storb, R., Prentice, R. L., Weiden, P. L., Witherspoon, R. P., Sullivan, K., Noel, D. and Thomas, E. D. (1979). *Blood* **53**, 720-731.
Babb, J. L. and McGhee, J. R. (1980). *Infect Immun.* **29**, 322-328.
Barthold, D. R., Kysela, S. and Steinberg, A. D. (1974). *J. Immunol.* **112**, 9-15.
Bealmear, P. M. and Wilson, R. (1966). *Anat. Rec.* **154**, 261-274.
Berg, R. D. (1983). *Curr. Microbiol.* **8**, 285-292.
Berg, R. D. and Garlington, A. W. (1979). *Infect. Immun.* **23**, 403-411.
Bohnhoff, M., Miller, C. P. and Martin, W. R. (1964). *J. Exp. Med.* **120**, 817-828.

Bortin, M. M. (1984). *Exp. Hematol.* **12**, 199-204.
Bortin, M. M., Gale, R. P., Kay, H. E. M. and Rimm, A. A. (1983). *J. Am. Med. Assoc.* **249**, 1166-1175.
Brinton, C. C. (1967). *Acta Odont. Scand.* **22**, 441-455.
Brockman, D. E. and Cooper, M. D. (1973). *Am. J. Anat.* **136**, 455-462.
Bull, D. M. and Ignaczak, T. F. (1973). *Gastroenterology* **64**, 43-50.
Bullen, C. L., Tearle, P. V. and Willis, A. T. (1977). *J. Med. Microbiol.* **9**, 325-333.
Carter, P. B. and Collins, F. M. (1974). *J. Exp. Med.* **139**, 1189-1203.
Chase, M. W. (1946). *Proc. Soc. Exp. Biol.* **61**, 257-259.
Chiller, J. M., Skidmore, B. J., Morrison, D. C. and Weigle, W. O. (1973). *Proc. Natl. Acad. Sci. U.S.A.* **70**, 2129-2133.
Cooper, W. C., Mariani, T. N. and Good, R. A. (1975). *In* "Immunodeficiencies in Man and Animals" (Bergsma, D., Good, R. A., Finstad, J. and Paul, N. W., eds), pp. 223-228. Sinauer Associates, Sunderland, Mass.
Cottier, H., Schaffner, T., Chanana, A. D., Joel, D. D., Sordat, B., Bryant, B. J. and Hess, M. W. (1975). *In* "Gram-negative Bacterial Infections and Mode of Endotoxin Action" (Urbaschek, R. and Neter, E., eds), pp. 80-85. Springer-Verlag, Berlin.
Craig, S. W. and Cebra, J. J. (1971). *J. Exp. Med.* **134**, 188-200.
De Vries, M. J., Van Bekkum, D. W., Van Putten, L. M., Van der Waaij, D. and Balner, H. (1964). *Recherche Scient.* **147**, 115-117.
Dubos, R., Schaedler, R. W., Costello, R. and Hoet, P. (1965). *J. Exp. Med.* **122**, 67-76.
Dutton, R. W. (1973). *J. Exp. Med.* **138**, 1496-1505.
Ehrenkranz, N. J. (1970). *J. Pediatr.* **76**, 839-847.
Eickhoff, J. (1979). *In* "New Criteria for Antimicrobial Therapy: Maintenance of Digestive Tract Colonization Resistance" (Van der Waaij, D. and Verhoef, J., eds), pp. 5-11. Excerpta Medica, Amsterdam.
Emmelot, C. H. and Van der Waaij, D. (1980). *J. Hyg.* **84**, 331-340.
Ferretti, J. J., Shea, C. and Humphrey, M. W. (1980). *Infect. Immun.* **30**, 69-73.
Foo, M. C. and Lee, A. (1972). *Infect. Immun.* **6**, 525-532.
Freter, R. (1972). *Infect. Immun.* **6**, 135-141.
Fubara, E. S. and Freter, R. (1972). *J. Immunol.* **111**, 395-403.
Gershwin, M. E. (1978). *In* "Animal Models of Comparative and Developmental Aspects of Immunity and Disease" (Gershwin, M. E. and Casper, E. L., eds), pp. 250-257. Pergamon Press, New York.
Gibbons, R. J. (1974). *In* "Anaerobic Bacteria: Role in Disease" (Ballows, A., DeHaan, R. M., Dowell, V. R. and Guze, L. B., eds), pp. 267-285. Thomas, Springfield, Illinois.
Gibbons, R. J., Van Houte, J. and Liljemark, W. F. (1971). *J. Dent. Res.* **51**, 424-435.
Gibbons, R. J., Spinell, D. M. and Skobe, Z. (1976). *Infect. Immun.* **13**, 238-246.
Grushka, M. and Lapp, W. S. (1974). *Transplantation* **17**, 157-163.

Heidt, P. J. and Van der Waaij, D. (1979). *Zbl. Bakt. Suppl.* **7**, 67–72.
Heit, H., Wilson, R., Fliedner, T. M. and Kohne, E. (1973). *In* "Germfree Research: Biological Effects and Gnotobiotic Environment" (Heneghan, J. B., ed.), pp. 477–483. Academic Press, New York.
Hentgens, D. J. (1967). *J. Bacteriol.* **93**, 1369–1373.
Heyworth, B. and Brown, J. (1975). *Arch. Dis. Child.* **50**, 27–33.
Holland, J. M., Mitchell, T. J., Gipson, L. C. and Whitaker, M. S. (1978). *J. Natl Cancer Inst.* **61**, 1357–1361.
Hughes, M., Machardy, S. M., Sheppard, A. J. and Woods, N.C. (1980). *Infect. Immun.* **27**, 576–588.
Joel, D. D., Hess, M. W. and Cottier, H. (1970). *Experientia* **26**, 694–697.
Joel, D. D., Hess, M. W. and Cottier, H. (1971). *Biol.* **231**, 24–25.
Joel, D. D., Hess, M. W. and Cottier, H. (1972). *J. Exp. Med.* **135**, 907–923.
Joel, D. D., Chanana, A. D. and Cronkite, E. P. (1974). *Semin. Hematol.* **7**, 464–481.
Johanson, W. G., Pierce, A. K., Sanford, J. P. and Thomas, R. N. (1972). *Ann. Intern. Med.* **77**, 701–706.
Johanson, W. G., Woods, D. E. and Chandhuri, T. (1979). *J. Infect. Dis.* **139**, 667–673.
Jones, J. M., Wilson, R. and Bealmear, P. M. (1971). *Radiat. Res.* **45**, 577–588.
Jutila, J. W. (1973). *J. Infect. Dis.* **128**, 99–103.
Kagnoff, M. F. (1978). *J. Immunol.* **120**, 1509–1513.
Kenny, J. F., Woleslagle, D. L., Gray, J. A., Michaels, R. H. and Pearson, M. A. (1970). *J. Infect. Dis.* **121**, 528–540.
Kohrshidi, M. and Mohagheghpour, N. (1979). *Infect. Immun.* **24**, 770–773.
Korngold, R. and Sprent, J. (1978). *J. Exp. Med.* **148**, 1687–1698.
Krakauer, R. S., Waldman, T. A. and Strober, W. (1976). *J. Exp. Med.* **144**, 662–673.
Laissue, J. A., Chanana, A. D., Cottier, H., Cronkite, E. P. and Joel, D. D. (1976). *Blood* **47**, 21–30.
Lake, A. M., Bloch, K. J., Neutra, M. R. and Walker, W. A. (1979). *J. Immunol.* **122**, 834–837.
Long, S. S. and Swenson, R. M. (1977). *J. Pediatr.* **91**, 298–301.
Maier, B. R., Onderdonk, A. B., Baskett, R. C. and Hentgens, D. J. (1972). *Am. J. Clin. Nutr.* **25**, 1433–1442.
Mattingly, J. A. and Waksman, B. H. (1978). *J. Immunol.* **121**, 1878–1881.
McGuirre, C. D. and Floyd, T. M. (1958). *J. Exp. Med.* **108**, 277–282.
Michalek, S. M., Kiyono, H., Wannemuehler, M. J., Mosteller, L. M. and McGhee, J. R. (1982). *J. Immunol.* **128**, 1992–1998.
Miller, J. F. (1962). *Proc. R. Soc. Biol.* **156**, 415–428.
Miller, J. F. A. P. and Howard, J. G. (1964). *J. Reticuloendothel. Soc.* **1**, 369–392.
Monier, J. C., Sepetjian, M., Czyba, J. C., Ortonne, J. P. and Thivolet, J. (1974). *In* "Proceedings of the First International Workshop on Nude Mice" (Rygaard, J. and Poulsen, C. O., eds), pp. 245–249. Gustav Fischer Verlag, Stuttgart.
Morgenstern, M. A. and Gorzynski, E. A. (1977). *Infect. Immun.* **17**, 36–42.
Munoz, J. (1964). *Adv. Immunol.* **4**, 397–440.

Mushin, R. and Dubos, R. (1965). *J. Exp. Med.* **122**, 745-757.
Nomura, T., Ito, T., Kagiyama, N. and Suzuki, T. (1974). *In* "Proceedings of the First International Workshop on Nude Mice" (Rygaard, J. and Poulsen, C. O., eds), pp. 215-219. Gustav Fischer Verlag, Stuttgart.
Ofek, I., Mirelman, D. and Sharon, N. (1977). *Nature* **265**, 623-625.
Okuda, S. and Weinbaum, G. (1969). *J. Immunol.* **103**, 869-871.
Okudaira, H., Suzuki, T., Choda, A., Ogita, T., Tadokoro, K., Mizushima, Y. and Horiuchi, Y. (1977). *In* "Proceedings of the Second International Workshop on Nude Mice" (Nomura, T., Ohsawa, N., Tamaoki, N., *et al.*, (eds), pp. 139-145. Gustav Fischer Verlag, Stuttgart.
Owens, W. E. and Berg, R. D. (1980). *Infect. Immun.* **27**, 461-467.
Parrot, D. M. V. (1962). *Transplant. Bull.* **29**, 102-104.
Parrot, D. M. V. and East, J. (1962). *Nature* **195**, 347-348.
Peavy, D. L., Baughn, R. E. and Musher, D. M. (1978). *Infect. Immun.* **19**, 71-78.
Pollard, M. and Sharon, W. (1970). *Infect. Immun.* **2**, 96-100.
Powles, R. L., Clink, H. M., Spence, D., Morgenstern, G., Watson, J. G., Selby, P. J., Woods, M., Barrett, A., Jameson, B., Sloane, J., Lawler, S. D., Kay, H. E. M., Lawson, D., McElwain, T. J. and Alexander, P. (1980). *Lancet* **i**, 327-329.
Raffi, M., Hashemi, J. N. and Mohagheghpour, N. (1977). *Clin. Immunol. Immunopathol.* **8**, 1-4.
Rich, R. R. and Pierce, C. W. (1974). *J. Immunol.* **112**, 1360-1368.
Rotimi, V. O. and Duerden, B. I. (1981). *J. Med. Microbiol.* **14**, 51-62.
Ruddle, N. H. and Waksman, B. H. (1968). *J. Exp. Med.* **128**, 1237-1254.
Salvin, S. B. (1958). *J. Exp. Med.* **107**, 109-114.
Savage, D. C. (1977). *Ann. Rev. Microbiol.* **31**, 107-133.
Savage, D. C. (1979). *Zbl. Bakt. Suppl.* **7**, 163-168.
Savage, D. C., Dubos, R. and Schaedler, R. W. (1968). *J. Exp. Med.* **127**, 67-76.
Schwartz, S. N., Dowling, J. N., Benkovic, C., De Quittner-Buchanan, M., Postko, T. and Yee, R. B. (1978). *J. Infect. Dis.* **138**, 227-231.
Stamey, T. A., Timothy, M., Millar, M. and Mihara, G. (1971). Calif. Medicin, *West. J. Med.* **115**, 1-19.
Stinson, M. W., Nisengard, R. J., Pelonero, L. and Drinnan, A. J. (1977). *Infect. Immun.* **24**, 532-538.
Storb, R., Epstein, R. B., Graham, T. C. and Thomas, E. D. (1970). *Transplantation* , 240-246.
Van Bekkum, D. W., Roodenburg, J., Heidt, P. J. and Van der Waaij, D. (1974). *J. Natl Cancer Inst.* **52**, 401-404.
Van de Rijn, I., Zabriski, J. B. and McCarthy, M. (1977). *J. Exp. Med.* **146**, 579-599.
Van de Merwe, J. P., Stegeman, J. H. and Hazenberg, M. P. (1983). *Antonie van Leeuwenhoek* **49**, 119-124.
Van der Waaij, D. (1969). *In* "Germ-free Biology" (Mirand, E. A. and Back, N., eds), pp. 181-189. Plenum Press, New York.

Van der Waaij, D. (1981). *In* "Recent Advances in Germ-free Research" (Sasaki, S., Ozawa, A. and Hashimoto, K., eds), pp. 387-395. Tokai University Press, Tokyo.
Van der Waaij, D. (1982). *In* "Action of Antibiotics" (Sabath, L. D., ed.), pp. 104-118. Hans Huber, Bern.
Van der Waaij, D. (1983). *In* "Antibiotic Choice: The Importance of Colonization Resistance". (Grüneberg, R. N., ed), pp. 67-94. Research Studies Press, Chichester.
Van der Waaij, D. and Berghuis, J. M. (1973). *J. Hyg.* **72**, 379-387.
Van der Waaij, D. and Heidt, P. J. (1977). *In* "Food and Immunology" (Hambraeus, L., Hanson, L. A. and McFarland, H., eds), pp. 133-141. Almqvist and Wiskell, Stockholm.
Van der Waaij, D. and Sturm, C. A. (1968). *Lab. Anim. Care* **18**, 1-10.
Van der Waaij, D. and Sturm, C. A. (1971). *Antonie van Leeuwenhoek* **37**, 139-151.
Van der Waaij, D., Berghuis-de Bries, J. M. and Lekkerkerk-van der Wees, J. E. C. (1971). *J. Hyg.* **69**, 405-411.
Van der Waaij, D., Berghuis-de Vries, J. M. and Lekkerkerk-van der Wees, J. E. C. (1972). *J. Hyg.* **70**, 335-342.
Van der Waaij, D., Vossen, J. M., Korthals Altes, C. and Hartgrink, C. (1977). *Am. J. Clin. Nutr.* **30**, 1887-1895.
Van der Waaij, D., Tieleman-Speltie, T. M. and De Roeck-Houben, A. M. J. (1978). *Antonie van Leeuwenhoek* **44**, 395-405.
Van Houte, J., Gibbons, R. J. and Pulkkinen, A. J. (1971). *Arch. Oral Biol.* **16**, 1131-1141.
Van Saene, H. K. F. and Van der Waaij, D. (1979). *J. Immunol. Meth.* **30**, 87-96.
Vos, O., De Vries, M. J., Collenteur, J. C. and Van Bekkum, D. W. (1959). *J. Natl Cancer Inst.* **23**, 53-73.
Wagemaker, G., Heidt, P. J., Merchav, S. and Van Bekkum, D. W. (1982). *In* "Experimental Hematology Today 1982" (Baum, S. J., Ledney, G. D. and Thierfelder, S., eds) pp. 111-118. Karger, Basel.
Welsh, J., Avakian, H., Ebringer, A. and Entwistle, C. C. (1980). *Br. J. Exp. Pathol.* **61**, 92-96.
Wilson, R., Sjodin, K. and Bealmear, M. (1964). *Proc. Soc. Exp. Biol. Med.* **17**, 237-239.
Wilson, R., Bealmear, M. and Sobonya, R. (1965). *Proc. Soc. Exp. Biol. Med.* **118**, 87-99.
Winston, D. J., Gale, R. P., Meyer, D. V. and Young, L. S. (1979). *Medicine* **58**, 1-31.
Woods, D. E., Straus, D. C., Johanson, W. G., Berry, V. K. and Bass, J. A. (1980). *Infect. Immun.* **29**, 1146-1151.

Chapter 8

Immunology of Adverse Reactions to Antimicrobial Agents

Kenneth W. Witte and Dennis P. West
College of Pharmacy, University of Illinois,
P.O. Box 6998, Chicago, Illinois 60680, U.S.A.

INTRODUCTION

A drug reaction based upon an immunological response is commonly called a 'hypersensitivity reaction' or 'drug allergy'. It is often difficult to determine if an adverse drug reaction is truly allergic, because mechanisms of immunologic adverse drug reactions are still not well understood, and routine confirmational immunological testing is not yet very specific or sophisticated. In most cases a distinction can be made between those adverse reactions which are dose-related and those which are immune-mediated. Dose-related adverse effects are predictable from the pharmacological action and toxicity profile, while allergic immune-mediated reactions are dose-independent and not generally predictable.

Dose-related adverse effects may be minimized by careful monitoring of organ systems where toxicity may occur. Thus, drugs with similar toxicity profiles that are known to cause adverse effects in the same organ system should be monitored carefully when used together. However, allergic drug reactions have certain features which distinguish them from toxic or idiosyncratic reactions which Parker (1980) defined as follows:

Antimicrobial agents and immunity
ISBN 0-12-383830-4

(1) Onset of the allergic state does not occur until sometime after initial exposure.
(2) Any route of drug administration may cause an allergic reaction.
(3) After an allergic state has been established, an allergic reaction may be precipitated by a minute amount of the offending agent.
(4) Clinical manifestations of drug allergy do not resemble the general pharmacologic effects of the drug.
(5) The symptoms of drug allergy are suggestive of known forms of allergic responses.
(6) Antibodies and/or T lymphocytes are demonstrated to react specifically with the offending drug and/or metabolite.
(7) The allergic reaction may be reproduced by administering a small amount of the suspected drug or drugs of similar chemical structure.
(8) Antiallergy agents may modify the allergic drug reaction.
(9) For some reactions, a sensitization or challenge test may be positive.
(10) Most allergic drug reactions are reversible when the offending drug is removed.
(11) The likelihood of an allergic drug response increases with the number of courses of therapy.
(12) When drugs are given chronically, the allergic reaction is greatest in the first 3 weeks of therapy.

Allergic drug reactions may comprise from 6 to 20% of all adverse drug reactions observed (Borda *et al.*, 1968; Caranasas *et al.*, 1974). An optimal approach to evaluating, preventing and treating a suspected drug hypersensitivity reaction includes:

(1) Obtaining a comprehensive drug history.
(2) Being aware of the various clinical manifestations of drug allergy.
(3) Understanding the factors that favour the development of allergic drug reactions.
(4) Understanding the immunological mechanisms involved in hypersensitivity drug reactions.

A. Drug History

A history of drug 'sensitivity' should raise a high index of suspicion towards a patient who may repeat an allergic reaction on re-exposure to the medication. Often, only a history of 'skin rash' may be available. This should indicate the necessity for caution and the patient should be regarded as potentially allergic to the drug or to drugs that are known to have cross-allergenicity.

If the patient reports a history of allergy to an unknown drug, certain laboratory tests may be useful in identifying the cause, but this is not frequently the case. The most reliable method of documenting an allergic drug reaction is to rechallenge the patient. However, this may produce an unacceptable clinical reaction and should generally be used only when benefit from treatment with the offending drug is high, risk to the patient is low, and there is no acceptable alternative treatment.

B. Clinical Manifestations of Drug Allergy

Symptoms of an allergic drug reaction usually have an acute onset, may last for a period ranging from minutes to months, or may occur periodically throughout an exposure period. Severity of symptoms may range from a mild cough to a fatal anaphylactic reaction. Some of the clinical manifestations of allergic drug reactions are listed in Table 1.

Table 1
Clinical manifestations of drug allergy

Skin eruptions
Urticaria
Maculopapular
Fixed drug
Erythema multiforme
Purpura
Exfoliative dermatitis
Vesico-bullous
Anaphylactic reactions
Lupus-like syndrome
Arthus reaction
Blood
Haemolytic anaemia
Granulocytopenia
Thrombocytopenia
Drug fever
Vasculitis
Serum sickness
Cytotoxic reactions involving individual organs
Kidney
Lungs
Skin
Liver

C. Predisposing Factors of Drug Allergy

Certain factors may predispose a person to develop an allergic reaction to a drug. Some of these factors are listed in Table 2. Antimicrobial agents are especially prone to cause allergic reactions because of their chemical structure, their capacity to act as or from an antigen, their intermittent use and the method of administration may be topical, oral or parenteral for the same drug. In addition, patients that receive antimicrobial agents may already have stressed immune systems that may affect their reactivity to the drug.

Table 2
Predisposing factors in drug allergy[a]

Factor	Effect
Age	Drug allergy is less frequent in young than in older individuals
Genetic background	Genetic make-up may alter (a) Drug metabolism (b) Capacity to respond to immune challenge (c) Sensitivity of tissue receptor sites (d) Elaboration of mediators
Sex	Females have a higher incidence of cutaneous reactions than do males
Concurrent host factors	Other diseases may increase incidence of reactions
Route of administration	Topical application of drug has the greatest capacity to induce allergy followed, in order of likelihood, by intravenous, intramuscular and oral routes of administration
Continuous *vs* intermittent exposure	Generalized reactions to certain drugs are more frequent with intermittent exposure
Nature of drug	Propensity to induce an immune response depends on the capacity of the drug to act as, or form, a complete antigen.
Dosage, duration of therapy	Prolonged courses of high doses are associated with increased reactions

[a]Adapted from Bellanti (1978).

D. Mechanism of Sensitization to Antimicrobial Agents

An antigen is a substance capable of inducing antibody formation or of producing sensitized lymphocytes. Large protein or large polypeptide drug molecules may act as a complete antigens. However, most drugs have fewer than seven amino acids and have a molecular weight of less than 1000 daltons. Such drugs only become antigens by chemical coupling to a larger molecular carrier (i.e. a tissue protein) and thus usually act as haptens. Covalent bonding of a hapten to a protein is usually required to render a stable hapten–protein immunogenic complex. Most drugs are unable to do this unless a more reactive metabolite is formed from the parent drug or an impurity of the drug is reactive. However, certain drugs (e.g. penicillins) form numerous reactive metabolites which have greater biochemical reactivity and a greater propensity to form covalent bonds with tissue proteins. Theoretically, any type of tissue protein may be involved in antigen formation. For example, when penicillin hapten binds to red cells, an immune haemolysis may occur.

Once formed, an antigen induces the immune system to react to bid the body of foreign material. This reaction manifests itself by production of specifically reactive antibodies (immunoglobulins) or specifically sensitized lymphocytes capable of reacting with antigen and may culminate with damage to tissues and organs. Such reactions were first classified by Gell and Coombs (1975).

Gell and Coombs's method of classification has limitations and many hypersensitivity reactions may fall into more than one category or remain unclassified. Simplistically, the classification of hypersensitivity reactions to drugs includes four main categories:

Type I—urticarial or anaphylactic reactions;
Type II—cytotoxic and cytolytic reactions;
Type III—immune-complex reactions;
Type IV—cell-mediated reactions (delayed hypersensitivity).

Types I, II and III are antibody-mediated and type IV is cell-mediated.

II. TYPES OF HYPERSENSITIVITY REACTIONS

A. Type I Hypersensitivity Reactions

The type I reaction is best known as immediate hypersensitivity. It occurs when a specific antibody (IgE) to an antigen is formed and attaches itself to a mast cell or basophil. On re-exposure, an interaction between attached antibody and antigen occurs, resulting in degranulation of the mast cell or basophil and release of pharmacologically active mediators.

Pharmacologic action of these mediators: histamine, serotonin, slow-reacting substance A (SRS-A) and vasoactive amines bring about increased capillary dilatation and permeability, bronchospasm and vasoconstriction. There may also be activation of the clotting mechanism with consumption of several components including fibrinolysins.

The tissues and organs involved are those with high concentrations of mast cells, such as skin, mucous membranes of the gastrointestinal tract and respiratory system, and bronchial smooth muscle. The most severe form of a type I hypersensitivity reaction is anaphylactic shock in which case several organs are involved.

Clinical manifestations of this reaction relate to mediator effects and the area in which they are released. For example, upper respiratory tract symptoms may include sinus headache, itching of eyes, tearing, sneezing, watery nasal discharge, itching of nose and throat irritation. These may occur within minutes of oral administration or by breathing in particles of the drug. Symptoms are often diagnosed as allergic rhinitis and conjunctivitis. Lung involvement may include asthma-like symptoms of wheezing, dyspnoea, dry cough and tightness in the chest.

Oral use of drug may lead to symptoms primarily affecting the gastrointestinal tract. Such symptoms may include glossitis, cardiospasm, nausea, vomiting, irritable bowel, diarrhoea, steatorrhoea and possible haemorrhage. The cause may be due to the drug or to additives in the dosage form to enhance drug stability or to give it colour.

Skin involvement is one of the most common manifestations of a type I hypersensitivity reaction. Clinical symptoms may include urticaria, pruritus, angio-oedema, weeping, erythema, and vesicopapular lesions. If any of these clinical manifestations occur shortly after administration of drug (minutes to a few days), a hypersensitivity reaction should be suspected.

Treatment of type I hypersensitivity reactions should be individualized according to the particular drug involved, route of administration, organ system or tissue involved, severity of reaction and clinical signs and symptoms. Treatment requires drugs that block mediator effects, such as antihistamines; drugs that reverse or counteract mediator effects, such as adrenergic agents; and drugs that inhibit mediator secretion, such as theophylline and corticosteroids. Another approach is to prevent the reaction by induction of hyposensitization. Using this mechanism, the immune system develops blocking antibodies (IgG) that bind to allergen and prevent binding to mast cells. This technique has been used in patients allergic to penicillin.

Table 3 lists antibiotics known to be capable of causing type I hypersensitivity reactions. Prevention of such reactions relies on careful drug history, skin testing if appropriate, and education of the patient on specific precautions to avoid trivial sensitization and re-exposure.

Table 3
Antimicrobial agents associated with anaphylactic reactions[a]

Amphotericin B	Aminoglycosides
Bacitracin	Penicillins
Cephalosporins	Sulphonamides
Clindamycin	Tetracyclines
Ethambutol	

[a]Adapted from Van Arsdel (1978).

B. Type II Hypersensitivity Reactions

Type II reactions are cytotoxic and include such clinical conditions as haemolytic anaemia, agranulocytosis, thrombocytopenia and vascular endothelium disorders.

Antigen or hapten attaches to some component of the target cell. The target may be erythrocytes, leucocytes, thrombocytes or endothelium of the vascular system. Specific antibodies (IgG or IgM) then react to antigenic constituents of the cell or to antigen bound to the cell which causes activation of complement. Activated complement, a complex group of serum proteins, increases capillary permeability, causes chemotaxis and promotes phagocytosis by polymorphonuclear leucocytes (PMN). This results in release of cellular enzymes causing cytotoxic or cytolytic injury to the cell.

Clinical manifestations are dependent upon the target cells involved and severity of reaction depends on the degree of immunologic destruction of these target cells. For example, involvement of erythrocytes, leucocytes, thrombocytes or vascular endothelium shows similar cytotoxic/cytolytic effects that result in haemolytic anaemia, agranulocytosis, thrombocytopenic purpura and vascular purpura respectively. Treatment consists of discontinuing the offending agent and treating the clinical manifestations.

C. Type III Hypersensitivity Reactions

Type III reactions are known to be immune complex-mediated. Classic examples are the Arthus and serum sickness reactions.

Immune complexes are formed when antigen binds to antibody (usually IgM or IgG). Instead of being cleared from the circulation by phagocytosis they deposit on target tissues and in vascular endothelium. Complement is then activated, which leads to chemotaxis of PMN, and protein-digesting enzymes (lysozyme) are released that cause tissue injury.

The Arthus reaction occurs as a local reaction with haemorrhagic necrosis occurring at the site of injection within 12–24 h. This reaction usually involves large amounts of antigen in the target tissue and circulating antibodies which interact to cause complement activation, resulting in localized tissue damage.

A serum sickness reaction is a response that appears to be similar to the Arthus reaction and is also mediated by immune complexes. However, instead of a localized reaction at the site of injection, circulating antigen-antibody complexes penetrate blood vessel walls and/or deposit in the basement membrane after which complement is fixed and activated. A systemic reaction results which involves target organs that are often highly vascular, such as the kidney.

Clinical features include pruritus, arthralgias with periarticular oedema, angio-oedema, low grade fever, enlarged lymph nodes and urticarial or maculopapular rash. Onset may range from a few hours (for the accelerated type) to as long as 3 weeks after drug is given. Laboratory determinations are generally not diagnostic. Hypergammaglobulinaemia and elevated erythrocyte sedimentation rate are commonly noted.

Treatment is generally accomplished with antihistamines and analgesics to control symptomatic complaint of pruritus and pain. If the reaction is severe, short-term corticosteroid therapy may be beneficial.

Penicillin is the most common cause of serum sickness but the frequency of this syndrome is relatively rare. Table 4 lists other causative antimicrobials.

Table 4
Antimicrobial agents associated with serum sickness[a]

Penicillins	Streptomycin
Erythromycin	Sulphonamides
Isoniazid	
Nitrofurantoin	

[a]Adapted from Van Arsdel (1978).

Clinical examples of immune complex-mediated reactions include: the Arthus reaction, serum sickness, vasculitis, rheumatoid disorders and certain types of nephritis. The type and severity of reaction is dependent on the quantity of immunoreactive complexes, the location and the presence of vasoactive amines.

D. Type IV Hypersensitivity Reactions

Type IV reactions are known as cell-mediated reactions. The pathogenesis has been established for localized allergic contact dermatitis but the mechanism of generalized cell-mediated reactions ('delayed' hypersensitivity) following ingestion or injection of antigen has yet to be determined.

A complete antigen is produced by binding haptens to various proteins in skin. It is known that NH_2 and SH groups of cystine and cysteine are binding sites for haptens (Elsens and Belman, 1953). The same allergen may conjugate with more than one type of protein. Thus, a clinical reaction may actually represent combined responses to binding of multiple haptens and multiple proteins simultaneously (Baer, 1964).

When T lymphocytes are exposed to allergen, there is blast transformation and proliferation of the clone of 'sensitized' cells, as well as 'elicitation' or release of lymphokines.

Clinical features include eczematous dermatitis. Acute contact dermatitis usually shows papulovesiculation, erythema and oedema. Chronically, the skin may show scaling and erythema, may be thickened or lichenified, and may be hypo- or hyperpigmented.

Treatment, as well as prevention, includes avoidance of allergen. In addition, topical corticosteroids, compresses and systemic and topical antipruritic agents are all non-specific and commonly used methods for managing allergic contact dermatitis.

III. ANTIMICROBIAL-INDUCED IMMUNOLOGICAL REACTIONS

Adverse reactions to antimicrobial agents based on an immune response cover a broad clinical spectrum. Drug-induced immune disorders may involve haematologic, hepatic, renal, skin, respiratory tract, vascular and other organ systems.

A. Anaphylaxis

Symptoms of acute anaphylaxis depend on the organ systems that are targeted by chemical mediators released in antigen–antibody interaction. Primarily affected are pulmonary, cutaneous and vascular systems. For example, an anaphylactic reaction to penicillin occurs only after an initial exposure has caused production of IgE antibodies. On second exposure, the patient may suddenly develop symptoms that may include pruritus, urticaria, dyspnoea, vomiting and angio-oedema. Oedema of the face, mouth and tongue often precedes laryngeal obstruction. Vascular collapse and death may occur within 15 min if treatment is not instituted.

Respiratory manifestations are secondary to obstruction of the airway and to circulatory failure. Circulatory failure occurs when there is a massive loss of fluids from the vascular system due to the vasodilating actions of the released vasoactive amines. The cardiac changes are particularly due to the effect of histamine on the myocardium. Urticaria is frequently associated with allergy to drugs.

Many antibiotics are reported to cause anaphylactic reactions (Table 3). In practice, the risk of anaphylaxis can be reduced by a careful drug history and reporting, the use of medical alert tags, avoidance of unnecessary drug therapy and the availability of resuscitation drugs and equipment.

B. Haemolytic Anaemia

Haemolytic anaemia caused by drugs is considered to be a type II hypersensitivity reaction. Table 5 lists antibiotics that have been implicated in this type of reaction. Clinical manifestations are usually mild until anaemia occurs, which may present as weakness and fatigue after having taken the drug for several weeks. Treatment consists of discontinuing the drug and treating the anaemia if severe.

Table 5
Antimicrobial agents reported to cause a positive antiglobulin test and/or haemolytic anaemia[a]

Cephalosporins	Streptomycin
Isoniazid	Sulphonamides
Penicillins	Tetracyclines
Rifampicin	

[a]Adapted from Garraty and Petz (1975).

Haemolytic anaemia is associated with a positive direct antiglobulin test (direct Coombs's test) as a result of immunoglobulins and/or complement adhering to red-cell membranes. Only in rare cases does the reaction lead to destruction of erythrocytes and haemolytic anaemia. When there is destruction of the cell, clinical disorders occur secondarily to loss of erythrocytic function or to the damaging effects of released cell contents (haemoglobulin).

There are at least four mechanisms involved in a drug-induced positive Coombs's test and/or haemolytic anaemia:

(1) Drug absorption,
(2) Immune complex,
(3) Autoantibody,
(4) Membrane modification.

The first three types are a result of an immune mechanism where antibodies are formed which react with the red blood cell (Petz, 1980). The membrane-modification type is caused by a non-immunological protein-adsorption mechanism in which no serum antibodies are found. To date, only cephalosporins have been reported to cause this type of reaction.

C. Agranulocytosis

Drug-induced agranulocytosis is a disorder characterized by a severe reduction in the level of circulating blood neutrophils (usually less than $200/mm^3$). The immunologic basis of drug induction is not entirely clear, but it has been classified under three headings (Young and Vincent, 1980):

(1) Immune suppression of granulopoiesis,
(2) Immune destruction of mature granulocytes,
(3) Association with autoantibody formation.

Onset of immune leucopenia usually occurs within 7-14 days after initial administration of drug. Fever, chills and arthralgias, along with pharyngitis and ulcerations of the mouth and anogenital area, may be the initial or early symptoms. Septicaemia is the major complication and may result in a mortality rate of 30% (Bottinger *et al.*, 1979). Drug-induced agranulocytosis is relatively rare and is often a self-limiting condition when the drug is promptly withdrawn. Supportive therapy with isolation and precautions, as well as antibiotics for infections in the presence of severe neutropenia, are important features of treatment. Table 6 lists antimicrobial agents associated with agranulocytosis.

Table 6
Antimicrobial agents associated with agranulocytosis[a]

Ampicillin	Chloramphenicol
Carbenicillin	Penicillins
Cephalosporins	Rifampicin
Sulphonamides	Nitrofurantoin

[a]Adapted from Pisciotta (1978).

D. Thrombocytopenia

Drug-induced thrombocytopenia is frequently produced via a type II hypersensitivity reaction. The drug or metabolite of the drug acts as a hapten with the thrombocyte. Lysis occurs in presence of complement and IgG drug-immune complexes which absorb to the platelet. In a previously sensitized patient, the platelet count may fall in minutes to hours on rechallenge. This reaction may occur when only very small amounts of drug (antigen) are given.

When the platelet count is too low, the patient may bleed spontaneously. Severity of bleeding may range from local effects (petechia or bleeding from mucous membranes) to lethal effects (extravastation of blood into tissues). Table 7 lists antimicrobial agents associated with thrombocytopenia.

Table 7
Antimicrobial agents associated with thrombocytopenia[a]

Cephalothin	Rifampicin
Chloramphenicol	Sulphonamides
Isoniazid	

[a]Adapted from Miescher (1973).

E. Drug Fever

Drug fever is defined as a febrile reaction resulting directly or indirectly from administration of a drug. Fever due to a drug should be expected when an elevated temperature cannot be attributed to an underlying disease process or to other complications occuring during therapy.

Drug fever is generally classified into three groups;

(1) Fever secondary to pyrogens or organisms in a contaminated drug,
(2) Fever related to the pharmacology of the drug,
(3) Fever secondary to a hypersensitivity reaction to the drug.

Drug fever due to allergic reactions is the most common cause of drug fever and may occur as the only symptom or in association with other allergic manifestations such as skin rashes, haematologic disorders, vasculitides and serum sickness reactions (Lipsky and Hirschmann, 1981). This fever may occur immediately but more commonly appears 7-10 days after the drug is started, especially when associated with other symptoms. The fever curve may be sustained or remittent as long as the patient is on the drug but usually returns to normal within 2-4 days after the drug is stopped (Cluff and Johnson, 1964).

Drug fever should be taken as a warning sign, because it may suggest a premonitory finding to a more serious adverse drug reaction such as a blood dyscrasia, anaphylaxis or vasculitis. Drugs that commonly cause an

Table 8
Antimicrobial agents implicated in allergic drug fever[a]

Cephalosporins	Penicillins
Chloramphenicol	Streptomycin
Erythromycin	Sulphonamides
Isoniazid	Tetracyclines
Nitrofurantoin	

[a]Adapted from Cluff *et al.* (1975).

allergic drug fever are listed in Table 8. Treatment includes discontinuing the offending agent. If the patient is on more than one drug, the drug most likely to cause fever should be stopped first.

F. Vasculitis

Drugs may produce reactions that primarily affect small vessels resulting in allergic vasculitis. Skin is the organ usually involved in small-vessel vasculitis, however, more complicated conditions occur when small vessels of the kidney, gastrointestinal tract, liver and other organs may be involved.

A type II or type III hypersensitivity mechanism affects the vascular endothelium in this reaction. Biopsy reveals a lymphocytic infiltrate of PMN cells, mononuclear cells and eosinophils. The infiltrate acts on blood vessels culminating in endothelial swelling, haemorrhage and thrombi.

In cutaneous vasculitis, haemorrhagic macules and papules of purpura may occur on lower extremities and dependent areas. This may be associated with a systemic reaction. In these patients fever, oedema, arthralgia, jaundice, haematuria and gastrointestinal bleeding may occur, depending on the organ involved. Laboratory determinations may show a decrease in renal function, proteinuria and haematuria in renal vasculitis, while elevated transaminases and bilirubin may occur in hepatic vasculitis.

Drug reactions are estimated to be responsible for about one-third of all vasculitis and about half the cases of systemic drug-induced vasculitis

Table 9
Antimicrobial agents implicated in vasculitis[a]

Penicillins
Sulphonamides
Tetracyclines

[a]Adapted from Fauci *et al.* (1978).

are potentially fatal. Table 9 lists some of the drugs that may cause vasculitis. Treatment with corticosteroids may be effective but failure rates are high with systemic vasculitis, especially with renal vasculitis.

G. Kidney Reactions

A drug (or metabolite) may act as an antigen or a hapten–protein and elicit an immune reaction that affects the kidney. This reaction may be caused by antigen–antibody complexes that circulate through the kidney or are bound to renal tissues. An immunological response ensues causing either direct injury to renal tissue (e.g. glomerulonephritis or interstitial nephritis) or ischaemic injury to renal tissue by affecting blood vessels to the kidney (e.g. acute necrotizing angiitis).

The mechanism of hypersensitivity may be a reaction of type II, III or IV or a combination. In most cases these reactions are not dose-related, do not occur immediately on exposure but after a period of time and usually abate upon discontinuation of drug. In addition, prior renal dysfunction increases the risk of reaction.

One of the most well documented renal immune reactions is acute interstitial nephritis. This reaction is characterized by an inflammatory response involving infiltrates of lymphocytes, macrophages and PMNs into the interstitium of the kidney. Histologic and functional tubular changes may also be present which may lead to a tubulointerstitial disorder. The distinguishing features are fever, rash, eosinophilia and eosinophiluria, haematuria and varying degrees of renal failure.

Interstitial nephritis occurs most commonly with semisynthetic penicillins, especially methicillin. Over 100 cases of acute interstitial nephritis secondary to methicillin have been reported. Data support the mechanism of this toxicity as immunologically mediated (Bennett, 1981; Maher, 1981). Some antimicrobial agents which have been reported to have caused acute immune-mediated interstitial nephritis are listed in Table 10. Onset is usually 10–20 days; however, it has been as little as 2 days or as much as 6 weeks.

Treatment includes drug withdrawal. Drug cross-sensitivity cases have been known to occur; therefore, it is best to give an antigenically unrelated antibiotic (Appel *et al.*, 1977*a*). In severe cases, supportive haemodialysis may be necessary and corticosteroids may be helpful; however, studies to support this are few. Other renal hypersensitivity reactions are rare in occurrence and include anaphylactic shock with acute tubular necrosis, anaphylactoid purpura leading to acute glomerulonephritis, polyarteritis nudosa leading to renal failure and acute necrotizing angiitis.

Table 10
Antimicrobial agents associated with acute interstitial nephritis[a]

Cephalosporins	Nafcillin
Penicillin G	Oxacillin
Ampicillin	Rifampicin
Carbenicillin	Sulphonamides
Methicillin	Co-trimoxazole

[a]Adapted from Appel and Neu (1977*a*, *b*) and Van Ypersele de Strilou (1979).

H. Lung Reactions

Adverse pulmonary reactions to drugs are relatively uncommon, but should be considered when the aetiology of a respiratory problem is unknown. In most cases, a correct diagnosis can be made if the clinician recognizes the clinical characteristics that correlate with the implicated drug. Withdrawal of the agent will usually result in resolution of the reaction but in certain situations corticosteroids may be necessary.

Some drugs such as acetylsalicylic acid and β-adrenergic blocking agents cause adverse pulmonary reactions that are not due to allergic mechanisms. Table 11 indicates pulmonary reactions caused by immunological mechanisms and indicates some antimicrobial agents that are implicated.

Table 11
Antimicrobial agents implicated in lung disorders[a]

Type of pulmonary reaction	Mechanism	Drug
Bronchoconstriction and asthma	Type I	Penicillins
		Cephalosporins
		Aminoglycosides
Systemic lupus erythematosus (SLE)	Type III	Isoniazid
		Penicillins
		Sulphonamides
		Tetracyclines
Generalized reactions:	Type III	Sulphonamides
Polyarteritis		Tetracyclines
Pulmonary eosinophilia II and III	Unknown, immune mechanism	Nitrofurantoin
		Sulphonamides
		Nitrofurantoin
		Penicillins
Pulmonary oedema and fibrosis	Unknown, toxic	Nitrofurantoin

[a]Adapted from Cole (1977).

1. Bronchoconstriction and asthma

In a majority of cases, this reaction is an allergic type I reaction; the classic example is that of penicillin. This reaction is secondary to the release of pharmacologically active mediators from mast cells in lungs that cause an imbalance in the cAMP/cGMP ratio resulting in bronchoconstriction and attendant clinical symptoms.

2. Systemic lupus erythematosus (SLE) involving the lungs

Several drugs are capable of provoking an SLE syndrome which affects the lungs. The offending agent may uncover a latent tendency to develop SLE and the reaction occurs more frequently in patients with a family history of rheumatic diseases. Type III hypersensitivity appears to be the reaction mechanism. Specific respiratory disorders attributed to this reaction may include pleurisy, dyspnoea with cough and disappearing lung (due to reduced respiratory movement). Lung symptoms may occur before general SLE symptoms and there is an associated presence of antinuclear antibodies in serum. Treatment includes withdrawal of the drug at which time symptoms usually revert; however, persistent cases have been reported to have occurred with isoniazid. Corticosteroids are commonly used to treat these persistent cases.

3. Polyarteritis involving the lungs

In these patients, drug-induced immune complexes may affect the small arteries and arterioles of the lungs. Pulmonary inflammation is often present and this commonly leads to respiratory problems.

4. Pulmonary infiltrates and eosinophilia

This may also be called Loeffler's-type syndrome. Because symptoms are minimal and improvement is rapid upon withdrawal of the agent, treatment is usually not necessary. However, on re-exposure, the reaction onset may be sudden and more severe and corticosteroids may be needed. The prognosis is usually good. Clinical signs are fever, cough and shortness of breath with wheezing.

5. Pulmonary oedema and fibrosis

Interstitial pneumonitis, which progress into pulmonary oedema and fibrosis, has been reported for certain drugs. Some cases are known to be caused by direct toxic effects, while others have been shown to be related to type IV hypersensitivity reactions. In the pulmonary lesion induced by nitrofurantoin, cough and dyspnoea usually occurs after 6 months or more of continuous treatment. This may result in a chronic fibrosis in which lung changes are irreversible.

J. Liver Reactions

Adverse drug reactions may cause hepatic injury in varying degrees. However, very few drugs are known to cause hepatic injury by an immune mechanism. In most cases, the immunological evidence to substantiate drug-induced hypersensitivity reactions in the liver is still questionable, since sophisticated methods of determination have yet to be developed.

If the reaction occurs in only a small percentage of patients taking the drug, and onset of reaction is consistent with the time scale of an immune response, and other symptoms such as skin rash, fever and oesinophilia occur, then the evidence favours an immune mechanism. Some types of adverse hepatic drug reactions to antimicrobial agents are listed in Table 12. The histological changes and biochemical effects related to the implicated drugs, as well as the clinical syndrome it resembles, are indicated.

Hepatocellular necrosis of both zonal and diffuse types leads to a viral-like hepatitis syndrome. Serum transaminases are often elevated from 10 to 200 times normal levels, while alkaline phosphatase levels are usually no more than three times normal. Gastrointestinal symptoms of nausea, vomiting and anorexia are common. Both direct and indirect bilirubin are

Table 12
Antimicrobial-induced hepatic injury related to hypersensitivity reactions[a]

Histological	Biochemical	Clinical	Drug
Hepatocellular necrosis, zonal or diffuse	Transaminases + + + Hyperbilirubinaemia Eosinophilia in 20–25% of cases Alkaline phosphatase +	Viral hepatitis	Isoniazid
Hepatocanalicular and canalicular injury	Alkaline phosphatase + + Bilirubin Transaminases + Eosinophilia in 20–25% of patients	Obstructive jaundice	Erythromycin estolate and ethylsuccinate
Mixed hepatocellular cholestatic injury	Transaminases Bilirubin Alkaline phosphatase + +	Atypical viral hepatitis	PAS Sulphonamides Nitrofurantoin
Chronic active hepatitis	Transaminases + + Alkaline phosphatase + Infiltrates	Autoimmune hepatitis	Sulphonamides Nitrofurantoin

[a]Difficult to determine if immunological, idiopathic or toxic reactions.

are elevated and may result in coagulation abnormalities and orange-yellow jaundice. Drugs are believed to cause immune-mediated hepatic damage only rarely but nevertheless may be associated with a high fatality rate when reactions do occur.

Hepatocanalicular damage resembles extrahepatic obstructive jaundice. Transaminases levels may be only moderately elevated and alkaline phosphatase levels may be eleveated threefold or more. Jaundice of a yellow-green colour and persistent pruritus are common. Serum bilirubin values are generally below 5 mg/dl. Mortality is low, hepatic injury is usually reversible and symptoms usually subside approximately 2–5 weeks after the drug is stopped.

Mixed hepatocellular cholestatic injury resembles atypical viral hepatitis. Signs, symptoms and clinical prognosis depend on the extent of cytotoxic damage and cholestatic injury caused by the drug.

Chronic active hepatitis is a syndrome identified more recently and is also called lupoid (autoimmune hepatitis). Clinical features include jaundice, anorexia, fatigue and hepatomegaly. Arthralgias and spider angiomas may also be present. Serum transaminases and alkaline phosphatase may be moderately elevated. Characteristic to the syndrome are hyperglobulinaemia and hypoalbuminaemia. Chronic active hepatitis often appears after months to years of drug exposure, but usually improves markedly after drug is discontinued.

K. Drug-induced Systemic Lupus Erythematosus

A number of antimicrobial agents have been associated with a syndrome resembling SLE. This syndrome differs in a few respects from idiopathic disease. Renal disease is less common and less severe, complement levels are more likely to be normal, and antibodies are likely to be against single-stranded rather than native double-stranded DNA.

The mechanism of induction of this syndrome remains unknown, but several antimicrobial agents have been implicated in altering the antigenicity of nucleoproteins (see Table 13).

Laboratory data may show evidence of an elevated erythrocyte sedimentation rate, antinuclear antibodies (ANA), anaemia and hypergammaglobulinaemia. Characteristically, the patient is on the drug a few weeks before the symptoms occur.

Clinical signs include malaise, lethargy, low-grade fever, headache and joint pain. A butterfly rash may also be noted. Clinical manifestations of the syndrome usually clear within a few weeks or months after drug is stopped.

Table 13
Antimicrobial agents associated with systemic lupus erythematosus

Isoniazid	Streptomycin
Sulphonamides	Tetracyclines
Penicillins	

L. Skin Reactions

Although most drug-induced cutaneous hypersensitivity reactions are due to unknown mechanisms, it has been shown that a drug may act as an antigen or hapten and trigger an immune-mediated hypersensitivity reaction in the skin. Antibody-mediated reactions that may demonstrate cutaneous involvement include urticaria, angiodema, Arthus reaction, serum sickness, thrombocytopenic purpura and vasculitides. Cell-mediated reactions that often involve the skin include allergic contact dermatitis. Some other cutaneous reactions that are theoretically immune-mediated include erythema multiforme, Stevens–Johnson syndrome, toxic epidermal necrolysis, erythema nodosum and fixed drug eruption.

The sensitization rate is known to depend on the route of administration of the drug. In the case of penicillin, it was shown that highest sensitization rates are produced by local application or by aerosol inhalation; oral administration produced the lowest rate, and parenteral routes (intravenous or intramuscular) gave intermediate rates. Concentration (dose) may have an effect, because higher concentrations give higher rates of cutaneous reactivity (Lindemayr, 1959).

In addition to previously described reactions which may produce cutaneous manifestations, maculopapular eruptions are next most common after urticarial reactions. Most maculopapular reactions are theoretically due to Type IV cell-mediated allergy (Marghescu, 1978). This supposition is based on clinical observations, on results of skin tests (patch and

Table 14
Antimicrobial agents implicated in allergic contact dermatitis

Aminoglycosides	Nitrofurazone
Bacitracin	Penicillins
Chloramphenicol	Polymyxin B Sulphate
Clindamycin	Streptomycin
Erythromycin	Sulphonamides
Gentamicin	Tetracyclines

intradermal) and on *in-vitro* lymphocyte transformation tests as well as macrophage migration inhibition tests (Girard, 1974). Since these tests are positive in only a small percentage of reactive patients, this mechanism remains theoretical.

The most common allergic skin disease caused by drugs is allergic contact dermatitis. Antimicrobial agents rank as one of the most common causes of this reaction. Table 14 lists antimicrobial agents implicated in allergic contact dermatitis.

IV. IMMUNOLOGIC REACTIONS DUE TO SPECIFIC ANTIMICROBIAL AGENTS

A. Penicillins

Penicillins are probably one of the most prescribed class of drugs worldwide, thus adverse reactions caused by penicillins pose a significant health problem (Erffmeyer, 1981). There are many forms of penicillin, but they cause similar hypersensitivity reactions due to their common β-lactam ring structure. However, the extent and severity of reactions vary.

Penicillin itself is a weak hapten, but becomes immunologically active when degraded into highly reactive metabolic breakdown products. For example, when benzylpenicillin is degraded, the β-lactam ring opens and reacts with tissue protein forming about 95% benzylpenicilloyl (BPO) group 'major determinants' and 5% other 'minor antigenic determinants'. Both types bind firmly enough with tissue protein to form immunogenic complexes (Parker, 1975).

These complexes are capable of eliciting an antibody response involving all the major immunoglobulins (IgG, IgM, IgA, IgD and IgE) (Van Dellen and Gleich, 1970). Presence of antibodies does not necessarily indicate an allergic response, because the latter also depends on the type and quantity of antibody and on hapten specificity. Type IV hypersensitivity reactions have also been produced by penicillin on the basis of activated lymphocytes (Sher, 1983).

Penicillin has been implicated in eliciting hypersensitivity in man corresponding to all four major classifications of Gell and Coombs (1975). Table 15 describes different adverse reactions to penicillin.

There have been numerous studies demonstrating the value of skin testing to detect penicillin hypersensitivity with penicillin natigens (Adkinson *et al.*, 1971; Sullivan *et al.*, 1981). However, skin testing does not always predict an allergic response. The skin-testing procedure can usually be carried out safely with minimal risk to the patient when simple precautions

Table 15
Immune-mediated hypersensitivity reactions to penicillins

Type of reaction	General Information
Anaphylactic	500–800 deaths/year (Valentine, 1979); incidence 1:10 000 (Idsöe, 1958); mainly occurs with parenteral administration
Urticaria	Causes may be hidden due to contamination of penicillin in certain foods
Serum-like sickness	Classical clinical picture of serum sickness (DeSwarte, 1980)
Haemolytic anaemia	A positive direct antiglobulin (Coombs) test develops in approximately 3% of the patients receiving i.v. penicillin $10–20 \times 10^6$ units/day (Abraham *et al.*, 1968); only a small percentage develop haemolytic anaemia (Garratty and Petz, 1975)
Leucopenia	Occurs mainly with high doses (Carpenter, 1980)
Thrombocytopenia (coagulation disorder)	Appears to be related to effect on platelet function (Aster, 1977); Most commonly reported with carbenicillin
Hepatitis	Reported with oxacillin and carbenicillin (Wilson *et al.*, 1975)
Kidney disorders	May be transient glomerulopathy or lead to interstitial nephritis; most common with methicillin; usually occurs in patients with a prolonged course of antibiotic; usually occurs with fever, eosinophilia and urinary sediment (Border *et al.*, 1974)
Vasculitis	Localized and diffuse types have been reported
Pulmonary	Type I reaction results in an asthma-like condition. Pulmonary infiltrates with eosinophilia have occurred; cause is unclear (Reichlin *et al.*, 1953)
Cutaneous manifestations	
Maculopapular	Rashes are common with type I reactions and serum sickness
Allergic contact dermatitis	Topical antimicrobials represent one of the most common causes
Fixed drug eruption, erythema multiforme, Stevens–Johnson syndrome, exfoliative dermatitis, toxic epidermal necrolysis	Pathogenesis unknown (DeSwarte, 1980)

are followed (Sher, 1983). The management of patients allergic to penicillin, who need penicillin and no other alternative is available, should be managed by those experienced in skin testing and penicillin-desensitization methods (Sher, 1983).

A careful drug history and selective intradermal skin testing are precautions to consider when penicillin is prescribed. Penicillins should be used with caution when there is a general history of allergies such as asthma, atopic dermatitis, hay fever or urticaria. If a patient is hypersensitive to one penicillin, he will have an increased risk of sensitivity to other penicillins.

B. Cephalosporins

In the last five years, there has been a great increase in the number of cephalosporin compounds. Despite the chemical similarity between cephalosporins and penicillin, there is a marked difference between the spectrum of action and the incidence of hypersensitivity. Up to 5% of individuals receiving cephalosporins experience some type of 'allergic reaction (Moellering and Swartz, 1976). In patients without a history of

Table 16
Allergic reactions to cephalosporins

Type of reaction	General information
Red-cell disorders	3% frequency of occurrence. Certain cephalosporins are known to modify chemically the red-cell membrane. One type is apparently non-immunological (Petz, 1971), while in a rare form antibodies are produced toward drug-coated red blood cells (Garratty and Petz, 1975)
Immediate hypersensitivity	Incidence is reported much lower than penicillins
Reactions similar to penicillin type	
Rashes	(Scheife *et al.*, 1976).
Maculopapular	
Morbiliform	
Urticarial	
Thrombocytopenia	(Gralnick *et al.*, 1972).
Granulocytopenia	(DiCato and Ellman, 1975).
Drug fever	(Scheife *et al.*, 1976).

penicillin allergy, the incidence of allergic reaction was less than 2% (Petz, 1971). In patients with a history of penicillin allergy, the incidence of cross-reaction varied from 5 to 15% (Mandell, 1973). In individuals with a positive history of penicillin allergy and a positive penicillin skin test, the incidence of allergic reactions to cephalothin was 50% (Thoburn *et al.*, 1968). Patients who have a history of life-threatening reaction to penicillin should be given cephalosporins with extreme caution. The incidence of hypersensitivity to the newer cephalosporins in relation to penicillin has not been well defined. Reported allergic reactions to cephalosporins are listed in Table 16.

C. Macrolides

The macrolide antibiotics have a very low incidence of immune-mediated adverse reactions. Only a few cases of urticaria and fixed drug eruption following therapy (Ketel, 1976) have been reported that could be considered an allergic reaction. A hepatic hypersensitivity reaction is now thought to be due to another mechanism (Braum, 1969). Only skin eruptions have been noted with any incidence (Kuder, 1960).

D. Lincomycins

As with the other macrolides, there is a low incidence of allergic reactions. Cases report of anaphylactic shock, acute urticaria and angio-oedema (Walker, 1969) have been reported. Coskey (1978) has suggested that clindamycin may act as a sensitizing agent and result in contact dermatitis. Transient abnormalities of liver functions, which are not dose-related and return to normal after the drug is discontinued, occur occasionally (Elmore *et al.*, 1974).

E. Vancomycin

There are limited data on vancomycin causing allergic reactions. However, anaphylactic shock and urticarial eruptions have been noted (Miller and Tausk, 1977).

F. Tetracyclines

Allergic reactions to tetracyclines range in frequency from 0·1 to 2%. (Weinstein and Welch, 1958). Specific types of hypersensitivity reactions are listed in Table 17.

Table 17
Allergic reactions to tetracyclines

Type of reaction	General information
Anaphylactic shock	The usual signs of anaphylactic shock have been noted following administration of tetracycline (Fellner and Baer, 1965)
Serum sickness-like reactions	Fellner and Baer (1966)
Immune haemolytic anaemia from tetracycline	Wenz *et al.* (1974)
Thrombocytopenia purpura with oxytetracycline	Kaunis (1975)
Acute interstitial nephritis with minocycline	Walker *et al.* (1979)
Fixed drug eruptions	Pasricha and Shukla (1979)

G. Aminoglycosides

Allergic reactions evidenced by eosinophilia, rash and fever occur in approximately 1–3% of patients receiving aminoglycoside therapy (Scheife *et al.*, 1976). More serious hypersensitivity reactions such as anaphylaxis and blood dyscrasias are extremely rare (Weinstein, 1975). Allergic reactions to aminoglycosides are listed in Table 18. Patients hypersensitive to one aminoglycoside may be hypersensitive to other aminoglycosides.

H. Sulphonamides

The overall incidence of reactions to sulphonamides is about 5%. The most common type of reactions are those affecting skin. In general, sulphonamides of any type should be used with extreme caution in patients with a previous history of severe allergy.

With decreased use of long-acting sulphonamides and discontinuation of sulphonamides in common dermatologic preparations, there has been an overall decrease in hypersensitivity reactions. However, with the increased use of the trimethoprim and sulphonamethoxazole combination, there has been an increase in reported adverse reactions to this particular combination. Table 19 lists allergic reactions to sulphonamides.

Table 18
Allergic reactions to aminoglycosides

Reaction	Drug	General information
Contact dermatitis	Streptomycin	Delayed-type reaction incidence reported 3–10% (Chakravarty and Sircar, 1961)
Immune haemolytic anaemia	Streptomycin	IgG antibodies were found by a positive direct and indirect Coombs's test (Martinez *et al.*, 1977)
Cutaneous eruptions Drug fever and eosinophilia	Streptomycin	In long-term treatment 11% of patients were found to have hypersensitivity reactions as described by Chakravarty and Sircar (1961)
Urticaria, maculopapular	Gentamicin	0.8% of patients (Hewitt, 1974)
Rashes and blood dyscrasias	Tobramycin	0·6% of patients (Speirs, 1976).
Cross-allergenicity	Kanamycin Neomycin Gentamicin Tobramycin	Allergic contact dermatitis may result in cross-sensitivity (Schorr *et al.*, 1973)

J. Nitrofurantoin

Allergic reactions to nitrofurantoin occur in the frequency range of 2–4%. These reactions may occur as exanthema, fever, allergic pulmonary infiltrates, angioneurotic oedema, anaphylactic shock or liver damage.

Pulmonary reactions to nitrofurantoin are classified into three types:

(1) Acute pneumonitis—sudden cough, fever and dyspnoea occurring hours to days after initiation of therapy. The reaction usually clears within 2–3 days after discontinuing the drug. This pneumonitis is probably allergic in nature and is often accompanied by eosinophilia (Simonson *et al.*, 1977).

(2) Subacute pneumonitis—more subacute may occur after the patient has been on the drug for up to a year. It is characterized by cough, dyspnoea and fever and may be associated with a lupus-like syndrome (Sollaccio *et al.*, 1966).

(3) Chronic pulmonary fibrosis has been reported to show interstitial infiltrate on chest X-ray and a non-specific interstitial fibrosis on biopsy specimen (Israel and Diamond, 1962). These changes manifest

Table 19
Hypersensitivity reactions to sulphonamides

Type	General information
Skin: common rashes are maculopapular or urticarial type. Less frequently are erythema nodosum, exfoliative dermatitis. Rarely Stevens-Johnsons syndrome, pemphigoid and Behcets syndrome. Contact dermatitis and photosensitivity less common today as a result of lower use of topical preparations containing sulphonamides	Drug eruptions may most often occur after the first week unless previously sensitized. Other symptoms of fever, malaise and pruritus may occur at the same time. Incidence has been reported by Koch-Weser, *et al.* (1971) to occur in 2·8% cases receiving sulphisoxazole and 3·0% for cases receiving sulphamethoxazole. Stevens–Johnson syndrome appears to occur more often with use of long-acting sulphonamides (Payles, 1970) and has been described after administering sulphonamide eye drops. (Gottschalk and Stone, 1976)
Serum-sickness reaction	Serum sickness-like reactions with rashes, fever and joint pain
Anaphylactoid-type reaction	In a patient previously sensitized, an immediate anaphylactoid reaction may occur
Drug fever	Incidence is approximately 3% with sulphisoxazole. More common with the long-acting preparations (Grieble and Jackson, 1958)
Haemolytic anaemia	Reported to occur in 0·05% of cases after sulphadiazine; has been related to lack of glucose-6-phosphate dehydrogenase
Agranulocytosis	Occurs in about 0·1% of the cases usually after 10 days of therapy and is not dose-related (Asmar *et al.*, 1981)
Trombocytopenia	A rare complication but has been reported (Claas *et al.*, 1979)

(Continued)

Table 19 (Continued)

Type	General information
Hepatocellular injury	Associated with mixed hepatocellular injury; more likely a toxic effect than a hypersensitivity reaction (Tonder *et al.*, 1974)
Pulmonary reactions	Sulphonamide-induced pulmonary reactions are rare; however, pulmonary eosinophilia reactions have been reported (Tydd and Dyer, 1976)
Systemic lupus erythematosus	Cases have been reported in patients using sulphonamides, especially the long-acting drugs, and in patients being treated with sulphasalazine for ulcerative colitis (Rallison *et al.*, 1961; Tonder *et al.*, 1974; Griffiths and Kane, 1977)
Allergic vaculitis	Allergic vasculitis with arthritis
Renal	Interstitial nephritis, nephrotic syndrome and renal problems have been associated with hypersensitivity reactions due to sulphonamides (Owens *et al.*, 1974; Appel and Neu 1977*b*

as a non-productive cough and dyspnoea with pulmonary function tests demonstrating restrictive ventilatory patterns. It usually develops after 6 months of being on the drug.

Hypersensitivity reactions to nitrofurantoin are considered mechanistically to be type III with mostly IgM or IgG antibodies reacting with antigen to form antigen-antibody complexes in target tissues. Neijer (1970) supports the postulate that allergic reactions in the lungs correspond to the Arthus phenomenon. Immunological abnormalities, including antinuclear antibodies have also been detected.

Nitrofurantoin rarely causes hepatic injury; however, there have been cases of chronic active hepatitis reported in females. Patients had used nitrofurantoin for 6 or more months before the onset of fatigue, anorexia and jaundice. Clinical and biochemical cure occurred within 12 weeks after drug withdrawal. Two fatal cases have been reported by Sharp *et al.* (1980); however, the mechanism is unclear.

K. Rifampicin

Adverse reactions tend to be mild and transient with daily administration of rifampicin. However, on intermittent administration or readministration, more severe reactions may occur. This may be a result of immunological mechanisms. IgE, IgG and IgM antibodies have been demonstrated and provide evidence that some adverse reactions to rifampicin may be immune-mediated Pujet *et al.*, 1974; Bassi *et al.*, 1976). Table 20 lists some reactions reported for rifampicin.

L. Metronidazole

The incidence of immune-mediated hypersensitivity reactions associated with metronidazole is low. Rissing *et al.* (1980) have reported erythematous and pruritic maculopapular rashes; however, the percentage of patients experiencing these reactions is small. Leucopenia is considered a possible but rare side effect, occurring in as many as 1-3% of patients (White *et al.*, 1980). The mechanism is not clearly defined. Most authors suggest that metronidazole might cause peripheral destruction of neutrophils, since marrow biopsies in a few of these patients have been normal or hyperplastic (Lefebvre and Hesseltine, 1965). The neutropenia lasts for the duration of therapy and reverses upon discontinuation of therapy; however, it may take 7-14 days to return to normal (McKendrick and Geddes, 1979). When the drug is used for prolonged periods and unexplained fever or sore throat is present, the possibility of metronidazole-induced leucopenia should be considered.

Table 20
Allergic reactions to rifampicin

Clinical types of reaction	Information
'Flu-like' syndrome (fever, chills, headaches, dizziness and myalgias)	Reported by Pujet *et al.* (1974); occurs with intermittent therapy
Blood dyscrasias (thrombocytopenia and haemolytic anaemia)	Both have been reported with intermittent doses of rifampicin (Girling, 1977). Cases of haemolysed red blood cells with or without renal failure have been observed (Kleinknecht *et al.* 1972). In some cases, antibodies to rifampicin have been detected
Exudative conjunctivitis	Cayley and Majundar (1976)
Stevens-Johnson syndrome	Nyirenda and Gill (1977)
Pemphigus vulgaris	Gange *et al.*, (1976)

Weart and Hyman (1983) have reported a case of serum sickness associated with metronidazole. Resolution of symptoms occurred upon withdrawal of drug.

M. Chloramphenicol

Hypersensitivity reactions to chloramphenicol are very rare; however, contact dermatitis, maculopapular rashes, urticaria, drug fever and even rarer instances of anaphylaxis and angioneurotic oedema have been reported.

The hypothesis that aplastic anaemia is caused by an immunologic mechanism has not been established. However, chloramphenicol-specific antibodies were found in patients who were in the acute phase of the disease (Kraft, 1983).

CONCLUSION

Adverse drug reactions to antimicrobial agents mediated by immunological or non-immunological mechanisms comprise a significant problem world-wide that may be both harmful and costly to the patient. When an undesired clinical event occurs, the clinician should have a high degree of suspicion that the event may be drug-related. A simple method to determine if an undesired event may be drug-induced is to stop the drug and observe whether the symptoms subside or disappear.

To lower the incidence of adverse reactions the clinician should:

(1) Establish the need for a drug by confirming the diagnosis.
(2) Select the most appropriate agent to treat the diagnosed patient.
(3) Prescribe the fewest drugs possible to meet the patient's therapeutic needs.
(4) Select drugs carefully in patients who give a positive history of hypersensitivity or undesired drug-related events.
(5) Evaluate the proposed therapy for potential cross-sensitivity to drugs to which the patient is known to be allergic.
(6) Monitor the patient's response closely for any undesired clinical event.
(7) If an undesired reaction occurs, stop the drug, evaluate for treatment and document the reaction.
(8) Documented reactions should be assessed clinically by ranking as (a) *probably*, (b) *possibly*, (c) *remotely* due to the suspected agent.

The clinician can minimize the risk by selecting drugs carefully and maintaining vigilance for adverse clinical events. This applies especially to antimicrobial agents because of their high propensity to function as immunomodulating agents and thus initiating hypersensitivity reactions as drug-induced.

REFERENCES

Abraham, E. N., Petz, L. D. and Fudenberg, H. H. (1968). *Clin. Exp. Immunol.* **3**, 343.

Adkinson, N. F., Thompson, W. L., Maddrey, W. C. and Lichtenstein, L. M. (1971). *N. Engl. J. Med.* **285**, 22–24.

Appel, G. B. and Neu, H. C. (1977*a*). *N. Engl. J. Med.* **296**, 663–670.

Appel, G. B. and Neu, H. C. (1977*b*). *N. Engl. J. Med.* **296**, 784–787.

Asmar, B., Maqbool, S. and Dajarai, A. S. (1981). *Am. J. Dis. Child.* **135**, 1100–1103.

Aster, R. H. (1977). *In* "Hematology" (Williams, W. J., Beutler, E., Erslev, A. J. and Rundles, R. W., eds) pp. 1290–1339. McGraw-Hill, New York.

Baer, R. L. (1964). *J. Invest. Dermatol.* **43**, 223–229.

Bassi, L., Di Berardins, L. and Silvestri, L. G. (1976). *Int. Arch. Allergy Appl. Immunol* **51**, 390–394.

Bellanti, J. A. (1978). *In* "Immunology II", pp. 365–369. W. B. Saunders, Philadelphia.

Bennett, W. M. (1981). *Semin. Nephrol.* **1**, 43–50.

Borda, I. T., Sloan, P. and Jick, H. (1968). *J. Am. Med. Assoc.* **205**, 99–101.

Border, W. A., Lehman, D. H. and Egan, J. D., Sass, H. J., Elode, J. E. and Wilson, C. B. (1974). *N. Engl. J. Med.* **291**, 381–384.

Bottinger, L. E., Furhoff, A. K. and Holmberg, L. (1979). *Acta. Med. Scand.* **205**, 457-461.
Braum, P. (1969). *J. Infect. Dis.* **119**, 300-306.
Caranasas, G. J., Stewart, R. B. and Cluff, L. E. (1974). *J. Am. Med. Assoc.* **228**, 713-717.
Carpenter, J. (1980). *S. Med. J.* **73**, 745-749.
Cayley, F. E. and Majundar, S. K. (1976). *Br. Med. J.* **1**, 199-200.
Chakravarty, S. and Sircar, D. K. (1961). *Acta Tuberc. Scand.* **41**, 144-148.
Claas, F. H., Van der meer, J. W. and Langerak, J. (1979). *Br. Med. J.* **2**, 898-900.
Cluff, L. E. and Johnson, J. E. (1964). *Prog. Allergy* **8**, 149-161.
Cluff, L. E., Caranasos, G. J. and Stewart, R. B. (1975). "Clinical Problems with Drugs" Vol. V. W. B. Saunders, Philadelphia.
Cole, P. (1977). *Drugs* **13**, 422-444.
Coskey, R. J. (1978). *Arch. Dermatol.* **114**, 446-450.
DeSwarte, R. D. (1980). *In* "Allergic Diseases, Diagnosis and Management" (Patterson, R., ed.), pp. 452-583. J. B. Lippincott, Philadelphia.
DiCato, M. A. and Ellman, L. (1975). *Ann. Intern. Med.* **83**, 671-672.
Elmore, M., Rissina, J. P. and Rink, L. (1974). *Am. J. Med.* **57**, 627-630.
Elsen, H. H. and Belman, S. (1953). *J. Exp. Med.* **98**, 533-549.
Erffmeyer, J. E. (1981). *Ann. Allergy* **47**, 288-300.
Fauci, A. S., Haynes, B. F. and Katz, P. (1978). *Ann. Intern. Med.* **89**, 660-676.
Fellner, M. J. and Baer, R. C. (1965). *J. Am. Med. Assoc.* **192**, 997-998.
Fellner, M. J. and Baer, R. C. (1966). *Arch. Clin. Exp. Dermatol.* **224**, 157-167.
Gange, R., Rhodes, E. L. and Edwards, C. O. (1976). *Br. J. Dermatol.* **94**, 445-448.
Garratty, G. and Petz, L. P. (1975). *Am. J. Med.* **58**, 398-407.
Gell, P. G. and Coombs, R. R. A. (1975). *In* "Clinical Aspects of Immunology" (Gell, P. G., Coombs, R. A. S. and Hachmann, P. J., eds), Blackwell Scientific Publications, Oxford.
Girard, J. P. (1974). *In* "Allergology", 8th International Congress of Allergology, Congress series no. 23. Excerpta Medica, Amsterdam.
Girling, D. J. (1977). *J. Antimicrob. Chemother.* **3**, 115-123.
Gottschalk, H. R. and Stone, O. J. (1976). *Arch. Dermatol.* **112**, 513-514.
Gralnick, H. R., McGinnis, M. and Halterman, J. (1972). *Ann. Intern. Med.* **77**, 401-404.
Grieble, H. G. and Jackson, G. G. (1958). *N. Engl. J. Med.* **258**, 1-7.
Griffiths, I. D. and Kane, S. P. (1977). *Br. Med. J.* **2**, 1188-1189.
Hewitt, W. L. (1974). *Postgrad. Med. J.* **50** (*Suppl. 7*), 55-62.
Idsöe, O. (1958). *Bull. World Hlth Org.* **18**, 323-344.
Israel, H. L. and Diamond, P. (1962). *N. Engl. J. Med.* **266**, 1024-1026.
Kaunis, N. G. (1975). *J. Am. Med. Assoc.* **231**, 734-735.
Ketel, W. G. (1976). *Contact Dermatitis* **2**, 363-364.
Kleinknecht, D., Homberg, J. C. and Decroix, G. (1972). *Lancet* **i**, 1238-1239.
Koch-Weser, J., Sidel, V. W. and Dexter, M. (1971). *Arch. Intern. Med.* **128**, 399-404.

Kraft, D. (1983); *In* "Allergic Reactions to Drugs" (De Weck, A. L. and Bundgaard, H., eds), pp. 480-523. Springer-Verlag, New York.
Kuder, H. V. (1960). *Clin. Pharmacol. Ther.* **1**, 604-609.
Lefebvre, Y. and Hesseltine, H. C (1965). *J. Am. Med. Assoc.* **191**, 126-130.
Lindemayer, W. (1959). *In* "Dermatologie and Venerologie" Vol III/1, (Gottron, H. A. and Schonfeld, W., eds), p. 327. Thieme, Stuttgart.
Lipsky, B. A. and Hirschmann, J. V. (1981). *J. Am. Med. Assoc.* **245**, 851-853.
Maher, J. F. (1981). *Semin. Nephrol.* **1**, 27-35.
Mandell, G. L. (1973). *Ann. Intern. Med.* **79**, 561-565.
Marghescu, S. (1978). "Allergische Arzneiexantheme". Perimed-Verlag D. Straube, Erlangen.
Martinez, J., Lletona, L., Barbolla, L., Frieyro, E., Bouza, E., Eilsanz, F. and Fernandez, M. N. (1977). *Br. J. Haematol.* **35**, 561-571.
McKendrick, M. W., and Geddes, A. M. (1979). *Br. Med. J.* **2**, 796.
Miescher, P. A. (1973). *Semin. Hematol.* **10**, 311-325.
Miller, R. and Tausk, H. C. (1977). *Anesth. Analg. (Cleve.)* **56**, 870-872.
Moellering, R. C. and Swartz, M. N. (1976). *N. Engl. J. Med.* **294**, 24-28.
Neijer, A. (1970). *Acta Allerg.* **25**, 63-68.
Nyirenda, R. and Gill, G. V. (1977). *Br. Med. J.* **2**, 1189.
Owens, C. J., Yarbrough, P. R., III and Brackett, N. C. (1974). *Arch. Intern. Med.* **134**, 332-338.
Parker, C. W. (1975). *N. Engl. J. Med.* **292**, 511, 732, 957.
Parker, C. W. (1980). *In* "Clinical Immunology" (Parker, C. W., ed.), pp. 1219. W. B. Saunders, Philadelphia.
Pasricha, J. S. and Shukla, S. R. (1979). *Br. J. Dermatol.* **101**, 361-362.
Payles, C. V. (1970). *Med. Clin. North Am.* **54**, 1077-1089.
Petz, L. D. (1971). *Postgrad. Med. J.* **47**, 64-69.
Petz, L. D. (1980). *Clin. Hematol.* **3**, 455.
Pisciotta, V. (1978). *Drugs* **15**, 123-143.
Pujet, J. C., Homberg, J. C. and Decroix, G. (1974). *Br. Med. J.* **2**, 415-418.
Rallison, M. L., O'Brien, J. and Good, R. A. (1961). *Pediatrics* **28**, 908-917.
Reichlin, S., Loveless, M. G. and Kane, E. G. (1953). *Ann. Intern. Med.* **38**, 113-120.
Reykes, M. P., Palutke, M. and Lerner, A. M. (1973). *Am. J. Med.* **54**, 413-418.
Rissing, J. P., Moore, W. L., Newman, C., Crockett, J. K., Buxton, T. B. and Edmondson, H. T. (1980). *Curr. Ther. Res.* **27**, 651-663.
Scheife, R. T., Levy, M. and Greenblatt, D. J. (1976). *In* "Drug Effects in Hospital Patients" (Miller, R. R. and Greenblatt, D. J., eds), pp. 229-235. John Wiley, New York.
Schorr, W. F., Wenzel, F. J. and Hegedus, S. I. (1973). *Arch. Dermatol.* **107**, 533-539.
Sharp, J. R., Ishak, K. G. and Zimmerman, H. J. (1980). *Ann. Intern. Med.* **92**, 14-19.
Sher, T. M. (1983). *Med. Clin. North Am.* **30**, 161-176.
Simonson, W., Stennett, D. J. and Hall, C. A. (1977). *Drug. Intell. Clin. Pharm.* **11**, 654-656.

Sollaccio, P. A., Ribaudo, C. and Grace, W. J. (1966). *Ann. Intern. Med.* **65**, 1284-1286.
Speirs, C. T. (1976). *Scott Med. J.* **21**, 178-181.
Sullivan, T. J., Wedner, H. H., Shatz, G. S., Yecies, L. D. and Parker, C. W. (1981). *J. Allergy Clin. Immunol.* **68**, 171-184.
Thoburn, R., Johnson, J. E. and Cluff, L. E. (1968). *J. Am. Med. Assoc.* **198**, 345.
Tonder, M., Norday, A. and Elgyo, K. (1974). *Scand. J. Gastroenterol.* **9**, 93-96.
Tydd, T. F. and Dyer, N. H. (1976). *Med. J. Aust. Nal.* **1**, 570-573.
Valentine, M. (Chairman) (1979). *In* "NIAID Task Force Report, Asthma and Other Allergic Diseases." Department of Health, Education & Welfare, Public Health Serivce NIH Publication 79-387, 501.
Van Arsdel, P. P. (1978). *In* "Allergy, Principles and Practice' (Middleton, E., Reed, C. E. and Ellis, E. F., eds), Vol. II, pp. 1394-1395. C. V. Mosby, St. Louis.
Van Dellen, R. G. and Gleich, G. J. (1970). *Med. Clin. North Am.* **54**, 997-1010.
Van Ypersele de Strilou, C. (1979). *Kidney Int.* **16**, 751-765.
Walker, R. G., Thomson, N. W., Dowling, J. P. and Ogg, C. S. (1979). *Br. Med. J.* **1**, 524.
Walker, W. R. (1969). *Can. Med. Assoc. J.* **101**, 763-765.
Weart, W. C. and Hyman, L. C. (1983). *S. Med. J.* **76**, 410-411.
Weinstein, H. I. and Welch, H., (1958). *Antibiot. Annu.*, 643-646.
Weinstein, L. (1975). *In* "The Pharmacological Basis of Therapeutics" (Goodman, L. S. and Gilman, A., eds), 5th edn, pp. 1167-1180, Macmillan, New York.
Wenz, B., Klein, R. L. and Alezari, P. (1974). *Transfusion* **14**, 265-269.
White, C. M., Price, J. and Hunt, K. M. (1980). *Br. Med. J.* **1**, 167.
Young, G. A. and Vincent, P. C. (1980). *Clin. Hematol.* **9**, 483-491.

Chapter 9

Antimicrobial Agents in the Immunocompromised Host

Kenneth V. I. Rolston, Gerald P. Bodey and Victor Fainstein

Section of Infectious Diseases, Department of Internal Medicine, University of Texas, M.D. Anderson Hospital and Tumor Institute, 6723 Bertner Avenue, Houston, Texas 77030, U.S.A.

1. INTRODUCTION

Some of the major components of host defence are humoral and cell-mediated immunity, as well as polymorphonuclear leucocytes. Defects in each of these components increases the risk of infection caused by a specific group of organisms. Knowledge of these defects plays an important part in the selection of antibiotics for the treatment of infections in the 'immunocompromised host'. During the last two decades, many highly effective antimcirobial agents have been discovered or synthesized in the laboratory. These agents have enabled us to make substantial progress in the treatment of infections. However, the battle against infection is far from over. The ability to treat most bacterial infections successfully has led to the development of therapeutic modalities such as intensive chemotherapeutic regimens and bone marrow transplantation, with greater risk for immunosuppression. Indwelling vascular catheters and other access devices are being employed with ever increasing frequency and for a wide variety of indications in such patient populations, thereby increasing the susceptibility for infection in patients already at considerable risk. In addition, microorganisms which were regarded as non-pathogenic and which are frequently resistant to antimicrobial agents are emerging as

Antimicrobial agents and immunity
ISBN 0-12-383830-4

'opportunistic pathogens', highlighting the ever-changing nature of the aetiology of infections and the need for newer strategies for their management. Many of these strategies are directed towards bolstering the host defence system. However, antimicrobial agents have a major role to play in the treatment of infections in immunocompromised patients.

II. INFECTIONS ASSOCIATED WITH IMMUNOSUPPRESSION

The factors causing immunosuppression and the organisms commonly associated with defects in each group are listed in Table 1. It is evident from this list that a wide variety of microorganisms are capable of inflicting damage upon the immunocompromised host. This chapter will focus primarily on the management of infections in neutropenic patients. Information about some of the newer antimicrobial agents will be presented along with a discussion of the potential advantages and/or disadvantages they might have over the older agents.

Table 1
Host factors predisposing to infection and associated pathogens

Humoral immune dysfunction	Cellular immune dysfunction	Neutropenia
Haemophilus influenzae	Bacteria	Bacteria
Streptococcus pneumoniae	Mycobacteria	*Escherichia coli*
	Listeria monocytogenes	*Pseudomonas aeruginosa*
	Salmonella	*Klebsiella pneumoniae*
	Norcardia spp.	*Staphylococcus aureus*
		Staphylcoccus epidermidis
	Fungi	Corynebacteria (CDC-JK)
	Cryptococcus neoformans	
	Histoplasma capsulatum	Yeasts
		Candida spp.
	Protozoa	*Torulopsis glabrata*
	Pneumoncystis carinii	
	Toxoplasma gondii	Filamentous fungi
	Cryptosporidium spp.	*Aspergillus* spp.
		Phycomycetes
	Viruses	
	Cytomegalovirus	
	Herpes simplex virus	
	Varicella-zoster virus	
	Helminths	
	Strongyloides stercoralis	

Neutropenia (both quantitative and qualitative) is probably the most important factor responsible for the increased frequency of bacterial infections in cancer patients. An inverse correlation between the number of circulating neutrophils and the frequency of infection was demonstrated by Bodey *et al.* (1966). The frequency of infection starts to increase at neutrophil levels of less than $1000/mm^3$ and rises markedly when levels of less than $100/mm^3$ are reached. A sharp decline in the neutrophil count, as well as the protracted duration of profound neutropenia, are also associated with an increased risk of infection.

Approximately 70% of all infections that develop in neutropenic cancer patients are caused by enteric Gram-negative aerobic bacilli (*Escherichia coli*, *Klebsiella pneumoniae* and *Pseudomonas aeruginosa*) and Gram-positive cocci (*Staphylococcus aureus* and *S. epidermidis*). In recent years several other organisms have emerged as important pathogens, including *Enterobacter* spp., *Serratia marcescens* and *Acinetobacter calcoaceticus* among Gram-negative, and *Corynebacterium* spp., CDC-JK diphtheroids, *Bacillus* spp. and Enterococci among Gram-positive organisms. Local differences in microflora exist with different organisms predominating in different institutions.

The most common infections occurring in neutropenic patients are pneumonia, septicaemia, skin and soft-tissue infections and gastrointestinal infections (oral mucositis, pharyngitis, oesophagitis and perianal lesions). Since neutropenic patients are unable to mount an adequate inflammatory response, infection can disseminate rapidly. This mandates the commencement of 'empiric antimicrobial therapy' directed against a variety of Gram-negative and Gram-positive organisms as soon as a neutropenic patient becomes febrile. Failure to institute antibiotics immediately has an adverse effect on survival particularly when dealing with Gram-negative bacillary infections. In a recent survey of bacteraemia caused by *P. aeruginosa*, Bodey *et al.* (1984) found a 73% response rate when appropriate antibiotic therapy was started on the same day that the patient became febrile. A 24–48 h delay resulted in a 46% response rate and this fell even further (22%) when appropriate antibiotics were not started until 3–4 days later.

III. FACTORS INFLUENCING ANTIBIOTIC SELECTION

Several factors influence the selection of antibiotics used in empirical regimens in neutropenic patients (Table 2). The regimen should provide a broad spectrum of activity against a wide variety of Gram-positive and Gram-negative organisms (Table 1). A single antibiotic is not likely to

Table 2
Factors influencing choice of antibacterial regimens

1. Antibacterial spectrum
2. Bactericidal activity
3. Potential for synergy
4. Pharmacokinetic properties
5. Efficacy in neutropenic patients
6. Therapeutic index (serum concentration/inhibitory concentration ratio)
7. Toxicity/safety factors
8. Cost

provide such broad-spectrum coverage, although some newer agents possess remarkably wide antibacterial spectra and might be considered for single-agent therapy. Two-drug regimens do not provide universal coverage either, but the addition of a third drug does not seem to increase efficacy in clinical trials.

Bactericidal antibiotics seem to be superior to bacteriostatic agents in patients with neutropenia. This is due to the fact the neutropenic patients must rely entirely upon antibiotics to eradicate the infection. Recently, Sculier *et al.* (1984) demonstrated that serum bactericidal activity was predictive of the outcome of Gram-negative bacillary bacteraemia in both neutropenic patients and those with adequate neutrophil counts. In neutropenic patients a peak serum bactericidal titre of 1 : 8 or less was associated with failure in 83%, while a peak serum bactericidal titre of 1 : 16 or more was associated with clinical success in 87%. The significant peak bactericidal titre in patients with adequate neutrophil counts was 1 : 8 with no successes below this level and a 98% success rate at or above this level.

There is evidence to suggest that antibiotic combinations that interact in a synergistic manner *in vitro*, provide greater serum bactericidal activity and are more effective clinically than non-synergistic combinations. In a retrospective study, Klastersky *et al.* (1972) found that synergistic combinations were associated with an 80% cure rate (80 of 100 patients) while non-synergistic combinations were effective in only 49.5% (52 of 105). The effect of antibiotic synergy on the outcome of Gram-negative sepsis was also studied by Anderson *et al.* (1978). They observed that synergism was particularly important in patients with 'rapidly fatal' underlying disease who developed Gram-negative sepsis. Of such patients, 77% responded to synergistic combinations, whereas only 52% responded to non-synergistic antibiotic combinations. Synergistic combinations probably increase efficacy by lowering the minimal inhibitory concentrations (MICs) of both drugs for the offending pathogen, thereby providing greater antibacterial activity in the blood and tissues. This may be particularly true of aminoglycosides where achievable serum and tissue levels are much lower than with β-lactam agents.

Combinations should only be considered 'synergistic' when both antibiotics are individually active against the organism and using them together enhances the activity of both. Conversely, combinations should only be regarded as 'non-synergistic' if both antibiotics are active against the organism, but their activity is not enhanced when used together. For instance, gentamicin and carbenicillin, both of which are active against *P. aeruginosa*, may be expected to interact synergistically, whereas gentamicin and cephalothin may not. Since cephalothin is not active against *P. aeruginosa*, a comparison of these two regimens is not that of a 'synergistic' *vs* a 'non-synergistic' one, but that of one active antibiotic *vs* two. Several investigators have shown that results are better when the infecting organism is susceptible to both antibiotics in a particular regimen than when it is susceptible to only one (Anderson *et al.*, 1978; Fainstein *et al.*, 1984).

Certain pharmacokinetic properties might influence the selection of antibiotics. These are serum protein-binding, diffusion into target tissues, serum half-life and major excretory pathway. Extremely high protein-binding leaves less 'free drug' to exert its activity. Diffusion into target tissues is particularly important in infections such as meningitis, where the antibiotic must traverse the blood–brain barrier, and pneumonia, where poor diffusion into lung and bronchial secretions might produce unsatisfactory results. Since neutropenic patients seldom form abscesses, diffusion of antibiotics into abscess cavities is not of much concern. A long serum half-life results in therapeutic serum levels of the drug for sustained periods of time. The major excretory pathway becomes important when dealing with patients who have renal or hepatic insufficiency.

It has been shown by Bodey *et al.* (1972) and other investigators that aminoglycosides are not very effective against Gram-negative bacilli in the presence of neutropenia and should not be used alone in such circumstances. On the other hand, the carboxypenicillins (carbenicillin, ticarcillin) retain their efficacy despite the presence of neutropenia and can be used either in combination with other β-lactams or with aminoglycosides.

The therapeutic index, i.e. the ratio of the serum concentration of an antibiotic to the concentration required to inhibit the growth of an organism (MIC), might play an important role particularly in neutropenic patients. A wide therapeutic margin is preferable to a narrow one. Serum levels of the newer β-lactam agents are often several hundredfold higher than the inhibitory concentration. This is frequently not so with aminoglycoside therapy where far lower serum levels are obtained. This fact might account for the poorer efficacy of the aminoglycosides. For example, in a study of netilmicin alone conducted by Yap and Bodey (1979), the response rate was 89% when the MIC was $\leqslant 0\cdot025\ \mu g/ml$, but was only 33% if the MIC was $0\cdot78$–$1\cdot56\ \mu g/ml$.

Antibiotic selection should also be influenced by the potential toxicities of various agents. Aminoglycosides have long been associated with nephro- and ototoxicity and require frequent monitoring of serum levels which can be expensive and time-consuming. The nephrotoxicity of aminoglycosides can be potentiated by antibiotics such as cephalothin and by antitumour agents such as cisplatin. These factors must be considered when selecting empiric antibiotics. In general the β-lactams are much safer antibiotics.

Neutropenic patients rely primarily on antibiotics for control of infections as they are unable to mount an adequate inflammatory response of their own. To obtain maximum killing of infecting organisms, it is likely that the serum concentration must be higher than the MIC at all times. Conventional, intermittent, 6–8 h dosage schedules can result in intervals between doses when the antibiotic concentration is subinhibitory. This is particularly true of the aminoglycosides since achievable serum levels of these agents are far lower than the β-lactams. It is possible that, in neutropenic patients receiving intermittent schedules of aminoglycoside therapy, the infecting organisms are able to multiply during such intervals, when the concentration is inadequate. Continuous therapy, resulting in sustained antibiotic levels, might prevent such an occurrence and improve the response rates in neutropenic patients. Therefore, the schedule of antibiotic administration might be of considerable importance and further studies are needed in this area.

Antibiotic selection is also influenced by experience in the local hospital. Certain pathogens may be endemic in a particular hospital and must be borne in mind when empiric regimens are designed. For example, at our institution, vancomycin has been incorporated into recent antibiotic regimens because of the increased frequency of infections caused by methicillin-resistant, coagulase-positive and coagulase-negative Staphylococci, Enterococci and JK diptheroids. Amikacin should be the aminoglycoside of choice in hospitals which have a greater frequency of gentamicin- or tobramycin-resistant isolates. The routine use of amikacin does not increase the frequency of resistance to it. Conversely, the use of amikacin reduces the incidence of resistance to other aminoglycosides. Therefore it is not necessary to 'save' amikacin for use against resistant isolates only. All other factors being equal, the least expensive antibiotics should be employed.

IV. ANTIBIOTIC REGIMENS IN NEUTROPENIC PATIENTS

The introduction of carbenicillin provided the clinician for the first time with an antibiotic that had significant activity against *P. aeruginosa*. Prior to the availability of this drug, neutropenic patients with *P. aeruginosa* bacteraemia did no better with antibiotic therapy than without it. Since then, several agents, including the carboxy- and ureidopenicillins, aminoglycosides, cephalosporins and cephalosporin-like compounds, have appeared on the scene and strengthened the armamentarium available for use in the febrile, neutropenic patient. Several drugs have been used either alone or in combination in major studies conducted at cancer research centres both in the United States and in Europe.

A. Single-agent Therapy

1. Carboxypenicillins

Carbenicillin is a semisynthetic carboxypenicillin with antipseudomonal activity. Its major drawback is a lack of activity against *Klebsiella* spp. Bodey *et al.* (1969) used this agent as therapy for Gram-negative infections in netropenic patients. A total of 91% of patients with *P. aeruginosa* infections responded. Other infections did less well with response rates of 59, 0 and 0% for *E. coli*, *Klebsiella* spp. and *Serratia* spp. In another study, Klastersky *et al.* (1973) compared carbenicillin and gentamicin alone to gentamicin plus carbenicillin in cancer patients. Carbenicillin alone was successful in 50% of patients. Ticarcillin is similar to carbenicillin in its *in-vitro* spectrum but is more potent on a weight basis, enabling a lower dose to be given without a reduction in efficacy. It has also been used as single-agent therapy by Rodriguez *et al.* (1973) with an overall response rate of 43%. The response rate for Pseudomonas infections was 80% but much poorer responses were seen with the *Enterobacteriaceae*. These data demonstrate the usefulness of the carboxypenicillins in treating infections in neutropenic patients. However, their use alone is suboptimal as they lack a broad Gram-negative spectrum.

2. Ureidopenicillins

The ureidopenicillins (mezlocillin, piperacillin and azlocillin) possess a broader antibacterial spectrum than the carboxypenicillins. Mezlocillin is equivalent to ticarcillin as an antipseudomonal agent, while piperacillin and azlocillin have been shown consistently to be more active *in vitro* against this organism. All three agents have significant activity against *Klebsiella* spp. and Enterococci and the overall activity of piperacillin *in vitro* is superior to that of the others.

Mezlocillin, 3 g intravenously over a 2-h period every 4 h, was used by Issell and Bodey (1980) for the treatment of 92 episodes of documented infections in 75 myelosuppressed cancer patients. The overall response rate was 49%, while the response rate in 59 evaluable bacterial infections was 46%. Only 35% of septicaemic patients responded and the response rates of infections caused by *P. aeruginosa*, *K. pneumoniae* and *E. coli* were 42, 64 and 70% respectively.

Similar results were obtained when Wade *et al.* (1980) used mezlocillin as a single agent. Two dosing regimens were used (260 and 45 mg/kg/day) with overall response rates of 52%. Ten of 17 infections in the low-dose group and eight of 17 infections in the high-dose group improved. Only one of six bacteraemias and three of six pneumonias improved with mezlocillin therapy. Although mezlocillin was well tolerated in both studies, results indicate that it cannot be recommended for use as a single agent for the treatment of infections in febrile, neutropenic patients.

3. *Aminoglycosides*

Gentamicin alone was used by Bodey *et al.* (1972) to treat 67 patients and was used in combination with either carbenicillin or cephalothin in an additional 55 patients. An overall response rate of 45% was achieved in infections caused by organisms susceptible only to gentamicin. Patients with profound neutropenia at commencement of therapy had a response rate of only 22%. Response rates of 75, 60 and 40% were seen in infections due to *E. coli*, *Klebsiella* spp. and *Pseudomonas* spp. Schimpff *et al.* (1971) used gentamicin in eight patients with Pseudomonas bacteraemia, seven of which continued to be bacteraemic while on therapy. The patient who recovered had a rapidly rising neutrophil count.

Tobramycin, introduced in 1974, has greater *in-vitro* antipseudomonal activity than gentamicin. It was evaluated by Valdivieso *et al.* (1974), who achieved an overall response rate of 54%. However, as with gentamicin, the response rate with profound neutropenia ($< 100/mm^3$) was only 24%.

Amikacin, a kanamycin derivative has activity *in vitro* against tobramycin- and gentamicin-resistant Gram-negative bacilli. A 69% response was seen in patients treated with amikacin who had previously failed to respond to cephalothin plus carbenicillin (Valdivieso *et al.* 1975). Continuous infusion of amikacin rather than the routine technique of intermittent infusion might have contributed to the improved response.

In a similar study by Feld *et al.* (1977), patients not responding to therapy with carbenicillin and a cephalosporin received sisomicin either intermittently or via continuous infusion. An overall response rate of 54% was seen in patients where a pathogen was cultured. Of patients on continuous infusion 61% responded compared to only 46% receiving intermittent sisomicin. Only 46% of patients with initial neutrophil counts of less than $100/mm^3$ responded to sisomicin therapy.

Netilmicin has an *in-vitro* spectrum similar to gentamicin but is considered to be less nephrotoxic. Yap and Bodey (1979) evaluated netilimicin in cancer patients. Patients with adequate neutrophil counts received an intermittent schedule of drug while neutropenic patients ($<1000/mm^3$) received netilmicin via continuous infusion. An overall response rate in 100 episodes of documented infection was 60%. The response rates for infections caused by *E. coli*, *Klebsiella* spp. and *P. aeruginosa* were 100, 55 and 42% respectively.

These data (Table 3) demonstrate that the aminoglycosides alone are not optimal therapy for Gram-negative infections in neutropenic patients. They also suggest that, in this setting, continuous infusion therapy might be superior to intermittent infusion.

Table 3
Results obtained with single agents in infections in neutropenic patients

Reference	Antibiotic	Overall response (%)
Bodey *et al.*, 1969	Carbenicillin	59
Klastersky *et al.*, 1973	Carbenicillin	50
Rodriguez *et al.*, 1973	Ticarcillin	43
Issell and Bodey, 1980	Mezlocillin	59
Wade *et al.*, 1980	Mezlocillin	52
Bodey *et al.*, 1972	Gentamicin	51
Valdivieso *et al.*, 1974	Tobramycin	54
Valdivieso *et al.*, 1975	Amikacin	69
Feld *et al.*, 1977	Sisomicin	54
Yap and Bodey, 1979	Netilmicin	60
Fainstein *et al.*, 1983*a*	Ceftazidime	76
Piccart *et al.*, 1984	Cefoperazone	77

4. Cephalosporins

Cephalosporins have been used most commonly in combination with other antibiotics. However, ceftazidime and cefoperazone, two new 'third-generation' cephalosporins with broad antibacterial spectrum including *P. aeruginosa*, have been used as single-agent therapy. Fainstein *et al.* (1983*a*) compared ceftazidime alone and in combination with tobramycin as initial therapy for infections in neutropenic and non-neutropenic cancer patients. The response rate for both regimens was

72% in microbiologically proven infections. Of infections caused by Gram-negative bacilli including all *P. aeruginosa* infections, 94% responded to ceftazidime alone. This compared favourably with the 95% response rate seen with the combination of ceftazidime and tobramycin. Infections caused by Gram-positive organisms did less well with response rates of 50% for ceftazidime and 60% for the combination. This study suggests that ceftazidime alone is an effective new antibiotic for the treatment of Gram-negative bacillary infections, even in neutropenic patients, and the addition of an aminoglycoside is probably not necessary. Since ceftazidime is less effective against Gram-positive organisms, it should probably be combined with an agent such as vancomycin in order to provide broader initial coverage.

Piccart *et al.* (1984) compared cefoperazone alone to cefoperazone plus amikacin as empiric therapy for febrile cancer patients. In neutropenic patients, cefoperazone was effective in 17 or 22 patients (77%) and a cure was achieved in 16 patients (73%). The combination of cefoperazone and amikacin was effective in 16 of 22 patients (73%), but cured only 13 of 22 (59%). A higher rate of superinfection accounted for this lower cure rate. Cefoperazone was effective in eight of 11 episodes of Gram-negative rod bacteraemia and the combination in eight of 12 episodes. All three cefoperazone failures had *P. aeruginosa* bacteraemia, although two were polymicrobial. These results indicate that cefoperazone was as effective alone as it was when combined with amikacin and could be used as monotherapy in neutropenic patients. However, results with polymicrobial and *P. aeruginosa* infections need to be improved.

Other investigators have evaluated moxalactam and ceftazidime as monotherapy, but their results are yet to be published. More clinical experience is needed before monotherapy with broad-spectrum agents can be recommended routinely in neutropenic patients.

B. Combination Antibiotic Therapy

Antibiotic combinations offer several advantages over single-agent therapy in the treatment of infections in neutropenic patients. Primarily, antibiotic combinations provide a wider antibacterial spectrum than single agents making it possible to cover a greater number of potential pathogens. Other advantages over monotherapy are:

(a) the potential for a synergistic reaction and enhanced bactericidal activity;
(b) the prevention of the emergence of resistant organisms;
(c) the possibility of reducing the dosage of potentially toxic drugs.

Many antibiotic combinations have been evaluated in neutropenic patients. Most contain an aminoglycoside in addition to an antipseudomonal penicillin or a cephalosporin. Several newer agents, such as the extended-spectrum penicillins, cephalosporins, monobactams and imipenem, have recently become available and are likely to have an impact both as single agents and in combination with other antibiotics in neutropenic patients.

1. Aminoglycoside plus antipseudomonal/ extended-spectrum penicillin

Several recent trials employing combinations of an aminoglycoside with antipseudomonal or extended-spectrum penicillins are summarized in Table 4. In general, response rates of between 55 and 85% were obtained regardless of the antibiotic combination used. Carbenicillin and ticarcillin possess a similar spectrum of activity (*P. aeruginosa*, *E. coli*, *Proteus*) and the choice between them is largely a matter of personal preference or experience. However, ticarcillin is more active *in vitro* against isolates of *P. aeruginosa*, allowing lower dosages to be administered, possibly reducing the occurrence of hypokalaemia, and may be preferred over carbenicillin.

Table 4
Results obtained with an aminoglycoside plus an antipseudomonal/extended-spectrum penicillin in infections in neutropenic patients

Reference	Antibiotics[a]	Overall response (%)
Lawson *et al.*, 1984	Tob+T	67
	Tob+M	69
De Jongh *et al.*, 1982	A+T	72
Wade *et al.*, 1981	A+T	56
	A+P	58
Love *et al.*, 1979	G+T	97
	N+T	95
	A+T	91
Issell *et al.*, 1979	Tob+C	70
Keating *et al.*, 1979	G+C	68
	S+C	72
	A+C	70
EORTC, 1978	G+C	71
Schimpff *et al.*, 1971	G+C	55
Rodriguez *et al.*, 1969	G+C	50

[a]Abbreviations: A, amikacin; C, carbenicillin; G, gentamicin; M, mezlocillin; N, netilmicin; P, piperacillin; S, sisomicin; T, ticarcillin; Tob, tobramycin.

However, comparative clinical trials have not demonstrated any therapeutic superiority of one drug over the other. Similarly, no significant difference has been found between combinations containing these two drugs and those containing newer extended-spectrum penicillins (mezlocillin, piperacillin), despite differences in the spectrum of activity of the latter, especially against *Klebsiella* spp. and Enterococci. For example Lawson *et al.* (1984) obtained overall response rates of 67 and 69% using combinations of tobramycin with ticarcillin and mezlocillin respectively. Wade *et al.* (1981) achieved an overall response rate of 56% with amikacin and ticarcillin and 58% with amikacin and piperacillin in febrile neutropenic patients.

The choice of the aminoglycoside depends largely upon the pattern of resistance seen at individual institutions. Since the occurrence of gentamicin- and tobramycin-resistant isolates is fairly widespread, most institutions now use amikacin as their aminoglycoside of choice. Rather than increase the occurrence of resistance to amikacin, this manoeuvre has resulted in a decrease in resistance to other aminoglycosides (Ristuccia and Cunha, 1982). Therefore amikacin does not need to be held in 'reserve' only for use against resistant organisms. The relative toxicity of individual aminoglycosides might also govern their choice in empiric regimens. Although some studies have suggested that tobramycin and netilmicin may be less toxic than the other aminoglycosides, most investigators have found no significant differences in the toxic potential of the various aminoglycosides in neutropenic patients. For example, in the study conducted by Love *et al.* (1979), there were no significant differences in toxicity when regimens combining ticarcillin with gentamicin, netilmicin or amikacin were compared. Similarly, Keating *et al.* (1979) found the toxicity of gentamicin, amikacin and sisomicin to be equal when used in combination with carbenicillin.

2. *Aminoglycoside plus extended-spectrum cephalosporin*

Several recent studies (Table 5) have evaluated combinations of an aminoglycoside with an extended-spectrum or 'third-generation' cephalosporin in the treatment of infections in neutropenic patients. Fainstein *et al.* (1984), achieved an overall response rate of 64% using moxalactam plus tobramycin in neutropenic cancer patients. The respective response rates for urinary tract infection, septicaemia and soft-tissue infections were 100, 75 and 76%. Pneumonias responded poorly (39%). No serious side effects were seen. In another trial, Fainstein *et al.* (1983*a*) used a combination of tobramycin and ceftazidime and achieved an overall response rate of 73%. However, 95% of Gram-negative rod septicaemias responded including all four caused by *P. aeruginosa*. A response rate of 60% was seen in septicaemia caused by Gram-positive organisms. Winston

Table 5
Results obtained with an aminoglycoside plus an extended-spectrum cephalosporin in infections in neutropenic patients

Reference	Antibiotics[a]	Overall response (%)
Piccart *et al.*, 1984	Cef+A	73
Fainstein *et al.*, 1984	Tob+M	64
Winston *et al.*, 1984	A+M	79
Fainstein *et al.*, 1983*a*	Tob+C	73
De Jongh*et al.*, 1982	A+M	71

[a]Abbreviations: A, amikacin; C, ceftazidime; Cef, cefoperazone; M, moxalactam; Tob, tobramycin.

et al. (1984) used a combination of moxalactam and amikacin and were able to demonstrate improvement in 79% of their patients. Seven of nine patients with *P. aeruginosa* responded and a 72% response rate was seen in septicaemias. Bacteraemic enterococcal superinfections occurred in seven patients. No antibiotic related haemorrhage occurred. These results compare favourably with those obtained with aminoglycoside–penicillin combinations.

Studies in the past have shown that cephalothin potentiates the nephrotoxicity associated with aminoglycosides (Klastersky *et al.*, 1975; Wade *et al.*, 1978). This does not seem to occur when third-generation cephalosporins are combined with aminoglycosides. It is clear from these data that both cephalosporins and extended-spectrum penicillins, when combined with an aminoglycoside, offer adequate protection against bacterial infections when used as initial therapy in febrile neutropenic patients. As mentioned before, however, there are several drawbacks with aminoglycoside therapy. As a class, aminoglycosides are not very effective in neutropenic patients. They are potentially nephro- and ototoxic and require frequent monitoring of serum levels which are expensive, time-consuming and uncomfortable for the patient. Also, the therapeutic margin provided by aminoglycosides is narrow as levels achievable in the serum are fairly low. With the availability of the extended-spectrum penicillins and cephalosporins, which possess broad antibacterial activity, are fairly non-toxic and achieve serum levels that are sometimes several hundredfold the MIC of the most commonly isolated Gram-negative bacteria (Bodey *et al.*, 1981; Eliopoulos and Moellering, 1982), it has become possible to combine these two classes of drugs and eliminate the aminoglycosides altogether.

3. Double β-lactam combinations

Combinations of two β-lactam agents have been used for more than 10 years (Middleman *et al.*, 1972), but with the recent availability of broad-spectrum agents, interest in such combinations has been rekindled. Two studies have recently been published (Table 6) in which double β-lactam combinations were used to treat febrile neutropenic patients. A total of 65% of infections treated with moxalactam plus ticarcillin responded in the study conducted by Fainstein *et al.* (1984), compared to 64% of those treated with moxalactam plus tobramycin. The respective response rates for septicaemia, urinary tract infections, soft-tissue infections and pneumonia were 85, 100, 66 and 41%. Side effects included skin rashes, coagulation abnormalities and superinfections due to Enterococci and fungal elements. Winston *et al.* (1984) achieved a 77% response rate with moxalactam and piperacillin compared to a 79% response rate with moxalactam and amikacin.

Coagulation abnormalities have been reported in patients receiving agents such as moxalactam and cefoperazone (Fainstein *et al.*, 1983*b*). These abnormalities can be reversed by using vitamin K and the prophylactic use of this agent is recommended in patients receiving these antibiotics. Other third-generation cephalosporins (cefotaxime, ceftazidime) may not be associated with coagulation abnormalities because of structural differences and may be used instead of moxalactam or cefoperazone. Superinfections with organisms such as Enterococci and fungi have also been observed with the use of broad-spectrum antibiotics such as moxalactam (Yu, 1981) although colonization seems to occur more frequently.

Table 6
Results obtained with double *β-lactam combinations in infections in neutropenic patients*

Author	Antibiotics[a]	Overall response (%)
Winston *et al.*, 1984	M+P	77
Fainstein *et al.*, 1984	M+T	65
Bodey *et al.*, 1979	C+Cef (continuous)	57
	C+Cef (intermittent)	65
EORTC, 1978	C or T+Cep	72
Klastersky *et al.*, 1975	T+Cep	55
Middleman *et al.*, 1972	C+Cep	60

[a]Abbreviations: C, carbenicillin; Cef, cefamandole; Cep, cephalothin; M, moxalactam; P, piperacillin; T, ticarcillin.

Although the idea of using double β-lactam combinations is an attractive one, caution must be exerted until more clinical data are available. These agents might interact in an antagonistic manner. The coverage against Gram-positive organisms (coagulase-negative Staphylococci, CDC-JK diphtheroids, *Bacillus* sp.) may not be optimal and may require the addition of agents such as vancomycin in institutions where these organisms abound. Double β-lactam combinations may also increase the chances of the development of resistant organisms. Thus, more clinical studies evaluating such regimens are required before their role in the treatment of infections in neutropenic patients can be fully established.

4. Other combinations

Various other antimicrobial combinations have been evaluated in neutropenic cancer patients. Some of these regimens are summarized in Table 7.

Table 7
Results obtained with miscellaneous antibiotic combinations in infections in neutropenic patients

Reference	Antibiotics[a]	Overall response (%)
Keating *et al.*, 1981	TMP-SMX+T	77
Jadeja *et al.*, 1984	V+P	72
Jones *et al.*, in press	$V+A_3$	68
	$V+A_3+A$	80

[a]Abbreviations: A, amikacin; A_3, aztreonam; T, ticarcillin; TMP-SMX, trimethoprim-sulphamethoxazole; V, vancomycin; P, piperacillin.

(a) Ticarcillin plus trimethoprim-sulphamethoxazole (TMP-SMX)

Keating *et al.* (1981) evaluated a combination of ticarcillin and TMP-SMX as initial empiric therapy in febrile episodes in patients with cancer. An overall response rate of 77% (79 of 102 infections) was achieved. Major sites of infection responded as follows: septicaemia 89%, urinary tract infections 100%, soft-tissue infections 85% and pneumonia 52%. Gram-negative bacillary infections were associated with a response rate of 87%. The initial neutrophil count did not have much influence on response rates but a higher response rate (84%) was seen in patients in whom the neutrophil count increased during therapy than in those (72%) in whom it decreased or remained stable. Since TMP-SMX has a broad antibacterial spectrum including activity against Gram-positive organisms and good penetration into most body tissues (Salter, 1982), it is a promising agent especially when combined with an antipseudomonal agent such as ticarcillin. Its use as a therapeutic agent might be limited because of widespread use in prophylaxis.

(b) Piperacillin plus vancomycin

In a recent study, Jadeja *et al.* (1984) used piperacillin plus vancomycin as initial therapy for febrile episodes in cancer patients. The response rate in 95 episodes of documented infection was 72%. Various sites of infection responded as follows: bacteraemia 78%, soft-tissue infections 71% and pneumonias 38%. A 73% response rate was obtained for infections caused by Gram-negative organisms with only six of 10 *P. aeruginosa* infections responding to therapy. Twelve of 14 infections caused by Gram-positive organisms responded, due mainly to the activity of vancomycin which had been included because of an increased number of infections due to coagulase-negative Staphylococci, CDC-JK diphtheroids and *Bacillus* spp. at that institution. The overall response rate with this combination was comparable with other regimens for neutropenic patients. However, four of 10 patients with *P. aeruginosa* infections failed despite *in-vitro* susceptibility to piperacillin. Several factors may influence this unsatisfactory *in-vivo* response. One may be the slow and incomplete *in-vitro* killing of *P. aeruginosa* by piperacillin. Some investigators have also demonstrated differences between bactericidal and inhibitory concentrations with the new ureidopenicillins (Winston *et al.*,1978; Eliopoulos and Moellering, 1982). Piperacillin has been shown to be less effective than ticarcillin in the treatment of endocarditis due to *P. aeruginosa* (Reyes and Lerner, 1983). These data suggest that piperacillin should be used in combination with another antipseudomonal agent when treating *P. aeruginosa* infections.

(c) Monobactam (aztreonam) plus vancomycin

Aztreonam is a synthetic monobactam with activity against aerobic Gram-negative bacilli including *P. aeruginosa* (Sykes *et al.*, 1982). This drug was recently evaluated (Jones *et al.*, 1985) alone and in combination with amikacin as initial empiric therapy in neutropenic patients. Vancomycin was added to provide coverage against Gram-positive organisms. The overall results with aztreonam plus amikacin plus vancomycin (80%) were slightly superior to those with aztreonam plus vancomycin (68%). Fourteen of 16 (88%) Gram-negative infections responded to aztreonam plus vancomycin, the two non-responders being Pseudomonas infections, whereas all 17 episodes of Gram-negative infections responded to aztreonam plus amikacin plus vancomycin including all five Pseudomonas infections. Aztreonam is adequate for the treatment of Gram-negative bacillary infections in neutropenic patients, although more clinical experience is needed to determine its efficacy against *P. aeruginosa*. Since it is not active against Gram-positive organisms, a specific agent providing Gram-positive activity should be added.

C. Length of Therapy

The duration of antimicrobial therapy in the febrile neutropenic patient is still a controversial issue. Pizzo *et al.* (1984) recommended the continuation of antibiotic therapy if the patient remains febrile and neutropenia persists. Since the chances of developing fungal infection were high in patients receiving prolonged parenteral antibiotics (Pizzo *et al.*, 1982), modification of coverage to include antifungal agents in such patients seems indicated. Joshi *et al.* (1984) were able to discontinue antibiotic therapy in febrile neutropenic patients in whom infection was doubtful, and thereby reduce the incidence of fungal infections, but recommend continuing antibiotic therapy whenever the slightest possibility of infection exists. It has been our general policy to continue antibiotics for 4 days after signs and symptoms of infection have resolved, to a minimum of 7 days. Infections such as pneumonia require longer treatment. This approach seems to be associated with a low relapse rate and a low frequency of superinfection (Bodey, 1984).

V. SUMMARY

It is evident, from the multiplicity of regimens discussed above, that no single regimen is appropriate under all circumstances. From studies conducted at this institution and at others, we can conclude that aminoglycosides are not very effective in the face of neutropenia. The questions of whether or not synergistic combinations offer an advantage over non-synergistic regimens needs further clarification. Studies using only one effective agent against Gram-negative bacilli and achieving cure rates comparable to regimens with potentially synergistic combinations seem to indicate that synergism may not be a major therapeutic factor, except perhaps agaisnt *P. aeruginosa*. Although monotherapy appears adequate for most Gram-negative infections, no single agent has a sufficiently broad spectrum also to cover the Gram-positive organisms that occur frequently in neutropenia. Three-drug regimens have not been more effective than those with two drugs.

Current experience indicates that combination antibiotic therapy should be instituted promptly when a neutropenic patient becomes febrile.

Antibiotics should be continued until signs and symptoms of infection have cleared. Selected patients might benefit from granulocyte transfusions and antifungal therapy might be required in patients whose fever does not respond to antibacterial agents. Newer modalities such as passive immunization might improve outcome when used in conjunction with antimicrobial therapy.

REFERENCES

Alavi, J. B., Root, R. K., Djerassi, I., Evans, A. E., Gluckman, S. J., MacGregor, R. R., Gverry, D., Schreiber, A. D., Shaw, J. M., Koch, P. and Cooper, R. A. (1977). *N. Engl. J. Med.* **296**, 706–711.

Anderson, E. T., Young, L. S. and Hewitt, W. L. (1978). *Chemotherapy* **24**, 45–54.

Bodey, G. P. (1982). *In* "The Aminoglycosides" (Whelton, A. and Neu, H. C., eds), pp. 557–583. Marcel Dekker, New York.

Bodey, G. P. (1984). *Arch. Intern. Med.* **144**, 1845–1851.

Bodey, G. P., Buckley, M., Sathe, Y. S. and Freireich, E. J. (1966). *Ann. Intern. Med.* **64**, 328–340.

Bodey, G. P., Rodriguez, V. and Luck, J. K. (1969). *Am. J. Med. Sci.* **257**, 408–414.

Bodey, G. P., Middleman, E., Umsawasdi, T. and Rodriguez, V. (1972). *Cancer* **29**, 1697–1701.

Bodey, G. P., Ketchel, S. J. and Rodriguez, V. (1979). *Amer. J. Med.* **67**, 608–616.

Bodey, G. P., Fainstein, V. and Hinkle, A. M. (1981). *Antimicrob. Agents Chemother.* **20**, 226–230.

Bodey, G. P., Jadeja, L. and Elting, L. (1985). *Arch. Intern. Med.* **145**, 1621–1629.

Bolivar, R., Weaver, S. S. and Bodey, G. P. (1984). *Diagn. Microbiol. Infect. Dis.* **2**, 255–260.

Collins, M. S. and Roby, R. E. (1984). *Am. J. Med.* **76** (3a), 168–174.

de Jongh, C. A., Wade, J. C., Schimpff, S. C., Newman, K. A., Finley, R. S., Salvatore, P., Moody, M. R., Standford, H. C., Fortner, C. L. and Wiernik, P. H. (1982). *Am. J. Med.* **73**, 89–96.

Eliopoulos, G. M. and Moellering, R. L., Jr. (1982). *Ann. Intern. Med.* **97**, 755–760.

EORTC International Antimicrobial Therapy Group (1978). *J. Infect. Dis.* **137**, 14–29.

Fainstein, V., Bodey, G. P., Elting, L., Bolivar, R., Keating, M. J., McCredie, K. B. and Valdivieso, M. (1983*a*). *J. Antimicrob. Chemother.* **12** (*Suppl. A*), 101–110.

Fainstein, V., Bodey, G. P., McCredie, K. B., Keating, M. J., Estey, E. H., Bolivar, R. and Elting, L. (1983*b*). *J. Infect. Dis.* **148**, 745–750.

Fainstein, V., Bodey, G. P., Bolivar, R., Elting, L., McCredie, K. B. and Keating, M. J. (1984). *Arch. Intern. Med.* **144**, 1766–1770.

Feld, R., Valdivieso, M., Bodey, G. P. and Rodriguez, V. (1977). *Amer. J. Med. Sci.* **274**, 179–188.

Fuchs, P. C., Barry, A. L., Thornsberry, C. and Jones, R. N. (1984). *Chemotherapy* **25**, 392–394.

Herzig, R. H., Herzig, G. P., Graw, R. G., Jr., Bull, M. I. and Ray, K. K. (1977). *N. Engl. J. Med.* **296**, 701–705.

Issell, B. F. and Bodey, G. P. (1980). *Antimicrob. Agents Chemother.* **17**, 1008–1013.

Issell, B. F., Keating, M. J., Valdivieso, M. and Bodey, G. P. (1979). *Amer. J. Med. Sci.* **277**, 311–318.

Jadeja, L., Bolivar, R., Fainstein, V., Keating, M. J., McCredie, K. B., Hay, M. and Bodey, G. P. (1984). *Antimicrob. Agents Chemother.* **26**, 295–299.

Jones, P., Rolston, K., Fainstein, V., Elting, L. and Bodey, G. P. (1985). *Rev. Infect. Dis.* **7** (*Suppl. 4*) 5741–5746.

Joshi, J. H., Schimpff, S. C. Tenney, J. H., Newman, K. A. and de Jongh, C. A. (1984). *Am. J. Med.* **76**, 450–457.

Keating, M. J., Bodey, G. P., Valdivieso, M. and Rodriguez, V. (1979). *Medicine (Baltimore)* **58**, 159–170.

Keating, M. J., Lawson, R., Grose, W. and Bodey, G. P. (1981). *Arch. Intern. Med.* **141**, 926–930.

Klastersky, J., Cappel, R. and Daneau, D. (1972). *Antimicrob. Agents Chemother.* **2**, 470–475.

Klastersky, J., Cappel, R. and Danaeu, D. (1973). *Cancer* **31**, 331–336.

Klastersky, J., Hengsen, C. and DeBusscher, L. (1975). *Antimicrob. Agents Chemother.* **7**, 640–645.

Lau, W. K., Young, L. S., Black, R. E., Winston, D. J., Linne, S. R., Weinstein, R. J. and Hewitt, W. L. (1977). *Am. J. Med.* **62**, 959–966.

Lawson, R. D., Gentry, L. O., Bodey, G. P., Keating, M. J. and Smith, T. L. (1984). *Am. J. Med. Sci.* **287**, 16–23.

Love, L. J., Schimpff, S. C., Hahn, D., Young, V. M., Standford, M. C., Bender, J. F., Fortner, C. L. and Wiernik, P. H. (1979). *Am. J. Med.* **66**, 603–610.

Middleman, E. A., Watanabe, A., Kaizer, H. and Bodey, G. P. (1972). *Cancer* **30**, 573–579.

Piccart, M., Klastersky, J., Meunier, F., Lagast, H., Van Laethem, Y. and Weerts, D. (1984). *Antimicrob. Agents Chemother.* **26**, 870–875.

Pizzo, P. A., Robichaud, K. J., Gill, F. A. and Witebsky, F. G. (1982). *Am. J. Med.* **72**, 101–111.

Pizzo, P. A., Commers, J., Cotton, D., Gress, J., Hathorn, J., Heimenz, J., Longo, D., Marshall, D. and Robichaud, K. J. (1984). *Am. J. Med.* **76**, 436–449.

Reyes, M. P. and Lerner, A. M. (1983). *Rev. Infect. Dis.* **5**, 314–321.

Ristuccia, A. M. and Cunha, B. A. (1982). *Med. Clin. North Am.* **66**, 303–312.

Rodriguez, V., Whitecar, J. P. Jr. and Bodey, G. P. (1969). *Antimicrob. Agents Chemother.* **9**, 386–390.

Rodriguez, V., Bodey, G. P., Horikoshi, N., Inagaki, J. and McCredie, K. B. (1973). *Antimicrob. Agents Chemother.* **4**, 427–431.

Salter, A. (1982). *Rev. Infect. Dis.* **4**, 196–236.
Schimpff, S. C., Satterlee, W., Young, U. M. and Serpick, A. (1971). *N. Engl. J. Med.* **284**, 1061–1065.
Sculier, J. P. and Klastersky, J. (1984). *Amer. J. Med.* **76**, 429–435.
Sykes, R. B., Bonner, D. P., Bush, K. and Georgopapadakau, N. M. (1982). *Antimicrob. Agents Chemother.* **21**, 85–92.
Valdivieso, M., Horikoshi, N., Rodriguez, V. and Bodey, G. P. (1974). *Am. J. Med. Sci.* **268**, 149–156.
Valdivieso, M., Feld, R., Rodriguez, V. and Bodey, G. P. (1975). *Am. J. Med. Sci.* **270**, 453–463.
Wade, J. C., Smith, C. R. and Petty, G. B. (1978). *Lancet* **i**, 604–606.
Wade, J. C., Schimpff, S. C., Newman, K. A., Fortner, C. L., Moody, M. R., Young, V. M. and Wiernik, P. H. (1980). *Antimicrob. Agents Chemother.* **18**, 299–306.
Wade, J. C., Schimpff, S. C., Newman, K. A., Fortner, C. L., Standford, H. C. and Wiernik, P. H. (1981). *Am. J. Med.* **71**, 983–990.
Winston, D. J., Wang, D., Young, L. S., Martin, W. J. and Hewitt, W. L. (1978). *Antimicrob. Agents Chemother.* **13**, 944–950.
Winston, D. J., Barnes, R. C., Ho, W. G., Young, L. S., Champlin, R. R. and Gale, R. P. (1984). *Am. J. Med.* **77**, 442–450.
Yap, B. and Bodey, G. P. (1979). *Arch. Intern. Med.* **139**, 1259–1262.
Yu, V. L. (1981). *Ann. Intern. Med.* **94**, 784–785.
Ziergler, E. F., McCutcan, J. A. and Fierer, J. A. (1982). *N. Engl. J. Med.* **307**, 1225–1230.

Index